UP TO MY ARMPITS

UP TO MY

ARMPITS

ADVENTURES
of a
WEST TEXAS
VETERINARIAN

by

CHARLES W. EDWARDS, JR., D.V.M.

illustrations by Wayne Baize

IRON MOUNTAIN PRESS
Marathon, Texas
2003

Third Printing

October 2003

ISBN 0-9657985-6-9 (hardback)

ISBN 0-9657985-7-7 (trade paper)

Printed and Bound by Capital Printing Company
Austin, Texas

Cover Design - Leisha Israel, Blue Sky Media
Austin, Texas

Cover Artwork - Wayne Baize
Fort Davis, Texas

Iron Mountain Press
P.O. Box 325
Marathon, Texas 79842

www.ironmtnpress.com

To my wife, JoAnn,
And to my daughters, Nancy Edwards and Janet Edwards Franklin,
And to all those cows I treated.

Table of Contents

Prologue: Introduction   *i*

Chapter 1: Background   *1*

Chapter 2: Arrival   *5*

Whirlwind During Caesarean Section 9 • Embarrassing Events 10 •
Two Calls to the Reid Brothers Ranch 13 • Smokey Babb at Rough
Creek Ranch 20 • Eating Preferences of a Cow Belonging to S.S.
"Ted" Harper 22 • Sleeping Sickness Vaccination 23 • First Vehicles
25 • Buck Pyle and Chorizo 27 • Banky Stocks at Cole and Alf
Means' Y6 Ranch 27 • Blas Payne 30 • Revelation 31

Chapter 3: The Early Years   *35*

Working in the Rain at the Kincaid Ranch 35 • Calf Delivery at the
Post 38 • Louie Weinacht Ranch Call 41 • My First Ranching
Experience 42 • Learning Lessons 43• "Wet" Mexicans 45 •
Around the Campfire near Gomez Peak 47 • Bob Sproul's Ranch 49
• The Proposal 50 • The Wedding 51 • A Strong Back and Weak
Mind? 53 • Rings 54 • W.W. "Walter" McElroy Sr. 55 • Brucellosis
58 • Frank Warren at the Allison Ranch in the Glass Mountains 58 •
Murphy Bennett and King Hines 60 • An Injured Colt 63 •
Screwworms 64 • Auction Ring Calves 68 • The Breakdown 68 •
Some Aspects of Early Day Practice 71 • Kerr Mitchell's Calving
Shed 74 • The Over Zealous Ranch Hand 75 • Frances and S.S.
"Ted" Harper 76 • Calf Meningitis 77 • W. E. "Bill" Bunton 78•
Chow Dogs 80 • The Bashful Bull 81 • Castration Infection in Calves
83 • Fayette Yates' Poodle 85 • Cancer Eye - Pinkeye Seminar 85•
Punkin 88 • Clay Espy's Horse Guante 88 • A Very Late Night 91 •
The Holstein Bull at Lobo 92 • The Calf Puller 93 • Late Spring Frost
in 1952 94 • Lechuguilla 95 • Lechuguilla in South Brewster County
100 • Mr. Matthews, Elsinore Cattle Company 101 • J.M. "Manny"
Fowlkes and the Lion Dogs 103 • Rabies 104 • F. C. (Frank
Courtney) Mellard 112 • Roping a Cow from a Pickup 118 • First-
Class, High-Quality Sotol 119 • George Jones and Angus Bulls 120 •
General Boatner 121 • Purchase of the Hospital 122 • Ben's Goat
Dogs 122 • Harry's Goats 123 • Lynn "Crit" Crittendon 123 • My
Mashed Finger 124 • Drenching Sheep 126 • Cavin Woodward's
Pay Day Dandy 128

Chapter 4: Drouth - Drought   *133*

Robert Edward Lee Tyler **136** • Struggles Through the Drouth **140** • The Struggle for Water **142** • C. K. "Kenneth" Smith **143** • Spaying Heifers **144** • Postmortems **146** • Hollywood Comes to Marfa **147** • Another Side of Veterinary Medicine **150** • More Drouth Stories **150** • Dilemma **153** • Pressure to Practice Human Medicine **154** • Birth Defects **155** • Stargazers **156** • Unusual Problems with Plants **156** • Supplemental Feeding **162** • Hay **165** • My Efforts to Cope **167** • Ralph Lowe and the Bar C Ranch Horses **172** • The X Ranch Horses **173** • Morgan and Frances Chaney's Horses **175** • Other Thoroughbred Horses **176** • Hogs **177** • The Joe Bishop Cow **180** • Off-Duty **182** • Visiting **183** • Hunting Rabbits **184** • Reading **185**

Chapter 5: Shortly After the Drouth   *187*

Electronic Ejaculator **187** • A Not-So-Typical Work, Thankfully **188** • Brucellosis Testing for Eradication **190** • The Wooden Headgate **191**

Chapter 6: Up to My Armpits   *193*

While I Was Working **194** • 35 Head All Day **197** • My first 1000-Cow Day (Late 1950s) **198** • Ted Gray **201**

Chapter 7: Some Memorable Workdays   *203*

Faith Cattle Co. **203** • Maureen Godbold **204** • Graveyard Pens **205** • Charlie Donaldson **206** • Jim Phillips **207** • Cole and Alf Means **209** • Testing Without a Squeeze Chute or Headgate **211** • The Mix-up **212** • Procaine Penicillin in Aqueous Suspension **213** • Morumide **214** • Dick Swartz and the Grasshoppers **214** • Heat at Carrizo Springs Ranch **215** • On the Spot **217** • The Tranquilizer Gun **218** • C.C. "Coley" Means and the Angus Cows **220** Cockleburs **221** • Dick Henderson **222**

Chapter 8: The Veterinarian's Family Pets   *225*

Nanny Goat **225** • Zeke, Abe, and Boots **226**

My Pickups **234** • Toyah Cow Work 1960 **238** • A Complicated C-Section **246** • Horses and Colic **247** • Snow and −15° F **248** Trouble with Blood Samples **252** • Dry Spell at the Six Bar Ranch **253** • Rust Largent **253** • Sanderson Flood in 1965 **256** • One Memorable Postmortem Event **257** • Grass Seed **258** • Preston Johnson **258** • The Inconsiderate Cow **259** • Kick in the Chest **260** • Cold and Colder Weather **261** • The Ranchwomen **268** • Dr. Bonsma's Demonstration **269** • Pine Country of New Mexico **270** • A.R. Eppenauer, Sr. and the $5,000 Chickens **271** • Texas Veterinary Medical Diagnostic Laboratory **272** • Venezuelan Equine Encephalomyelitis **273** • Jim's Cow **277** • Charlie Gregory and the Old Mule **278** • John P. Searls, MD, Tetanus Vaccinations **279** • Some Airplane Trips **281** • The Cotton Gin Scales **284** • Horse Castration **285** • Bob War **287** • And the Rains Came **288** • Mutilations **291** • Horse Gore at the X Ranch **293** The Easter Eggs **294** Cold and Hot Hands **296** • The Newcomer's Bull **297** • The Carpets Versus the Rancher's Boots **297** • Grass Fires **298** • High Lonesome **302** • Poochie Quigg **308** • Copperheads **311** • Ken Rolston and the New Mexico Snowstorm **311** • Horse Gore at Chinati **315** • Blue Norther **315** • Removing Porcupine Quills **316** • Lorena Ann Kelly and Shannon **318** • F1 Tiger Stripe **319** • Braford Bull **320** • The Pregnancy Testing Horse **321** • Bodie's Teeth **321** • Jon Means **322** • Lizzie Means **323** • Mrs. Ron "Janet" Helm **324** • Sue (Keeling) and Dan C. "Topper" Frank Jr. **325** • Topper's Lion Hunt **328** • Topper Frank and the Cow on Fire **328** • A Boy's Pet Turtle **330** • Aubrey Lange's Helicopter **330** • Big Bend Ranch **331** • Wind **333** • Ted Harper **334** • Arm Injury **335**

Chapter 10: Shadows and Hints of Retirement 337

Heat Exhaustion at Altuda **337** • Blue Norther at the Barlite Ranches **339** • The Ribs **341** • Wind at the Arnold pens **342** • Heat Exhaustion at Presidio Stockyards **344** • Ike Roberts **347**

Chapter 11: Reflections 349

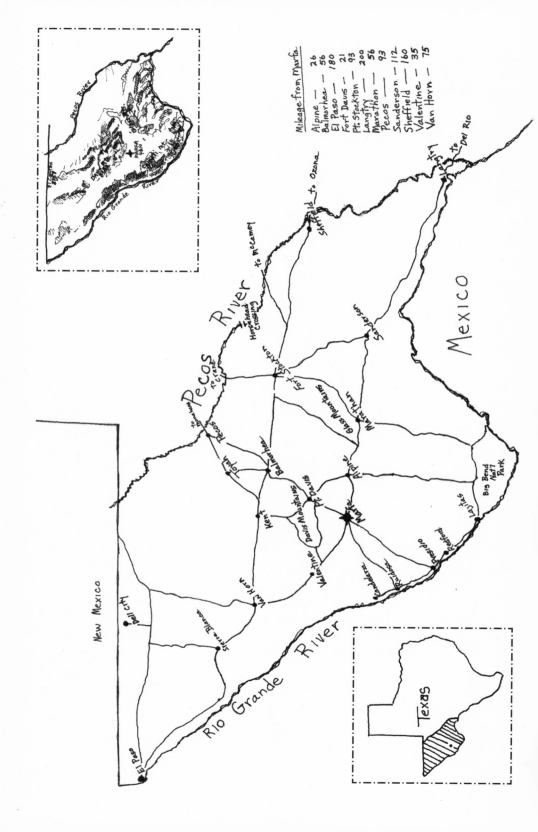

Prologue

Introduction

This is a collection of notes about my experiences. Included are a few stories I heard that particularly impressed me. I began writing at the suggestion of Lee Bennett, my daughters' history teacher. I continued with the encouragement of numerous persons, especially my wife, JoAnn, and my daughters, Nancy Edwards and Janet Edwards Franklin. The writing allowed me to while away the time after my retirement. Also, I wanted to give my grandchildren, and perhaps their children, some idea of where I lived, the type of practice I had and some of the people who influenced my life.

I retired from full-time practice at the age of 70 caused by emphysema, more correctly chronic obstructive pulmonary disease (COPD), but perhaps more so due to heat intolerance. My thermostat either wore out or was burned out by episodes of heat exhaustion because it became increasingly difficult for me to tolerate heat. I suffered with cold, but heat would cause me to melt.

I was reluctant to retire because I didn't think I could cope with inactivity after 46 years of going seven days a week, twenty-four hours a day. However, my last cow work was a hot summer day with bright sunshine. I had to stop, hunt shade, and rest four times while pregnancy palpating and blood testing only thirty-six cows. I realized then my decision to retire was not premature. A few months later I suffered a heart attack that really took the wind out of my sails. Writing these notes and doing some reading seem to satisfy my intellect. A heart walk in the early morning takes care of my physical needs. However, I did continue with a limited practice for another 6½ years.

I feel truly blessed and privileged to have lived in this beautiful area, been of service to such wonderful people, practice the profession I love, and yet make a comfortable living for my family. Actually the ranchers, cowboys, ranch hands and "wet"

Mexicans were all of a special breed that made my life so enjoyable. They faced adversity with a philosophical approach and a can-do attitude that was contagious.

The ranchwomen were truly remarkable. Many of them were good cowhands and worked along side of us. All were good cooks who fed us a banquet* at each meal. Some would cowboy until mealtime, then fix the groceries and often return to the work. Some would travel long distances over poor roads and in adverse weather to bring us our meal. Although these women worked hard, I never heard any complain. All were gracious ladies that were treated with respect.

How fortunate I was to have known and worked with such fine people, both women and men, white, brown, and black. I wonder if the area attracted this caliber of people or does it mold them this way?

My practice was never a hurried, impersonal relationship with my clients. They were my friends. I was usually able to have a relaxed, pleasant visit but there were times, of course, when this was not possible. The names mentioned were actual people. Some names were omitted to save possible embarrassment; other names have faded from my memory.

I thoroughly enjoyed most of my practice, working with capable, congenial people in pleasant weather. There was a high percentage of success although much of the surgery was under poor conditions, and many of the problems were in an advanced stage due to the difficulty of finding the animal in a timely manner. This recovery rate gave me a great sense of satisfaction, and my clients were generous with their praise.

Much of what I have written is about adverse conditions, inclement weather, difficult cases, and uncooperative patients that resulted in the things that were either traumatic or embarrassing. Some were even a little humorous. These instances are probably remembered because they were unusual.

There were some injuries that came with the territory and some stressful times that often occur in a large animal practice. I am fortunate to have escaped serious injury.

My practice was never sophisticated as many became with the advancements in equipment and techniques. It was a "fire engine

---

* A good meal when you're tired and hungry is truly a banquet.

practice." This was the term used in the profession for those that went from place to place, day and night to alleviate the pain and suffering of animals. It was a practice often of blood, sweat, and tears. Most of the livestock were raised as a means of livelihood; therefore, my treatments and fees were based on economics tempered by compassion.

There were a few house calls in towns to see pets, but by far the majority were ranch calls to attend to large animals. This is cow country, so I was primarily a cow doctor, resulting in most of my stories having to do with cattle.

When I first arrived, almost all the cattle were Herefords and the area was well known for the high quality cattle promoted by the Highland Hereford Breeders' Association. The only cattle that I can remember that were not Herefords were those crossbred by Cole and Alf Means, some mixed breeds belonging to Jimmy Livingston, and those owned by Cecil Rourk. Cap Yates and his son, Fayette, had a herd of purebred Longhorns and soon acquired Charolais which were considered exotic at that time. Of course, most ranchers kept milk cows, usually Jerseys, and then there were the cattle scattered along the Rio Grande River that were a mixture of milk stock, beef cattle, and the nondescript *corriente* from Mexico.

In later years, there were still more Herefords than any other single breed, but the crossbreed Hereford-Brahma and Angus-Brahma had become popular. There were also a number of Angus, Charolais, and Limousin, as well as a few purebred Brahmas and Longhorns. I learned to accept all the breeds and enjoyed working with them. The baby calves of all were a joy to watch as they romped around their mothers or chased each other, kicking up their heels with the tail straight up in the air. The stocking rate for cattle varies from as few as three or four up to as many as twenty or twenty-five head per section (640 acres), extremes of 20-200 acres per cow.

My practice territory for many years encompassed the part of West Texas known as the Trans-Pecos. It extended from the Pecos River to the east, the Rio Grande River to the south and west, and the New Mexico state line to the north. There were a few times that it spilled over into adjacent areas. From Marfa, it is about 180 miles northwest to El Paso, 200 miles southeast to Langtry, 60 miles south to Presidio on the Rio Grande River and 150 miles east to Sheffield on the Pecos River.

The elevation of the Trans-Pecos varies from 1500 feet to over 8000 feet. However, most of my practice was in the Davis Mountains-Big Bend area. Most of the ranches had an elevation between 3000 and 6000 feet. My hospital in Marfa was about 4600 feet.

It was in the geographical area known as the Chihuahuan Desert. We would joke about this, but we really didn't appreciate outsiders calling it a desert. We would say that the water was only 50% relative humidity and a two-inch rain was one where the drops were two inches apart. It was said that the time it rained 40 days and 40 nights this area got a half-inch.

There was a year when we received over 30 inches of rainfall and the country really put on its Sunday clothes. One fellow's comment was, "Wouldn't this be a great country if we got that much rain every year?" My father spoke up and said, "No, if we did, farmers would come in and dig up all the beautiful grassland and ruin it."

The high dry plateau in which Marfa lay surrounded by mountains caused radiation cooling during the night which produces some downright cold early mornings, many times the coldest in the state. When the sun came up, the weather quickly warmed to a very pleasant temperature. Sometimes, trying to dress properly presented a challenge.

Presidio and the adjacent lowland are hemmed in by bare rock mountains that are close by on all sides. The area has relatively little vegetation. The elevation is much lower, and the temperature is much higher. The summertime temperature is often the highest in the state, but the winters are hard to beat.

The Davis Mountains have a few ponderosa pine and even a little grove of aspen. There is some piñon pine but most of the trees are mountain cedar or juniper or oak. The foothills and flats (plains) are mostly open grasslands while the lowlands have primarily desert plants.

My practice territory was so large that it necessitated lots of driving. That wasn't so bad because I enjoyed it. Especially impressive were beautiful sights of fat cattle on green grass that turned golden after frost. It would look like a wheat field when waving in the breeze. The majestic mountains looked purple when viewed from a distance. On long calls, I would often travel a different way going and coming. But even when this was not possible, seeing the same area from a different direction at a different time of day would be equally scenic. Sometimes I would enjoy the return trip more because I might not be in such a hurry or, as quite often was the case, it would be daylight going home, whereas it had been dark initially. Often we had a beautiful sunrise and an equally beautiful sunset. A big white-topped cloud producing a thunderstorm followed by a rainbow was a sight to behold. Perhaps it made such an impression because it was not a very common occurrence. When time permitted, I would sometimes stop by the side of the road to enjoy the view. Actually the traveling gave me quality quiet time to recharge my batteries as I communed with God while contemplating his handiwork with wonder and awe.

Some of the sights that I always enjoyed were of the big mule deer, especially in the fall when they were fat with their coats dark and shiny and the bucks with their antlers that they carried so majestically. The antelope are properly called *pronghorns*, although that name was never used locally. They would race you when driving on a country road, often outrunning your vehicle, then passing in front. Sometimes they would circle around and attempt to re-cross in front.

Other scenes: An old buck antelope working a doe like a cutting horse working a steer. I'm not sure what was taking place but I never saw the doe regain the herd nor did I see the doe escape. A big long-eared, lanky jackrabbit running and dodging, jumping some bushes while skirting others. The golden eagle soaring high in the blue sky but a buzzard soaring in a thermal, equally graceful. You just didn't want to think how ugly they were while feeding on a roadkill skunk.

I have written of factual events as I remember them. Much of what I have written occurred in the early days of my practice, so only a few things were found in my ledgers to remind me of dates and details because most of the case histories of these early happenings had been discarded. I'm sure I remember more of the earlier years because I was more impressionable at that age. Also, I believe the poor roads and rather crude facilities caused more memorable wrecks. My choice of vehicles and clothing and the lack of proper equipment and available medicines also contributed to a more colorful practice.

There is much slang and vernacular. My original notes were written in long hand because I do not type. When my daughter, Nancy, offered to type them on a word processor, I asked her to correct my grammar. She encouraged me to leave it because that is the way I think and talk. "Be yourself, Dad."

A fellow U.S. Marine, John Mikus of Ohio, and I began corresponding on the 55th anniversary of our hitting the beach on Iwo Jima during World War II. We related our experiences since then. I sent him a few of my stories to give him an idea of where I was located and what I had been doing. He answered that I sure didn't talk like they do up there. I told him, "Mikus, I never did talk like you, but perhaps my speech has been influenced somewhat by my working fifty years on West Texas ranches with cowboys, ranch hands and 'wet' Mexicans."

Lee Bennett told me that once, when she was telling a tale, she was interrupted by someone correcting her. She stopped, turned to the person, and said, "This is my story, I'll tell it like I want!"

Now my memory is as good as it ever was, just a whole lot shorter. Actually, this is not altogether the case because I can remember many things that happened forty or fifty years ago, but I can't remember where I put my car keys.

Come join me. Get a cup of coffee, hunker down on your haunches by a campfire, or pull up a chair to a kitchen table. Listen to some stories. Very informal. Don't expect the grammar to be correct. It's written like I talk.

Chapter 1

Background

I was born on a ranch near Sanderson, Texas, on January 7, 1925 and lived my early years on various ranches near the border with Mexico. I had a wonderful childhood hunting, fishing, horseback riding, and playing with puppies, dogie calves, and lambs. I thought of myself as a real cowboy and ranch hand although at that early age I am sure that I was more a pest than a help. But my parents were patient with me, letting me do things that I could and allowing me to watch while they explained what they were doing at other times.

I had no playmates on the isolated ranches. My older sister spent most of the time with our maternal grandparents, the Barnetts, in town.

When I started school in Del Rio, Texas, I kinda shied away from other children not knowing how to play with others, but I gradually gentled down and acclimated to civilization, making friends.

The drouth (drought) and depression of the 1930s caused my father to go bankrupt in the ranching business and I had to learn to live in town. I finished grammar school and high school in El Paso, Texas.

I spent summers on the ranches of friends and relatives where I learned the fine arts of building fence, especially digging post-holes and shoeing horses. I learned to do these chores, but I didn't learn to like them. One summer was spent on the ranch of my cousins, F.O. "Buster" and Alicia Edwards, on Liveoak Creek near Uvalde, Texas. This was truly a vacation and was one of the most memorable times of my life.

My father bought me a horse that was kept at the stockyards where I began to help a little with the stockyard work and finally they put me on the payroll. The cattle handled in these yards were almost all steers imported from Mexico. Many of them came by railroad and often there would be a downer in one of the stock cars. The policy was to destroy these because they were in such pitiful condition. I began to take these and care for them. Mostly it was tender-loving care, propping them upright, then hand feeding and watering them.

When one recovered a rancher would buy it from me to add to his group. My success rate was very low until a veterinarian who came to the yards to test the imported steers for tuberculosis began to take an interest in me and my project. He started giving me advice and a few crude drugs. Nux vomica was the only one I remember. It helped so much that I used it in my early practice.

This was my first experience with a veterinarian. In fact, I didn't know there was such a thing as an animal doctor. We rarely went to a physician ourselves. He invited me to visit him at his veterinary hospital but I was too busy because I was making big money at the stockyards whenever I had any spare time. Jobs were pretty scarce in those days and twenty-five cents an hour was not to be ignored.

My parents and I inquired into the veterinary curriculum at Texas A&M College and were referred to one of the system's junior colleges. Therefore, I took my pre vet studies at John Tarleton Agricultural College in Stephenville, Texas, and left the Rio Grande — Mexican border for the next few years. Dr. Verne Scott, the elder who was one of the professors and the college veterinarian, took me under his wing. He also had a limited private practice and I got my first real introduction into the profession. I transferred to Texas A&M to begin the veterinary medical studies.

World War II was in full swing and I joined the U.S. Marine Corps in June 1943. I was wounded on Iwo Jima and spent the rest of my tour of duty in hospitals.

I returned to Texas A&M in January 1946. The first semester back was really hard for me. That summer, a full semester course load was offered to get the class back on a regular schedule. The hot summer in classrooms, laboratories, and dormitory rooms without air conditioning was uncomfortable but the studies were about to get me down. I was sorely tempted at times to give up and quit as other veterans had done but when I thought that the only two things I could do very well were digging postholes and shoeing horses, I would go back to studying with renewed vigor.

2

I graduated in June 1949. I had managed to squeeze a five-year course into 7½ years by attending college two summers. However, I did take a little time off for a Pacific island cruise, courtesy of the U.S. Marine Corps.

Dr. Ben Gearhart, veterinarian and rancher at Marfa, Texas, was building a veterinary hospital and was looking for someone to run it. He offered me the position that I eagerly accepted over the telephone. He hired me sight unseen.

Everyone in the dormitory had left at the end of the semester but I was still on campus taking the State Board examination to obtain my veterinarian's license to practice. I packed and loaded my car as soon as the test results were known and I left the next morning for Marfa.

Chapter 2

Arrival

I arrived in Marfa June 11, 1949, and took a room in the Crews Hotel. Mary Martha, Dr. Gearhart's wife, met me the next morning and I followed her to the ranch. I stayed with them at the ranch the next month, supposedly for the hospital to be finished but probably for my indoctrination and acclimation.

Mary Martha mothered me and fed me up. She told me who was related to whom, all the in-laws and outlaws, and that almost all the people in the area were related. She cautioned me to be careful what I said and to whom, also to be careful about agreeing or disagreeing. A person may cuss his kinfolks or friends but he doesn't want any outsider making disparaging remarks about either. She gave me some pointers on social graces but having been born and grown up within throwing distance of the Rio Grande, they were not much different than my own values. The newspaper and local news were important. When men exchange information in a coffee or barber shop it is 'news,' when women do so in a beauty parlor it is 'gossip'.

Ben had accumulated a number of choice cases at the ranch for me to cut my teeth on. I am not sure if his purpose was to test me, give me experience and confidence, or to break me in before turning me loose on the public. Perhaps it was all of these things. Cancer eye surgery was a major part of it, both excision (shaving) and treatment of superficial (surface) growths and ablation, or total removal, of the eye. Castration of the horse was emphasized, especially of the cryptorchid. The testicle is retained within the abdominal cavity and can be located only by feel. There is some skill to finding it immediately upon entering the abdomen but if it is not where it is supposed to be then there is a problem. Ben would repeatedly hide it among the intestines and I would *puddle guts* until it was found. At the time I thought the practice was being carried to an extreme but in later years the skill and confidence I acquired proved to be invaluable.

While I was still in my indoctrination phase, Dr. Ben Gearhart took me to his neighbors', Cole and Alf Means', Y6 Ranch. Ben had recently been expounding the virtues of Hereford cattle, in general, and his, in particular. Cole and Alf were doing some crossbreeding. They had bought some high-powered Brahma bulls from Hudgins in south Texas and were breeding them to their Hereford cows. Now Ben was a lot of things, but I don't think anyone ever accused him of being bashful. He blurted out right in front of them, God and everybody, "Charlie, look at those long-eared, long-legged, long-headed cows. They could drink out of a milk bottle. They're messing up a good set of Hereford cows!"

(Now I want you to know at the time of this writing, Ben's herd of cows has consisted of those long-eared, long-legged, long-headed cows, and he made disparaging remarks about the Hereford breed before his passing.)

The Means' crossbreeding program was 25 or 30 years ahead of the demand. These cattle later became very popular.

I worried at night about some of my patients. Ben said I would be O.K. in a few years. Do my best and go to the next case. When I retired after 46 years I was still taking patients to bed with me. Sometimes it became pretty crowded: dogs and cats, horses and cows, and an occasional sheep or goat.

When the hospital was finished or Ben and Mary Martha felt safe in turning me loose, I moved to town and lived in the Robinson apartments (site of the present day fire station) across the street from the courthouse and next door to Ben's mother. She was a dear lady and took over Mary Martha's duties of mothering me.

Each night I would call Ben to discuss cases that I had seen that day. His guidance and encouragement were invaluable.

I had been cautioned in college not to be too technical when talking to ignorant farmers and ranchers. Many would think I was just covering up with big words for my lack of knowledge. I was called to C.K. "Kenneth" Smith's 101 Ranch to postmortem a bull. I opened him up and had pieces scattered over half the hillside, when Kenneth became impatient, took out his pocket knife, cut the liver and said in disgust, "cirrhosis of the liver, that ———— ole senecio* again," and started walking back to his car. I gath-

---

* The common name is groundsel but it was rarely used in this area although the name senecio was sometimes confused with ceniza, the beautiful purple sage and also with chamisa, the four-winged saltbrush which was a desirable plant for grazing.

ered up my instruments and followed, very subdued. I did take time to cut the liver and discover how hard it was. So much for those poor dumb hicks. I told my boss, Dr. Gearhart, of my embarrassment. He laughed and cautioned me to look for the obvious before looking for the needle in the haystack. Also it might be time well spent to study the poisonous plants as they were a major problem locally.

Soon after I began practice, Jimmy Livingston brought a yearling heifer. She was of mixed blood having lots of ear, showing that there was a fair amount of Brahma blood. These cattle have a tendency to have a short fuse especially when they are raised in a big ole country, rarely seeing a human. She was fighting mad, bellowing, loud, fast breathing, shaking her head, charging and hitting the fence, mouth open, and with profuse salivation. She was tucked up in the abdomen showing she was neither eating nor drinking. I had seen a few rabies cases while in college and had taken a series of 21 injections from a cute little biting puppy. I knew this heifer had rabies and I didn't want any part of her.

Jimmy loaded her and took her to Dr. Dollahite, another veterinarian in town. Shortly, Jimmy brought me a length of mesquite limb that had been extracted from her throat. I was really perplexed and upset. I talked to Ben that night. He wasn't very sympathetic. He told me five conditions could look very similar: rabies, calf diphtheria, mesquite limb in the throat, some forms of pneumonia, and some loco poisonings. She had probably been upset by rounding up and hauling to town. He also said this was a good time to decide whether I wanted to practice in this area. I went into a corner and had a long, soul-searching talk with myself. I never refused another case for fear of contracting a disease. I did, however, take rabies treatments so many times that I lost count. A certain amount of risk comes with the territory. I'm not counting my refusals to treat rattlesnakes.

My first experience with rabies was in El Paso during the summer of 1948. I was working for Drs. Siemer and Broadwell at the El Paso Veterinary Hospital between semesters while I was still a student.

I was given a little more rope towards the middle of my second summer and was being allowed to examine some selected patients and treat a few under supervision. A Mexican lady brought a small puppy three weeks of age complaining it was not eating. It was very aggressive, growling and biting. I questioned the owner thoroughly who stated that the bitch (mother) and all the other pups were healthy, eating and acting normally, and this one had not been out of the house. She requested that we hospitalize the pup as it was the pick of the litter and had been promised to the owner of the sire. I should have suspected something was wrong as it appeared to be only a smooth haired mongrel. Later that day, Dr. Broadwell said that he suspected rabies. I assured him it could not be and related the history that had been told me. He was not convinced and said I could not always depend on the accuracy of history or even symptoms people relate. Sometimes it was caused by ignorance of the facts but often times the known facts were related incorrectly for one reason or another. He thought sometimes it was an intentional effort to mislead.

The pup died the next day. I removed the brain and hand carried it to the laboratory. I told them I was a veterinary pathologist and wanted to confirm the diagnosis regardless of whether it was positive or negative. We had studied the rabies positive brain and compared it to the normal healthy brain during the previous semester, so I knew what to look for. We just didn't have the sophisticated equipment at the hospital to prepare the specimen. Also a licensed pathologist was required for public health reasons. My purpose in wanting to confirm the diagnosis was because a rumor had circulated in our class that private labs often would report results as positive regardless of their findings to cover their tracks. I had numerous bites from the needle-like teeth so I felt I had maximum exposure, yet I was not anxious to take the 21 injections in the abdomen that was the prescribed prophylactic treatment at that time. They were reported to be very painful with rumors of abscesses and sometimes nerve involvement side effects. I had become accustomed to the needle from the many penicillin injections I had taken, but I also had acquired a fear of cold steel in the belly.

The lab reported a positive test, and I repeated my request to hold the specimen, that I would be right down. I hot footed it to the lab and confirmed the diagnosis to my satisfaction. I went to the owner's address and was told neither owner was home. I asked to see the bitch and the other pups and was told all had died. The one taken to the hospital was the last survivor. I was so infuriated that I didn't trust myself to have further contact with them, so I reported the case to the city-county health department for them to notify the owners and make recommendations.

I went to a local physician who insisted on giving the injections in the abdomen. When I refused, he consented to write a prescription for them. I then administered them to myself. They were subcutaneous injections and I had no problem going from arm to arm, then leg to leg. The injection sites did become larger and larger until I skipped the very last one, the twenty-first.

Whirlwind During Caesarean Section

One of my very first cases was a young heifer about 16 or 17 months old that had been accidentally bred. She was much too young and besides the calving would be out of season with the other heifers. Now this breeding was an accident according to the rancher's plans, but I think the bull did it on purpose.

She was trying to calve but was too small, there not being nearly enough room. A caesarean section was decided on. The heifer was snubbed to a post, laid down and rolled on her back. The front legs were tied together and up to the fence. The hind legs were also tied and up to the fence kinda stretching her out.

I used scissors to clip the hair on her midline from the navel to the udder. I scrubbed her belly, also my hands and arms, with tincture of green soap. The instruments were put in a tray with Quseptic solution, a Norden Lab quaternary ammonium disinfectant. This disinfectant didn't have the good strong odor of saponated cresol solution, but it had the advantage of being transparent so that the instruments could be seen. Groping around in a cloudy solution for a scalpel can be hazardous to your health. Also it had a nice cherry red color that looked like Kool-Aid which really impressed the wet Mexicans. On occasion I have had one to gag and spit with a distorted face. The Quseptic had a very bitter taste but sometimes the temptation to drink a little on a hot day was irresistible.

I was making every effort to perform clean surgery according to our standards at that time and in that place. Sterility is out of the question in a cow pen, even in this day and time, but our best efforts then were crude compared to later standards.

I infiltrated the midline with procaine anesthetic and made a generous incision. It heals from side to side, not end to end. The length provided more room but necessitated more suturing. The uterus was exposed and opened. A big, beautiful, lively calf was delivered. Not many brand-spanking newborn are pretty, but a baby Hereford calf with his red body and white face, big black eyes, and pink nose, is a sight to behold.

While the ranch hand assisting me rubbed it down with a tow sack, I started putting the heifer back together. I was proceeding carefully to close the uterus when a big whirlwind, that some call a dust devil, hit, carrying dust, dirt, hair, and powdered dry manure into the incision. I had been taught that the proper exclamation in the face of adversity was to say "Ah-ha" instead of "Uh-oh." I don't recall my comment at that time, but I have a faint suspicion that it may have been somewhat stronger.

My attempts to clean only resulted in causing the debris to become embedded in the tissue. I did the best I could, finally working sulfanilamide powder in so I couldn't see the dirt. I continued suturing, more to impress my audience than because I had much hope for her to survive.

I was deeply distressed and called my boss, Dr. Gearhart, that night. I guess I was looking for sympathy. Ben consoled me, saying that she would be all right because there were so many bacteria they would fight and kill each other off. Sure enough, she lived! Never looked back. I don't know if Ben truly thought she would live or was only trying to keep me from worrying and becoming discouraged.

Embarrassing Events

I've experienced a couple of embarrassing moments, maybe three. Some of them were caused by an attack of foot-and-mouth disease, I would stick my foot in my mouth, talking when I should have been listening. Sometimes things happened that I didn't earn — they were a gift.

*   *   *   *   *

Soon after my arrival in Marfa, I was driving around town with a girl telling me who lived where. I was driving slowly when a cat came running down the street straight for me with a good size dog in close pursuit. I stopped, the cat ran under my car with the dog just about to catch it. The cat was small enough, but the dog banged into the car and began the most God awful yelping you ever heard. He was kinda dazed and staggered around continuing to cry out.

It was a quiet Sunday afternoon in the summer. Air conditioners were few and far between, and people had their windows and doors open. The dog came through loud and clear; people poured out of their houses. I began to hear them calling to each other that the new vet in town had run over the dentist's, Dr. Nelson's, dog. I heard someone say, "What's he trying to do, drum up business?" The dog ran off. I didn't know what to do. I just sat there a moment, then tucked my head and drove off. It kinda put a damper on our relationship and ruined the good impression I was trying to make.

*   *   *   *   *

Shortly after I began practice, the phone was ringing as I walked in my office after a call to Joe Mitchell's Chastain Ranch across Alamito Creek. A honey-voiced young woman in Alpine said her horse was sick. I told her I would be right over. There was no veterinarian in Alpine at that time. I had on khakis that were bloody from cancer eye surgery so I changed into a pair of white overalls that I had from college surgery class. I still wore them occasionally to impress people of my newly acquired professional status. I scraped the mud and blood off my boots, washed my face and hands again, and combed my hair.

I drove to Alpine going up and around the Sul Ross College hill to Gene Benson's house and pens. A pretty young thing was on the far side of the pen with her arms around a big roan horse. "Sugar doesn't feel good. He keeps pawing and looking back." She was dressed in a white riding habit and had long golden hair. When she fluttered her eyelashes at me, I became all thumbs. I managed to dissolve some chloral hydrate crystals in some water and mix a little Turcapsol with mineral oil. This product was a combination of turpentine, capsicum, and ginger. This combination of herbs and spices is not generally accepted now, but it served me well for many years in colic cases.

I had not acquired many skills at this early time in my practice, but tubing, the passage of a stomach tube through the nostril down the esophagus to the stomach of a horse, was my claim to fame. I would probably have performed this procedure to impress the young lady regardless of what was wrong with the horse.

I gathered up my goodies and stumbled across the rocky pen, gliding along over, between, and around the big rocks with all the grace and charm of a camel. I managed to accomplish the feat without spilling anything although I was somewhat embarrassed because I thought I was agile in my youth, only exhibiting two left feet on the dance floor.

That big ole horse looked at the stomach tube and shied at that snake. He bowed his neck, danced sideways and rolled his eyes, showing way too much white for my comfort. If ever there was a misnomer, the name of Sugar for this horse was it. We sparred around a little and I finally started in his nostril with the tube and my chest began to swell with self-satisfaction until suddenly he slung his head violently, threw out the tube and snorted blood all over my pretty white overalls. I looked sheepishly over at the girl to see her nice white riding habit was now polka dot and she had the most distressed look on her face.

I'm not sure how I finished, I was in a daze. I was in such a state of shock and embarrassment that I didn't get her name and address to send a statement. I just wanted to get away. Maybe I didn't think I deserved a fee.

* * * * *

George Jones was a prominent rancher but when working cattle he didn't act or dress accordingly. I had met him at least once when I first arrived in the area but didn't recognize him when I was called to his ranch the first time. He was down in a pen sorting cattle, speaking Spanish to another man. He had on a sweat-stained, beat-up straw hat, and wore dusty Levi blue jeans slung low under his belly and run-over boots decorated with cow manure. I could distinguish no difference in the accent of the two men. Both were dark-skinned and weather-beaten. George's big belly was the only distinction between them. He soon came over to the fence and I attempted to talk to him in Spanish, having mistaken him for a Mexican ranch hand. I have been able to stick my foot in my mouth on any number of occasions but rarely have I been so embarrassed as I was that time. His comment was, "I hope you can treat cows better than you speak Spanish."

George Jones was a very special person to me. He had a great deal of influence in my life and was responsible to a large degree in what success I had in my practice. I will always remember my first meeting with him at the McElroy Stockyards in El Paso. It was 1939 or 1940. I'm not sure whether I was on the payroll yet or not. I hung around helping (maybe just getting in the way) for some time before I was actually hired. The ranchmen, cow buyers, and traders all impressed me with their big white hats, shiny boots, and nice cars. Someone introduced me as the son of U.S. Customs Inspector Edwards. Mr. Jones shook my hand and said, "If you make half the man your daddy is, you will be all right."

This made my failure to recognize him on my first call to his ranch even more embarrassing.

*   *   *   *   *

George Jones once called me to see a sick cow in his Quebec pens. There were two cows in there. One looked pretty thin and the other was in good flesh. No one was there to help, but this was not uncommon and not a problem as I often examined and treated without assistance. I put the sorry cow in the chute and began poking and prodding, finally discovering an enlarged uterus and a low grade fever. I began treating her for metritis (infected uterus) when George drove up. "That's the cow I just brought home from your place that you've been treating for the last week." George just shook his head and I was embarrassed that I had not recognized her.

Two Calls to the Reid Brothers Ranch

Roy and Wade Reid were two older ranchers. Their place was in the Barrilla Mountains in the northeast edge of Jeff Davis County, possibly part of the ranch was in Pecos and Reeves Counties. Dorothy "Dot" Reid, Wade's wife, called and reported that the men had found a cow that was very thin, saliva stringing from her mouth, with her head in a water trough but unable to drink. My first thought was rabies. Shortly before, I had had the bad experience with the calf belonging to Jimmy Livingston that had a mesquite limb hung in the throat. My enthusiasm for a challenging new case was tempered by this thought. I collected a few instruments and drugs. I didn't have very many, but we didn't

13

know any better. We didn't know we had to have a lot of sophisticated equipment and medicines.

The drive down Limpia Canyon was spectacular, with many bridges across the winding creek with its running water and the big cottonwood trees lining the banks. Especially attractive were the palisade-type basalt rock bluffs along the canyon wall. Then to top it all off, the awesome view of the high, sheer cliff of Star Mountain when seen from Wild Rose Pass. It would take your breath away. I never tired of this sight, and I have been known to dawdle a little to enjoy it.

Where the dirt ranch road turned off the pavement there was a creek crossing. It was wide and had a gravel bottom with water running a few inches deep except for a couple of gravel bars that were dry and one fairly deep hole. It was kind of exciting when I dropped off into the hole, but I had up good momentum and kept on going. The ranch was about ten miles down this road and past the ranch headquarters of another ranch. The road was somewhat primitive. It had been part of the Army road from San Antonio to El Paso, the Butterfield Overland Stage road, and one route of the Chihuahua Trail. I don't think it had been worked since then. I was still driving my new Chevrolet sedan that I was so proud of, and I would wince when I hit high center. I would pull myself up off the seat to give a little more clearance. It doesn't do any good but it helps psychologically. I would hit a mud hole and splatter the car that I kept polished bright and shiny. I would later abandon this bit of appearance. The road went between the first ranch house and the barn and pens. I circled around there a time or two with dogs barking and dogie calves bawling until I finally discovered the road leading onward.

A couple of miles farther, I came to the ranch and Dot greeted me. I had coffee and cake and a nice visit. You didn't just dash up and go to work, besides this was my first call and we needed to get acquainted. They were so congenial that I'm afraid I always spent more time than I should have. Some would say I wasted time, but this was a different era. It is sad to remember those nice, long visits and compare them with the way we now run around helter skelter. Our clients are more customers now instead of friends.

We finally got around to discussing the cow in question. She was up in the mountains, and the men said the road wasn't very good, that it might be better to go in their pickup. I thought of the road I had just traveled and they said the mountain road wasn't very good? I didn't argue and put my supplies in the back of their pickup. The three of us crowded into the cab. Pickups weren't very wide then. I was offered the middle seat but I declined preferring the outside. The person in the middle had nothing to hang onto as we bounced along. (These were the days before seat belts.) He also got elbows in his ribs from both sides, especially from the driver constantly turning the steering wheel. Also his left leg was continually being hit on the knee cap by the floor gear-shift stick. Wade wasn't much of a driver — he rode the clutch pretty bad. When he shifted gears it got real exciting.

Some old cowboys that spend most of their time in a saddle can make a pickup ride down a ranch road a real adventure. They don't really drive it, they just kinda herd it. Well, not that either exactly, it's more like letting a horse have his head to pick his way along. 'Course the dumb pickup doesn't watch where it's going, so the cowboy floorboards it and lets the chuck holes and rocks look out for themselves.

The outside position wasn't all roses because it was hot summer time with the window rolled down. Air conditioning in vehicles wasn't heard of and certainly not in a ranch pickup. Having three of us in the narrow cab forced me about halfway out the window to get smacked by brush. The real chore came as gate opener. The gates were wire gaps. This consisted of a post at each end connected by five strands of barbed wire. The hinges are wire and the latch consists of a wire loop at the base in which the post is inserted and a wire loop at the top to fit over the top of the post. A few sophisticated gates had cheater bars to assist in stretching the gate to fit the wire loop. The hame (curved part) of a horse harness made the best cheater. Most gates had to be closed by wrapping your arm around the fence post and grasping the gate post and squeezing. If an old shirt was worn, there usually wasn't much of a problem, but a good shirt would snag on a barb and you would have the devil trying to unthread it without a tear. Occasionally if you were real careful you would manage to get a little hide caught under that loop—it pinched pretty bad. The spontaneous exclamation would cause your companion to ask if you were hurt. To which you would invariably answer, "No," even as you bit your lip. These gates have caused many a man and a few women to lose their religion. There have even been some children that I strongly suspect may have had some unkind thoughts.

We finally arrived. It probably wasn't far in miles but it had seemed a long way. The cow was in a little 8×10 foot wire pen near a water trough. These pens were common when screw-worms were so bad. Minor worm cases were roped and treated where found. Others would be put in these small pens until they got well, fed hay and cottonseed cake and watered with a five gallon can. The cottonseed cake was later formulated to make a more complete supplement and was technically a range cube, although we called it cow cake.

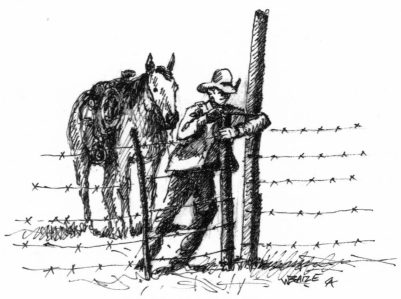

Struggling with a wire gap gate.

I had been hoping there would be mesquite trees around like there were near the house, but there weren't any in the hills, so that eliminated the chance of a mesquite limb in her throat. She was a gentle Hereford cow, pretty badly tucked up in the flanks, showing she hadn't eaten for several days. Usually a cow with rabies doesn't live long enough to get this bad. Also she was very lethargic instead of aggressive. However, this didn't rule out dumb rabies which is a form of the disease exhibited by having a vacant expression to the eyes and a complete lack of interest in the surroundings. We snubbed her to a post and I put nose tongs in place and pulled her head up causing her mouth to drop open. There was lots of grass packed in there with her cheeks pooched out like she had a good big chew of tobacco. I finally got her mouth clean and checked the tongue and teeth which seemed normal. I thought I was pretty clever to have fixed her up so promptly. I took my stomach tube and passed it down a nostril expecting it to go to the stomach so I could pump in a little water for showmanship. The blooming thing went only a little ways down her throat and stopped. I fiddled with it, took it out and put it down the other nostril. It still wouldn't go. I measured how far it went and felt of the neck. A bump, that I first thought was the larynx. It was down too far. I jiggled it and it wouldn't budge. I was at a loss. I put my arm beside the cow's head and measured. My hand should reach the object if I could get up enough nerve to put my hand down her throat without a speculum. While we were in school, I was told a recent graduate had lost a forefinger on his right hand to a horse while examining its mouth. The loss of that finger sure did cramp his style. The two old gents looked at me inquiringly.

I stalled, hoping they would say to let her go, it wasn't worth the risk. They didn't say a word, just looking back and forth at the cow and then to me. I finally picked up a little piece of wood and crammed it between her teeth and stuck my hand in gingerly. Deeper and deeper, farther and farther. I dug out a little grass and mucus that had a bad odor. I started back in and the cow coughed. Some of the loose material that had remained in her pharynx stimulated the cough which shot out into my face. I was blinded and gagging. I really felt sorry for myself. Roy and Wade didn't offer any sympathy or consolation. They didn't wrinkle up their noses or blink their eyes. As soon as I got my breath I went back in and finally removed all the grass from around the hard object, but I couldn't get a grip on it. I used my free hand to massage the outside of the neck and force the object up so that I could get a hold of it. It sure didn't want to come. Twisting and turning, pulling with one hand and pushing with the outside hand, it began to come. I forgot or at least ignored the sharp points on her teeth gouging my arm. I was afraid to let go, I might never again get such a good grip. At last it was out and so were all my fingers. I went to the water trough and washed the blood and crud from the object, my hand and arm. The object was a deer horn (properly antler), three prongs with sharp points. I don't see how she swallowed it as far as she had and I don't see how I was able to pull it out. I guess rats had gnawed an antler that had been shed recently to make this shape, although the cow could have helped by chewing on it. I was so proud of myself that I kept it. I still have it.

This was the first of many such removals of bones and deer horns. Some would be caught across the roof of the mouth, others across the bottom jaw teeth, under the tongue, a few between the upper and lower teeth that propped the mouth open. The cattle were trying to satisfy their need for phosphorus. Mineral mixes were few and expensive. Moorman's sold by Ben Pruett was the only one I knew of. It was usually fed only to registered stock when the grass was dry. A few ranches mixed bone meal and salt and fed it in troughs, as was some granulated Carlsbad salt which was red and looked really rich. However, it contained only potassium, no phosphorus. It was a by-product of the potash mines. Most fed white block or yellow sulfur salt. Happy Godbold soon began the Stock-Aid Mineral Company making a good economical mix that filled a great need.

The tooth scrapes on my hand and arm were oozing a little blood so I poured tincture of phenylmercuric nitrate over them. This stung like the mischief, but I guess it seared the bleeders or at least it was also red and blood didn't show. I put my shirt back on and the sleeve acted like a bandage. I wore heavy cotton khaki shirts and pants then. It seems that I had my arm down a cow's throat half the time in the first part of my practice and up the other end the later part, but there were no teeth back there.

I passed the tube again to make certain the esophagus was open. I admit I said a little prayer as it went down. I really hadn't felt safe until the tube went all the way and I breathed a sigh of relief. I pumped in a couple of gallons of water and removed the tube and nose tongs. Roy filled her water can and threw a chip of alfalfa and some cottonseed cake. Much to my disappointment, she just went over in a corner and stood there, showing no interest. They checked on her the next day and she had eaten all the feed and had drunk the water. Dr. Ben Gearhart and I talked almost every night as I discussed cases for guidance. I told of the experience, thinking he would be impressed. He didn't react — I guess he expected me to handle the situation.

*   *   *   *   *

A few weeks after my call to see the cow with the deer horn, I had another call to the Reid Brothers ranch. I about halfway dreaded this call, hoping those two old gents weren't such good cow doctors that they didn't need a vet except in really tough cases. However, they were so congenial, I anticipated a pleasant visit. It had continued to rain at regular intervals, and the water in Limpia Creek was still running at all the crossings but none high enough to cause any problem as there was a good gravel bottom.

I delivered a calf from a heifer that had been inconsiderate enough to get pregnant and calve out of season. Great effort was made to prevent calving during screwworm season, but this heifer and a yearling bull had gotten acquainted without benefit of a formal introduction.

I was in the kitchen, humbly accepting the praise for having delivered a live calf that was quickly up and nursing. I was drinking coffee and eating cake with Wade, his wife, Dot, and Roy Reid. I always enjoyed visiting with them and Dot baked a delicious cake. I may have dawdled. The telephone rang and Dot picked the receiver off the hook. It didn't seem like it was the same number of longs and shorts as it had been a while ago when she answered, but who's counting?

Suddenly, she told us there was an 8-foot rise coming down Limpia. This news threw me into a panic because of the crossings I had to make. Limpia was so long that it took quite a while for the creek to run down, and even then the crossings might be washed so badly they would have to be worked by a county road crew before they would be passable.

I left with Roy following to be sure I made it. The first crossing of the creek was about the same as coming out, just a little stream. But the big, wide one near the highway was up about 8 or 10 inches. That doesn't sound like much, but it was enough to cover the gravel bars that had been high and dry. There were also some pretty good ripples in the main channel.

I slowed down a little when I saw it, but remembered that he who hesitates is lost, so I gunned it. I had up a pretty good head of steam when I hit the water, which splattered up on the windshield in my face, blinding me.

Actually, being blinded didn't matter much because the water splashing had drowned out the engine. The momentum carried me out about halfway. I would have to stop in the deepest, swiftest place. Roy and I pulled off our boots and rolled up our pants legs and played in the water about an hour. Roy's snow white feet and legs were quite a contrast to his brown, weather-beaten face and hands. Roy's tender feet on that gravel caused him to tiptoe around like he was walking on eggs. He was quite a sight, but frankly, I wasn't in a mood to break out laughing. I was kinda panic stricken.

We dried off the spark plugs and distributor and anything else we could find, jiggling wires and hoses. Roy was almost as igno-rant as I was about what made a car go. I say almost, because nobody was as bad as I was. My standard first aid for a sick vehi-cle was to look in the gas tank, kick the tires, and start walking. Whatever we did to the engine worked, because it started. Of course, maybe the motor heat had dried out the necessary thinga-majig. The motor ran and the tires spun, but the car didn't go any-where. It just sat there and dug a hole. We cut a little seep-willow brush that we crammed under the tires, but most washed off by the fast running water about as fast as we put it down. We were working frantically with one eye up the creek, watching for that wall of water that had been reported.

We were plumb exhausted, and it looked hopeless when Roe Miller Sr. drove up in a butane truck. He told us that we were experiencing the rise in the water. The 8 inches had become 8 feet which may have been the normal and natural growth that comes with the passage of information by word of mouth. Some might call this exaggeration. On the other hand, there is a possibility that the crackle, snap, pop of the country telephone line may have been the culprit.

Roe had a winch on the front of his truck with a long cable that we hooked on the front of my car, and he pulled me out. What a relief!

Smokey Babb at Rough Creek Ranch

Mrs. Martin called me from Marathon early one morning saying her milk cow was sick and gave me directions to the ranch known as Rough Creek. It was south of Marathon in some rough country and a far piece from town. The directions made the trip interesting and a challenge to keep from going off on a pasture road or taking a wrong fork when the road divided at times. Now I heard it rumored that men aren't too good about stopping and asking for directions, but down along this road there wasn't anyone to ask, so I had a valid excuse to just keep going. I mean this was a *rural* road.

I was driving a Chevrolet sedan with poor clearance at the time and would often hit high center. This wasn't a car road and not a very good pickup one at that time. I learned later that one family down this road used a World War II Dodge Power Wagon to make the trip. Good thinking! The road showed to have been graded at one time but I had to straddle potholes and dodge rocks. My car was fairly new and still a little stiff but this loosened it up.

I finally arrived at the ranch to find Mrs. Martin's son-in-law, Smokey Babb, skinning a doe deer. It was summer and not deer season, besides it being a doe. However, there have been times when a permit has been issued to kill doe mule deer although I never heard of one issued to kill out of season. I didn't ask if he had a permit. Of course, this may have been an accident. I've heard of fellows claiming they were shooting at a coyote and this deer just happened to get in the way at the wrong time. Smokey had a two or three week black beard and long shaggy hair. He had on an old sweat stained, beat-up hat pulled low and bloody leather leggins (chaps) and run-over boots with only one spur. A half-smoked roll-your-own cigarette hung from the corner of his mouth. His 30-30 rifle was leaning handily against the tree from which the doe was hanging. The reputation of the Babb family was somewhat colorful and Smokey's involvement in his brother's, W.L. Babb's shooting of Stanley Jeffers in Lajitas added to the reputation. W.L. Babb's trial had not yet been held and rumors abounded. It seemed that Smokey was visiting W.L. who had a candelilla wax plant there in Lajitas and Stanley and Joe Jeffers were river riders. This was during the foot-and-mouth disease epidemic in Mexico. Horseback riders patrolled the river trying to keep cattle from Mexico out. This was the Aftosa Program.

The Jeffers and a visitor, Eugene Lefevre, were target shooting and apparently some of the bullets came close to Smokey and W.L., who decided to go visit them about this. Tempers flared, shots were exchanged, Stanley Jeffers was killed, and W.L. Babb was hit just below the shoulder.

Jim White told me he was on the panel to select a jury for the W. L. Babb trial. When questioned, he said he had known W. L.

in Del Rio and was excused from serving. He said he didn't know if the prosecution scratched him thinking he might be a friend, or the defense thinking he might know W. L. too well!

Smokey's appearance did little to allay my anxiety at this jumping off place. He made no comment regarding the deer and neither did I. I introduced myself, explained the purpose of my visit, and shook the bloody hand that he extended. He told me where to find the cow, suggesting that she was probably dead and continued with his chore. I went around behind the old lean-to shed and found the Jersey milk cow with a newborn calf by her side. She was in typical milk fever attitude, lying down with her head and neck kinked back to her side. She was cold to the touch with slow almost imperceptible breathing and heartbeat. She responded nicely to intravenous calcium gluconate which can produce the most spectacular recovery at times. However, if I assure the owner that the cow will soon be all right, she won't! Cattle seem to delight in making me look like a fool. It never ceased to amaze me how two cows with exactly the same history and symptoms can be so different in their response to medication.

The cow was on her feet eating and the calf nursing when Smokey came to the pen. He pushed his hat back with his thumb, scratched his head and said, "Well, I'll be ———!" We went to the house, drank some coffee and ate a cold biscuit. It doesn't take much water to make good coffee but this would have floated a horseshoe. We cussed and discussed the weather and stock prices. The doe was never mentioned.

These were tough times in a hard ole country. Ranch livestock were not killed and eaten, they were sold to raise cash to make a payment on the interest of the note at the bank. Maybe buy a few beans and some flour. This deer was not killed for sport, it was for sustenance. I suppose it is obvious that my fee for services was modest. I learned to know Smokey as a good cowboy and he became a friend.

Eating Preferences of a Cow Belonging to
S.S. "Ted" Harper

Soon after I began practice, Ted Harper brought a cow to my hospital from the southern part of the county between Casa Piedra and Presidio. This is a different world from that around

Marfa. The cow had metritis and was very sick. Ted left her with me when I told him the treatment I intended to give.

Her uterus was full of pus and the cervix was closed tightly so that it could not escape. A cow's cervix cannot be forced open manually so I gave her an injection of Stilbesterol, an estrogenic hormone, to relax the cervix and allow it to open. She had a high fever so I gave her sulfathiazole boluses by mouth. This was our best antibacterial agent at that time because penicillin was too expensive to use on range cattle. I gave the boluses with a balling gun which is an instrument to get them past the teeth and into the pharynx so that it would be swallowed without chewing or spitting it out. She wouldn't eat or drink so I gave her cottonseed meal and molasses mixed with water by a stomach tube and pump. I also gave dextrose and calcium gluconate intravenously. I then gently massaged the uterus by rectal palpation. This was repeated twice a day and the third day the cervix began to open and the purulent uterine material began to discharge. I irrigated the uterus with a stomach tube and pump using a special uterine catheter irrigator. I alternated the treatments using Quseptic disinfectant solution one day and acrifavine the next.

Her temperature returned to normal, the eyes and nose improved, but she still would not eat the cottonseed cake range cubes and alfalfa I had put on the ground for her. Ted came in from the ranch in a few days and I reported the situation to him. He took a chip of alfalfa and tied it about waist high on the fence with baling wire. To my astonishment, the cow immediately started eating it . Ted then told me that the pasture she had been in was hard old country and she had eaten only brush, dagger and lechuguilla blooms and didn't know to eat anything off the ground. He wasn't surprised she didn't eat range cubes because she had never been fed and didn't know what they were. He loaded her in the back of his pickup in the stock rack and hauled her to the ranch. He later reported that she made a slow but good recovery. I recommended that he sell her in the fall because these cases rarely become pregnant.

Sleeping Sickness Vaccination

I was told there had been plentiful rain in most of the area for the last few years. This was evident in the beautiful stands of grasses that were headed out and waving in the breeze, and the dirt tanks full of water.

The rainfall had been a mixed blessing, producing also a profusion of toxic loco weed, and an unusual batch of mosquitoes that had infected many horses with equine encephalomyelitis, commonly called sleeping sickness.

A number of horses had been poisoned with loco which produces a nervous disorder. There was no treatment and the only prevention was keeping animals away from the plant. The ones that were affected the worst had to be sold but many were kept if they could be used somewhat, especially the brood mares.

The sleeping sickness could be prevented by a vaccination. The dose was 1 cc (ml) given intradermally and repeated in 7 to 10 days. So far as was known, only the western strain of the disease was present in the area. This was substantiated by the fact that the disease was prevented when using only this strain in the vaccine. The eastern strain became a problem also in later years.

The intradermal injection was made by pinching up a small fold of loose skin on the neck just in front of the shoulder. A small syringe with a very fine needle was used. This somewhat delicate procedure had to be made with care to keep the vaccine from going under the skin or the needle going all the way through and out so the vaccine was squirted into the hair. .

Most horses didn't mind the shot too much if the fold of skin was pinched to numb it somewhat and a sharp needle inserted smoothly and quickly. A blunt needle, especially one with a hook on the end, was inviting trouble. There were no disposable needles at that time so care needed to be taken to protect the point. Many evenings were spent in sharpening needles on a whetstone.

Some horses seemed to be hypersensitive to the needle and this was particularly true of the ones affected with loco. They would shy and prance away and roll their eyes with so much white showing that they looked spooky. Just as the needle entered they might reach up with a forefoot attempting to paw your shirt pocket off or part your hair. It wasn't too bad to lose a pocket, but I sure didn't enjoy losing skin.

It was rumored that an accidental self-injection of the vaccine would give a person sleeping sickness. I personally never heard of anyone becoming sleepy, but some that had vaccinated themselves complained of chronic headaches. Because of the delicate procedure and the skittish horses, one often pricked the end of his finger. Many of the ranchers and all the ranch hands would rather have a veterinarian do the chore. I wasn't all that enthusiastic working with locos, but a certain amount of risk is expected when working with animals.

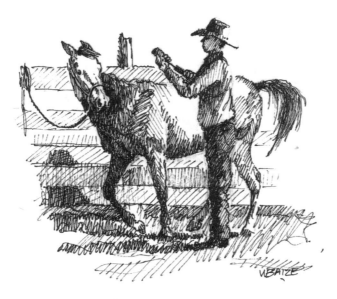

Preparing a vaccination.

I did stick my fingers a number of times. Maybe that's the reason I had a tendency to nod off when I went a day or so without sleep.

First Vehicles

When I first arrived in Marfa, I had a 1948 metallic blue Chevrolet sedan. You cannot imagine how proud I was of this vehicle. It soon proved to be impractical. A trip to Smokey Babb at the Martin Rough Creek Ranch and two to the Reid Brothers' Barrilla Ranch were especially memorable that first summer. It was too low to the ground and hit high center frequently. The soft springs for comfortable riding caused more problems. When loaded with medicine and equipment it was even lower and a little rough place would cause a bounce and it would hit bottom. The cloth seats would soil easily and stain badly besides absorbing odors, because many of the medicines of that day had strong smells, and often my clothes and boots would be pretty ripe.

Bubba Hord and I soon became friends and he talked me into buying a new type vehicle from his father, Herschel Hord, who owned the Chrysler-Plymouth dealership. It was a Plymouth station wagon that was all metal, had four doors and a good tailgate to use as a table. The seats were made of a smooth, impervious material, probably plastic. This material was hot in the summer and cold in the winter but easy to clean. The interior had more room, the springs were stronger and it had better clearance.

Several men had advised me to get a pickup, but having two vehicles was too rich for my blood. A used pickup was out of the question because at that time in this area a used pickup was really used up. The rancher drove the new pickup until it began to give trouble. His number one hired hand would get it next, followed by a flunky or it was used as a spare until it completely quit. The rough ranch roads and heavy loads caused this cycle to be relatively short because a two-ton load on a half-ton rated pickup was common.

Trading my car for a new pickup would have been the most practical solution, but I was single and dating. A man just didn't ask a girl on a date in a pickup at that time.

The Plymouth station wagon proved to be a fairly satisfactory practice vehicle if I drove slowly over ranch roads and did not load it too heavily. However, both of these were violated all too frequently.

If the ranch road was rough and I needed a heavy load such as phenothiazine drench, I would often go on the call with the rancher in his pickup. The phenothiazine drench dose was two ounces per sheep which meant a gallon would drench 64 head, theoretically. However, I always felt fortunate to drench 60 head with a gallon. A day's work consisted of at least a thousand head and usually considerable more. The weight wasn't so bad but the seventeen or so gallons would be bulky.

Buck Pyle and Chorizo

Buck Pyle was the managing partner of the West Pyle Cattle Co. He was always well dressed, even in a stockpen. Of course, he wasn't flanking calves. Buck's co-pilot, that helped him drive, was a really nice, well-mannered dachshund named Chorizo, which means sausage in Spanish. Chorizo stayed right by Buck's side even in the pens. Dr. Gearhart and I were at the Longfellow railroad stockpens inspecting Buck's calves that he was shipping. I don't remember why both of us were there; perhaps I was still on a leash as I had only recently come to work for Ben. Ben was trying to stop smoking and was chewing tobacco. He spit and it landed right on Chorizo's head. I'm not sure but what it was intentional. Buck got down on his knees, took out his mono-grammed handkerchief from his coat pocket, and wiped the juice off. Ben whispered, not too quietly, "That ole silly fool."

Years later Ben started carrying an English bulldog with him named Sissy. She was not nearly so nicely mannered as Chorizo. When going through Valentine, if a dog was on the street, Ben would say, "Sissy, look at that old common dog." Sissy would bark and run from window to window, almost becoming hysterical.

She loved to jump in water troughs to cool off. An exploratory oil well was drilled under the rim of the Sierra Vieja Mountains. No oil was found but a hot artesian water well remained. The water formed a pool with colorful mineral deposits in terraces. Ben stopped to look at it and Sissy jumped in to cool off. That water was scalding hot and immediately she began crying painfully. Ben waded in and carried her out but it was too late, the burns too bad. Ben's feet were badly burned, requiring a long, painful healing process. Ben took losing Sissy pretty hard.

Another English bulldog later rode the co-pilot seat, Nikki. She was much more dignified, fatter, and Ben was just as attached to her. Ben wouldn't stay in a motel unless his dogs could stay also. Rumor had it that he almost refused to go to the hospital for heart surgery because the dog was not allowed to stay with him.

Banky Stocks at Cole and Alf Means' Y6 Ranch

The fall of 1949 Alf and Cole Means called me one night from their Y6 Ranch near Valentine. They told me they had some sick calves, but they were having to leave for San Antonio to a cattle-man's meeting. I think it was a Texas and Southwestern Cattle Raisers Association meeting, and they both held offices. They said Banky Stocks was at the ranch and would help me. I had known Banky in El Paso. We both went to Austin High School but he went for only for a year. However, we had gone to several get-togethers and had become friends in a short time. I had a crush on his sister, Joan.

I arrived at the ranch bright and early the next morning. Actually it wasn't very bright but it was early. It was just getting daylight. I had gathered up all the sulfa drugs I had on hand. They were the only antibacterials I had for cattle then. I kept a little high-priced penicillin for dogs and cats but it was too expensive to use on cattle. We said our howdys and went to the pens to look at the calves. I had put in a couple of thermometers but they weren't needed. You could eyeball the sick. They had snotty noses, were drooling saliva, panting, coughing, and lying around. They were showing their illness plainly. I posted* a couple of dead ones to confirm my diagnosis of pneumonia. That 40 head of calves was the sorriest sight I had ever seen up to that time.

We went to the pasture where the calves had been turned out on arrival—a pretty good bunch, maybe 1000 head scattered out in a ten-section pasture. Banky drove the Jeep while I looked at the steers. Like the ones in the pen, the worst weren't hard to spot, nor were the ones off by themselves with their heads hanging down, but a few with only droopy ears were questionable. There were too many sick to try to gather and keep in the pen, so we decided to treat in the pasture.

We returned to the house and I telephoned Fort Worth for a new sulfamethazine bolus called Sulmet that I had just read about. It was a broader spectrum drug and only needed to be given once a day and the claim was made that it was easier on the kidneys because of slow excretion. The company agreed to put it on Trans Texas Airways which had recently begun commuter service and was landing in Marfa at the old Army Air Base. Then Banky and I went to the pens and started treating–giving the intravenous Disulfalac, a combination sulfathiazole-sulfapyridine to the sicker ones until it was exhausted, then the oral sulfathiazole boluses followed by the older sulfanilamide. I had chalked a

---

* Postmortem exam by opening the carcass and looking inside.

code for the drug given each so that I could repeat the same treatment when possible.

Some calves were already dehydrated so we caught these individually, passed a stomach tube and pumped in as much water as we felt safe in doing. This was especially important with sulfa drugs as they were bad about damaging the kidneys by forming crystals. I'll bet if those calves had known what was going to happen to them, they would have gone to the water trough and tanked up. I know I would have.

Late in the afternoon we gave the second dose of medicine and I went back to Marfa. I called Nathan Morris, the airport director. This was a pretty high-faluting name for the only airport employee. He sold tickets, wrestled baggage, and directed traffic (I guess that's what it was, he got out in front of the plane and waved his arms.) He also gave the airline their weather report. I found out that the plane I was hoping had my pills was due in about 8:30 in the morning. I was there waiting. I was very surprised to see Lynn Kern was the co-pilot. Lynn was from Ysleta and was in college with me. He quit and went in the Army Air Corps flying P-38 and P-40 fighters in North Africa and Italy. We both started back to Texas A&M after the war together but he couldn't keep his mind on vet medicine. I tried to study with him, but all he could think and talk about was airplanes. He finally gave up and went home, getting a job crop dusting. He tore up two or three planes hitting power lines but managed to walk away each time. Why in the world an airline would hire an ex-fighter pilot and crop duster was beyond me. I guess he settled down because he flew for them and their later line, Texas International, until he retired.

My Sulmet boluses were on board so I loaded up and went to the ranch. We treated the sick pen first and were pleased that we had lost only a couple of the worst ones. Banky had fed the sick cattle and cleaned their water trough and fed the pasture cattle cake. He had rigged up a saddle on the hood of the Jeep that he rode while I chauffeured. He would rope a steer and I would bail out, catch him, poke a pill down his throat with a balling gun, put a chalk mark on, take off the rope, climb back in the Jeep while Banky coiled his rope, and off we would go. I made a sudden turn and threw Banky off, so he rigged a safety belt to hold himself. He was a good roper and rarely missed, when I could put him in position. I wasn't a very good horse.

We worked in the pasture as long as we could see, then went to the ranch and tube-watered the calves that were tucked up the most, showing they hadn't drunk. We would cram in a few pieces of cake in their mouths which some would chew up and swallow. I wish that we had *Ensure* or a similar liquid nutrient at that time. It had to be the dark side of the moon, so we treated by headlights. I was not married at the time and I don't think Banky was either. We treated sick steers for five days, both of us staying at the ranch. Banky was a better cook than I was, but I was a mean bottle washer. However, we didn't eat very fancy.

We finally turned out almost all the sick pen before I left, leaving Banky with only a handful to nurse. He did have to drift in a few from the pasture that became sick or that we missed. When I first saw these cattle I thought they would all die, but if I recall correctly there were only 10 or 12 deaths.

I asked Alf Means if he wanted to read this to see if the facts were as he remembered them. He said, "No, you don't want to let facts mess up a good story."

Blas Payne

Blas Payne was a Negro cowboy working for the Combs Cattle Company. He was descended from a Seminole-Negro scout for the U.S. Army during the Indian wars. His grandfather was Isaac Payne, who had been awarded the Congressional Medal of Honor.

The fall of 1949 the Combs Cattle Company was shipping calves to the corn belt on the Southern Pacific Railroad in Marathon. The calves were being trucked in from the Kincaid, Post and Headquarters Ranches to the railroad stockpens, where they were unloaded, weighed, counted, and reloaded onto railroad cars. I was inspecting them for health and writing health certificates to accompany the calves to destination. My service was visual inspection which was relatively simple as the calves were originating on clean, healthy, ranch premises in this relatively recently settled area in a somewhat arid country. Joe Mitchell was a rancher from Marfa and was the commission man or agent for the midwestern corn belt buyer. David Combs was the Marathon rancher who was the owner of the Headquarters Ranch and the active manager of both the Kincaid and the Post Ranches that was selling the calves. Both were very knowledgeable and did not send any calf with questionable health problems or defects. We were standing around waiting for another truckload of calves when Blas questioned me, asking if I had just got out of college and knew all the latest things. I answered in the affirmative. He then asked if anything had been discovered to do anything about blackleg. This is a common name for *Clostridium chauvoei* infection, a highly fatal disease, primarily of calves. I told him no treatment had been developed. The vaccine to prevent it was very effective, but once contracted there was little or no hope, no cure had been found.* To this he looked sad, said he was sorry to hear that, pulled up his pants leg and said, "I sure got a bad case!" I was bewildered, especially when all the other cowboys started laughing. I finally managed a sheepish grin.

*   *   *   *   *

We were working cattle in the graveyard pens of the Post Ranch when a cloud built up and began lightning and thundering. Blas got in a pickup and left. I had noticed that he had done this on several other occasions. The first few times, I thought nothing of it, but then I began to think perhaps it was not just a coincidence. I asked one of the other cowboys if Blas was afraid of lightning. He told me a number of years before that Blas was horseback out in the pasture when a thunderstorm came up, and he was hit by lightning. The horse was killed, the saddle ruined, and Blas lay out in the pasture unconscious for several days before he was found. Yes, he is afraid of lightning, and no one criticizes him for going to the house when a storm comes up.

Revelation

My first six months was quite a revelation! The business end of running a practice had never entered my mind. I thought if I practiced good medicine and surgery, I wouldn't have anything to worry about. Was I in for a surprise!

Dr. Gearhart hired me on a percentage basis rather than a straight salary. Classmates who had shared their plans with me said they were going to receive a salary of $125 to $150 a month.

---

* Blackleg in a 1cc dose was the only vaccine given to cattle at that time, and it was given at branding time.

Positions (actually *jobs*, but *positions* sound more professional) were not very easy to find at that time. I didn't have a prospect when Dr. Gearhart called me, so I thought I had an exceptional arrangement, but by Christmas a regular paycheck began to sound really appealing, especially if I did not have the time consuming worry of running a practice.

I was to receive one-half of the net profits and devote full time to the practice. I was to be compensated at the rate of 8 cents a mile for the use of my car.

Dr. Gearhart was to furnish the facilities, the building and furniture, plus the goodwill that consisted of the introduction to the ranchers and consultation, both of which were very important to a new graduate and a newcomer to the community. He was to be relieved of the burden of having to practice for friends and relatives so he could devote full time to the ranch.

One of the first problems I faced was building an inventory. I had a few instruments from college classes in surgery and clinic where we treated animals brought to the college. Ben had a few instruments that he had used in his limited practice, but many he kept at the ranch to use on his own livestock.

Drugs and supplies were almost non-existent and had to have priority. I got initiated into searching the catalogs for their availability and the best prices. There was the dilemma of buying enough to get a quantity discount or keeping purchases to a minimum to preserve the bank account. Also I had to consider the length of time it took for them to reach me, as almost all came from Fort Worth.

Merchandise was sent out parcel post through the post office. It went on the Texas and Pacific train to El Paso where it was sorted and put on the Southern Pacific Railroad to Marfa. Sometimes it went on to Marathon, which was about sixty miles farther. The similarities of names caused some mix-ups; however, I never could understand why some went to Mexia because it was a whole different direction.

I was not only the purchasing agent, but the receptionist, paymaster, and bookkeeper. I kept the records, made the charges and sent the bills.

Most of Dr. Gearhart's practice had been *pro bono*, without charge, for relatives and friends so his fee schedule was pretty skimpy, and the one I had brought from college wasn't much better. I didn't even know how to mark up the prescriptions that I dispensed.

I had a sign in front and a diploma and license on the wall. Where were the patients? I discovered that a completely new practice is not inundated with clients beating on the door and the phone ringing off the hook[*].

Many people were surprised to learn I had gone to college to become a "vetinary." Most of the younger and middle-aged ranchers had gone to college, but I doubt if the old timers and most of the general public had been educated past the seventh grade, and there were quite a few that had got most of their knowledge in the school of hard knocks.

A few didn't realize that I expected a fee for my services, or at least they acted that way. One fairly prosperous rancher thought he was doing me a favor, I guess, by offering to let me treat his sick animals at no charge, for the experience. I was young, new in the area, and did not want to offend him, so it was a challenge to refuse the free service diplomatically. After I had declined his kind invitation a number of times and he persisted in his efforts, I finally let some very derogatory remarks slip out. I thought that I had made a bad mistake, but on the contrary, he became a good client.

My practice had been pretty quiet during the summer. The plentiful rainfall had produced a bumper crop of screwworm flies that resulted in many screwworm cases. Almost no elective surgery was performed because of the danger of screwworms.

I didn't get much chance to suture wirecuts and other injuries because of the damage caused by screwworms which occurred so quickly after the initial injury. I was able to hospitalize a few in my stalls which were screened in to prevent reinfestation after the worms had been killed with benzol or chloroform. The nasty old black Formula 62 used on cattle to prevent reinfestation was not used on horses as a rule because it caused severe irritation and often an infection.

The fall work had not been very lucrative, consisting primarily of inspecting and writing health certificates on the calves being

---

[*] The telephones at that time were upright with the earpiece resting on a hook on the side. When it was removed the phone was activated so it could be answered if it were ringing. Otherwise, the operator would ask, "Number, please" and she would connect you. My number was 79.

shipped north after weaning. This was not strenuous work, but it didn't pay very well either. My trip fee was 8 cents a mile at first, but soon it was increased to 10 cents a mile on pavement and 15 cents on dirt roads. The health certificate fee was a flat $5, regardless of the number of head inspected and the length of time I spent writing.

Cash on the barrelhead at the time of service was and still is completely unknown in a ranch practice. Formerly, it had been the policy of many ranchers to square up their accounts once a year in the fall when they sold their calves and old cows. There were still too many who paid once a year and caused hardships for someone like me who was operating on a shoestring.

Some just didn't get around to writing a check very promptly. Perhaps some were operating on borrowed money and used mine interest free as long as they could. Ben said that some put off paying part of their bills until after the first of the year for income tax purposes. I also learned that doctors were usually at the bottom of everyone's list when it came time to pay bills. Of course, I had a few of the deadbeats that always flock to a new business who run up a big bill until they are found out.

I probably had more than my share of charity cases, but then maybe our little town had more people who did not have the disposable income to spend on pets. (Medical services and pet food were considered luxuries at that time and a waste of money to spend on either.) However, who could resist a little tear-stained, sad face of a barefoot boy with a sick or injured puppy or kitten cradled in his arms? The smile that came on that face when the pet was returned after a successful treatment gave one a sense of satisfaction and fulfillment that is hard to describe. As I said before, by Christmas a regular paycheck would have looked mighty good.

Chapter 3

The Early Years

Working in the Rain at the Kincaid Ranch

January 1950 was the beginning of my first calving season. There had been a few calves to come too soon, and that had given me some self-confidence in my ability to handle difficult calving problems.

Jake Nutt was the foreman at the Kincaid Ranch, a division of the Combs Cattle Company. He was calving out a bunch of Hereford heifers and had penned the heavy springers[*] to check on during the night. Jake went to the pens, just before going to bed about 9:00. We didn't usually stay up late, there was no television, and the radio reception wasn't all that great in the mountains. Besides, *Fibber McGee and Molly, Red Skelton, Jack Benny, Amos and Andy, Inner Sanctum, The Shadow Knows* and other good programs, including the news broadcast, came on right after suppertime. Besides, everyone got up early. Sometimes we woke up the rooster so he could greet the new day. There were some older men who complained of waking up at 3:00 AM or so and not being able to go back to sleep. I would harass them by saying it was because they had a guilty conscience. This is one of the things that has come back to haunt me in my mature years.

One heifer was about ready to domino. She was restless with her tail up so he watched her a little while, and pretty soon the water bag appeared, shortly followed by a foot. She laid down, then got up, humped up and strained, but nothing else showed.

Jake was experienced at pulling calves so when he figured he had given her plenty of time he proceeded to check on things. He snubbed the heifer to a post, soaped up hand and arm, then explored the deep dark cavity. He could find neither the head nor the other leg. Jake knew enough not to pull on just one leg, so he

---

[*] Heifers whose abdomen had enlarged because they were in advanced pregnancy.

summoned me.

I had gone to bed and was sleeping "the sleep of the just" when the phone rang. I pulled on some clothes and drove to the hospital to load my equipment. I filled a war-surplus five-gallon water can with warm water and filled the gas tank from a storage tank on the hospital premises and was on my way.

Jake was still at the pens with his pickup running and the headlights on the heifer. He apologized for having continued to work on her after calling me, but his self respect wouldn't let him just sit back on his haunches and wait. However, rarely did anyone ever made any headway because they had given their best shot before calling me. It was a disadvantage for me, as often the tissues were damaged, the natural lubricant lost and the entire plumbing contaminated. It was difficult enough to keep things reasonably clean under the circumstances even for me, with all the emphasis that had been placed on it at vet school. The cowboys usually did a pretty good job, all things considered, but many times I wished they had called sooner. I didn't reprimand them because I understood they couldn't afford to call with every problem and because they were able to take care of most cases.

Jake hadn't hollered wolf by calling unnecessarily because this was a wooly-booger. Later on in my practice I probably would have performed a caesarean section as soon as I evaluated a case like this, but at that time it was only done as a last resort to save the cow.

I couldn't make any progress to straighten the head or retrieve the other leg. I pinched the calf's foot that was showing with no response. Then I made a small incision in it, no blood. The calf was dead.

It's rather surprising sometimes how long a calf will live after a cow goes into labor and how soon it will die at other times.

Lightning and thunder that had started in the northwest seemed to be getting closer. Jake said, "Doc, better hurry. It's going to rain." I answered, "Jake, I'm doing the best I can. I'm about to freeze, stripped to the waist with the wind blowing!"

Since the calf was dead, I proceeded to do an embryotomy. I first severed the calf's leg at the shoulder, then with the help of Jake and a block and tackle, I extracted it .

Jake was right, it started raining. It wasn't just a light winter drizzle. On the other hand, it wasn't a frog strangler. It was a pretty good rain, though, especially for the wintertime. It just doesn't thunder and lightning with a hard rain that time of the year. They say that if it thunders in February, it will frost in April. I didn't know what this goin's on in January was supposed to predict, but at that time it was sure enough wet and cold.

I finally got the head straightened out, and just then the heifer laid down. We untied her head, but she wouldn't get up even with encouragement from a hotshot and some verbal abuse. I wallowed around in the mud 'til I finally got ahold of the other leg and brought it out. With an OB chain attached, Jake and I pulled the calf by main strength and awkwardness. The heifer got up immediately and whirled around to check on her baby. She put us to flight and started licking the dead calf. It was a pitiful sight.

Jake invited me to spend the night, or what was left of it, but I had a cow work near Van Horn the next morning, so I declined.

Jake and I had a little trouble getting the mud chains on the car. I always hated to put them on. It was such a hassle to get them tight enough but not so tight they wouldn't latch. Jake insisted there was no way I could make the ten miles of dirt road back to Marathon without them, probably not even get to the Marathon-to-Fort Stockton highway that was not paved at that time but was a whole lot better than the ranch road.

I finally took off slipping and sliding, trying to keep the rear end back behind me, because it kept wanting to get in front. I crossed the cattle guard and drove onto the highway with a sigh of relief, maybe a little prematurely. I eased down towards town thinking that the rain seemed harder the farther I went. There were several swags that had water a few inches deep. A couple caused a little anxiety but no major problem. Jake hadn't exaggerated the road conditions.

I figured I ought to be getting close to Marathon and was beginning to breath a little easier when I arrived at a fair size draw that had a pretty good stream of running water. I didn't think too much about it because I had already crossed one kinda like it, or so I thought. Well, it turned out I thought wrong. I eased into the water, not wanting to cause it to splash up and drown out the engine. About halfway across I realized I had made a mistake when I felt my car being washed out of the road by the force of the water. I ended up almost against the lane fence and I thought I had had it. I guess there must have been some grass that allowed me to get enough traction to keep going forward, and eventually I was able to reach the other side and get back on the road.

It was only a short distance to the good gravel Iron Mountain Ranch road. I was on safe ground from there into Marathon and pavement. I was home free. I had made it.

Calf Delivery at the Post

The winter of 1949-50, I was called to the Post, south of Marathon. This was an abandoned U.S. Army Post, Camp Colorado. It is located about a mile north of Peña Colorado. In the past, this water hole had also been called Rainbow Cliffs. This is some 4 or 5 miles south of Marathon. After it was abandoned by the Army, it was used as an outpost by the Texas Rangers. Later, parts were used as ranch buildings. Blas Payne lived in the old army post headquarters building and took care of that division of the Combs Cattle Company. He had seen this two-year-old heifer in the pasture about a week before while he was feeding cake to cattle from a pickup. She had her tail up and one leg of a calf was showing. He went back to the ranch and saddled a horse to bring her in. She was nowhere to be found. Blas looked high and low for a week until he finally caught her at a watering. He drove her to the pens, snubbed her to a post and pulled that leg off. There was nothing else to latch onto so he called Jake Nutt, the ranch foreman who lived at the Kincaid division. Jake came and they took turns going in the cow. They finally pulled the calf's tail off but that was all they could get. They gave up after dark and called me. I arrived a little before midnight.

The big outside pen was unmortared rock about six feet high. Board cattle-working pens had been built inside. The crowd chute was facing the wrong way for access to her rear end, so she was snubbed to a post outside the chute. To make the work more challenging, there was nothing to prevent her from dancing from side to side, twisting and turning.

There was a cold north wind blowing and a light freezing rain falling. If it had been pouring down, no one would expect us to be out there, but it was just enough to be thoroughly miserable and not enough to put out the fire Jake and Blas were standing near to keep it warm so it wouldn't go out. That's what I accused them of doing. However, I did need it for light.

I could have kept the headlights on but that would have necessitated running the engine and wasting that high priced 18 cent-a-gallon gasoline. Occasionally, the wind would swirl a little, and I would get the benefit of the smoke. The wet wood didn't burn well to make much light, but it did a good job on smoke. Most of the time the brisk north wind kept the smoke and what little heat it was giving off away from me. Occasionally, one of them would come over to me wanting to help, but there wasn't room enough for one of my arms, much less both of them so there was nothing they could do except give me moral support and maybe a little sympathy.

At that time it was customary to strip to the waist to do obstetrical procedures. I couldn't explain why, that was just the way it was done. The calf being wedged in the birth canal had prevented the cow from urinating, so from time to time when I was least expecting it and had my arm in up to my shoulder, she would let go—all over me. It ran down my chest and into my pants. It was scalding hot. I'm sure she had a fever, but I think the reason it felt so hot was because I was so cold. If it just hadn't filled up my boots, it may not have been so bad. My toes were so cold, I had to concentrate on the calf to keep from moaning. I might have moaned a time or two anyway. There's a faint possibility I may have even thought harsh things about that cow, her ancestry, and maybe any future offspring. Soon the wet would become cold. I guess that part may not have been so bad because I was already wet from the drizzle. I would pull out a bone, some hair, then some hide—a little at a time. When a calf is delivered by dissecting it inside the uterus and bringing out a part at a time, it is called an embryotomy. There is no way one could dignify what I was doing by such a fancy scientific name.

All the natural lubricant had long been lost, and the soft tissues of the birth canal had not only lost their elasticity but had swollen, thereby further restricting the size of the opening. I guess what kept me going was determination, pride, or just plain bullheadedness. I used soapy water with a little disinfectant as long as it lasted, but eventually the supply was exhausted and all attempts at cleanliness were abandoned. Mineral oil was used as a lubricant.

Just as the sun was coming up, the last piece, the head, finally came out. Sulfanilamide powder was the only antibacterial product for intrauterine use that I had at that time. I stuffed in all I had, having serious doubts as to whether she would live. We didn't go through much ceremony in parting. I sure was glad when the engine started. At that time, there was still a little doubt when I stepped on the starter. Later, I would become a little aggravated if the motor didn't kick over immediately. It was about 65 miles back home and I sure wanted to stop in Marathon for a cup of coffee, but the only place that was open was the Gage Hotel dining room. It wasn't fancy by present day standards, but it was for those days. I just couldn't bring myself to go in there, looking like I did. Besides the dead calf had deteriorated in that week and had become pretty ripe. I hadn't noticed the odor was so bad in the cold wind, but now that I was beginning to thaw out, I wasn't sure I could ride with myself, much less go in the hotel. If it hadn't been necessary to go through the lobby, I might have opened the door and hollered for a cup. There was a greasy spoon down the street, but it wasn't open yet.

I made it home about 9:00 AM and looked up a high-priced, rubber, obstetrical suit in a catalog. I think it cost nearly $20. While in college we had seen one that a sales representative was trying to peddle. We laughed at the thick, clumsy outfit, didn't see how anyone could move in it; besides, what sissy would waste all that money. I found out what kind of sissy would. I ordered one before showering and going to bed. I was afraid if I didn't while the memory of the misery was so vivid, I might back out.

The suit turned out as I had expected. It was so thick and stiff it restricted my movements bad. Besides, it had cost so much I didn't want to ruin it, so I wouldn't wear it. Well, actually I did wear it some, but not while wallowing on the ground in the mud, manure and rocks — I wanted to save it. It went to pot pretty soon anyway. It was quite a conversation piece, having so much character with all the holes, cracks, and tears. I sure wish that I would have had duct tape then.

Jake reported that the heifer lived and was even fat when she was shipped that fall. It made it all worthwhile.

Louie Weinacht Ranch Call

JoAnn and I were on a date one night when a call came from Louie Weinacht. He had a heifer down in the·pasture about halfway between Balmorhea and Saragosa. She was having trouble calving. JoAnn decided to go with me.

Several men had give out trying to help her. This was typical of the times — after everything had been tried and all the men exhausted, the veterinarian was called just before shooting the animal. This was not true in all cases, but it was in a large percentage, especially those at a distance and this was about seventy miles away. I don't remember this particularly bothering me. It was just a fact of life, and I accepted it.

I tied the cow's tail to her neck with my tail rope to keep it out of the way. I stripped to the waist, washed her rear end and my hands and arms. I had forgotten my new rubber suit. She had lost all her natural lubricant and was sticky dry. I fixed a soapy solution with warm water—it had been hot when I left Marfa. I worked it inside with the help of a stomach tube and pump. I laid down on the ground wallowing out a little nest in the rocks and went to work. My soapy water didn't stay slick long, so I had to repeat it periodically. I didn't have much water, so I had to be sparing.

It was night, and a cold north wind was blowing. The men stayed over by a big fire they had built, kinda glancing over my way occasionally. JoAnn was furious at them. She wouldn't start the engine and use the heater in sympathy for me.

I was driving the Plymouth station wagon. There was more room for supplies, and the back tailgate could be used as a table. However, with the back end open and the wind blowing, JoAnn suffered almost as much as I did. At least I was busy concentrating on what I was doing instead of dwelling on my discomfort.

I finally delivered the calf which was dead, of course, and probably had been, even before those men had worked on her. The heifer lived, though, and I suppose my fee was reasonable, because I made a good friend and client that night.

The experience was very valuable for our relationship, because after our marriage JoAnn never doubted where I was or what I was doing out late at night. Although, perhaps, she did worry more about me.

My First Ranching Experience

I made many friends, and some of the ranchers kinda took me under their wing to get started in the ranching business.

A ranch came up for sale shortly after the first of the year about ten miles west of town. This didn't happen much in this country at that time. Most places were owned by old families. At that time and that place an old family was one that had been in the area thirty or forty years. This was 1950, and because of its isolation, the area hadn't been settled much until after 1910, although a few hearty souls had come as early as the 1880s after the railroad was built.

There were few places this size. It was only ten sections (6400 acres) which was the size of a pasture on a good many ranches. A small place like this wasn't considered an economical unit because the carrying capacity would be only about 200 cows. However, ranchers encouraged me to buy it because it was close to town, and I could take care of it in my spare time, using my hospital help.

Of course, I didn't have the purchase price or even a down payment, but several ranchers and Fred LaLanne, who managed the Federal Land Bank, figured out with co-signers, I could swing the deal on the land, and the Production Credit Association arranged to finance the cattle.

I got out a sharp pencil and a long piece of paper. I calculated the debt with the interest and taxes and compared that to what the place would produce. The best I could figure, it would take 101 years to pay it out. This was in the days when you figured the cost of land on a pay out of forty years so I passed on the deal. The fellow who bought it was from another part of the country, and he lost it during the drouth a few years later. I would have also.

I was then encouraged to buy stocker calves to pasture on different places. Dr. Gearhart took most of them. I bought some lightweight, long-legged, crossbred steer calves that were put in rough country. The Production Credit Association handled the loan, with ranchers as co-signers on the note. They were pastured on a weight-gain basis and did very well until the drouth and depressed prices hit.

Learning Lessons

My first encounter with Pat Mulloy was a disaster. Soon after beginning practice and while I was still single, I would sometimes go to the Little Red Bar or Ham's Drive-In at night for a beer and a few games of table shuffleboard. This is a waist high board about two feet wide and six feet long. Heavy metal discs about two or three inches in diameter are manually scooted towards a line.

I had met with Harry Langland who was also single and a couple of girls picked us up and led us astray, taking us to Ojinaga, Mexico, where a couple of nightclubs still were in operation.

Pat had a heifer in trouble, trying to calve, at the Jeff Ranch and had asked all over town for me. Finally, he located my car parked behind Ham's Drive-In, and the patrons there told Pat where I had gone. Pat sat in his pickup beside my car and waited and waited! He wasn't in the best humor when I returned, but he was determined. I picked up a few things and followed him to his ranch about 50 miles away.

It was a cold, windy night, and I nearly froze, stripped to the waist to deliver the calf. It didn't seem too awful cold when I left Marfa, so I didn't bring the new obstetrical suit. I thought I'd save it for when I really needed it. I really needed it this time. A nice lively bull calf was eventually on the ground. I gathered up my instruments and put on my shirt and coat and was admiring my handiwork as the calf wobbled around and latched onto a teat and began nursing.

I reached under my front seat and retrieved a half-pint bottle of bourbon to celebrate the successful procedure and offered Pat a nip. He must have been practicing on this speech all the time he waited for me at Ham's. Surely it could not have been extemporaneous, because it was the longest, most complete temperance lecture I ever received. I was cold, tired, and miserable and really wasn't in the mood for this. I threw the bottle as far as I could, got in my car, and left. I didn't think I was easily riled and was kind of self-satisfied that I had not answered. I never expected to see or hear from him again.

I was truly upset, but that lecture had the desired effect and may have been one of the best things that ever happened to me. I never carried a bottle again.

I had been cooling my heels a few days hoping for a phone call, and when it came, I nearly broke a leg answering. It was Pat Mulloy. I was shocked and didn't know what to expect. He was still giving forth on the evils of John Barleycorn when I had driven off, and I held my breath thinking perhaps he was going to pick up where he was when I left. He was very congenial and said he had another heifer in trouble, and would I please come. I did, the weather was nice, and it was daylight. I was able to deliver a live calf with a minimum of effort. The previous episode was not mentioned.

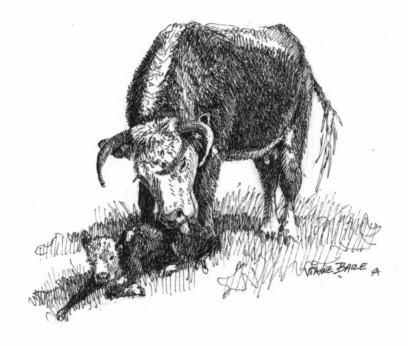

First bath.

The sight of the momma cow giving her baby its first bath while lowing softly is one of nature's greatest spectacles and one of my most rewarding experiences when I had helped in the birth process.

We went to the house for coffee and cake, having a nice visit that included his wife, Nellie, although I always called her Mrs. Mulloy. We became good friends, and he would often come by the hospital just for a visit during the slow years of the fifties. He also would come by after his wife died, and he sold the ranch to Bob McKnight. During the drouth, his ranch was one of the very few to get rain.

"Wet" Mexicans

In this area illegal aliens from Mexico were referred to as "wets," more than likely because Americans of Mexican descent and the legal aliens called the illegals, *mojadas,* which is the Spanish word for wets. They were called wetbacks in much of the border country. I understand the term originated because legal aliens crossed the Rio Grande River on a bridge, whereas the illegals slipped across the border either by swimming or wading. Below Presidio, where the Concho River from Mexico flows into the Rio Grande, the river was nearly always deep, and swimming was necessary; whereas, above this confluence, the river was often shallow and could be waded. Therefore, only the feet and legs were wet and not the back.

I understood that there was a quota on immigration, and the paperwork was somewhat complicated and relatively expensive for the poorer class. Conditions in Mexico were harsh and people crossed into the United States because the wages were better. Often much of their pay was sent to families in Mexico.

An example of the plight of these people was the fact that on several occasions, I had been performing a postmortem examination out in a pasture on a cow that was a little ripe when a group approached who cut off chunks of meat to eat. Their clothes would be typical. A beat-up, broad-brimmed straw hat and loose, ill-fitting, poorly bleached, or perhaps unbleached, white, coarse cotton shirt and pants, with a rope for a belt. The shoes would be huaraches (sandals) made from an old worn-out tire held on by leather thongs and often with no socks, regardless of the weather. A woolen serape thrown over the shoulder in warm weather or worn as a coat when it is cold. A small package wrapped with newspaper may contain a little food or personal effects, and in the early days, a glass jar for water which was later replaced by a plastic jug.

It was unbelievable how far they could travel in a night because often they would hide during the day. In times past, ranchers would feed any that passed their way and some would leave the house unlocked and leave food on the table when they were gone. Usually these isolated ranches would not be molested. Some would want to work permanently but others just a few days to get their strength. Most had a certain destination with family or friends and wanted to get far away from the border as soon as possible where they were not as likely to be discovered and deported.

These people have been badly maligned. Their inability to read and write, or even speak and understand the English language had sometimes been interpreted as a lack of mental capability. This resulted in poor communication, with it being said that the only thing a wet does not do backwards is digging a posthole. Their illegal status made them wary of being caught by chotas and returned to Mexico. *Chotas* is a slang term for border patrolmen, immigration agents.

Some Mexicans' ideas were interesting. It was thought that mastitis (an infection of the udder.) in a cow was caused by a coachwhip (red racer snake) crawling up her hind leg and nursing that teat. A horse with colic was caused by it eating a bug that was in the hay. I tried to explain to them that this is not what caused the colic. They nodded their head and said, "Sí, señor," but I could tell by attitude and facial expression that they were humoring me. I could tell they were thinking, "Poor old gringo, he don't know much." Many years later, it was discovered that blister beetles in alfalfa hay caused colic that often was so severe as to cause death.

Most of them were honest, hard-working men, and those that were raised on a ranch in Mexico were excellent ranch hands. Their powers of observation were usually acute and their memories, excellent. It was said that when one learns to read and write they lose their memory. They also said that the peon was not burdened with a lot of information that distracts his attention from the present.

Some wets have been known not to report any bad news such as a sick animal, broken windmill, or leaky trough. Perhaps it was because they didn't want to upset the boss who might throw a temper tantrum, but usually they were accused of negligence or trying to escape from having to do extra work.

Few of the first generation from Mexico learned English. It was difficult for me to be too critical of them, because I learned little Spanish in spite of the fact that I have been around it all my life. Those that have learned some English are often reluctant to use it as it may be misinterpreted. I was told that a Mexican ranch hand reported that he had been gone so long because he had trouble putting a cow in the pen. When asked why she had been penned, the man said, "She don't look so very good." The boss went to examine her. When walking around the pen he touched her and she spooked and ran over him. He got up, dusted himself off and exclaimed, "Hell, she's blind!" The Mexican answered, "That's what I said, 'She don't look so good.'"

But some can be exasperating. I was called to treat a downer cow[*] that had a complete uterine prolapse and was in shock. I treated her, giving injections, including intravenous fluids until she perked up and was stabilized. It was a cold, windy night on top of a rocky hill with only a wet Mexican to help me. I positioned the wet in front of her to watch her signs. I went behind and washed her, placing the uterus on tow sacks after giving her a spinal anesthetic. I grunted, groaned, and moaned. After a long, miserable time wearing only a t-shirt and wet pants, I finally replaced the uterus and sutured it in place after medicating it. I then went to her head to check on her condition and she was dead! I asked when she died and the man said almost immediately after I went behind her. He had let me work well over an hour on a dead cow. I guess I shouldn't have been so upset. My poor communication skills in the Spanish language had probably been the cause. He did what he was told, he <u>watched</u> her.

Around the Campfire Near Gomez Peak

I was at Dr. Connell's Bar C Ranch near Kent in the spring of 1950, drinking coffee at the chuck wagon, waiting for the herd to come in. This chuck wagon was the only actual wagon that I can remember. All the others were chuck boxes mounted on a pickup truck. Now, drinking coffee from a tin cup by a campfire may sound colorful and picturesque, but it's not all it's cracked up to be. Let me tell you about it.

---

[*] A downer cow is one that is lying down, unable to get to her feet. Most of these cases in range cattle are due to calving paralysis caused by a slow difficult birth.

First is the handle of the big heavy black coffee pot setting on the fire. Because it was so heavy I grabbed ahold with a firm grip. I did this kinda automatically because that's necessary to pour the coffee. Too late I remembered that the handle is the hottest place on the whole pot. Why, I don't know. It shouldn't be, but it is. I let go pretty sudden like and backed off, looking all around to see who all was watching. I blew on my hand, shook it a little and rubbed it on my pants. Then I looked at it. A person always has to inspect an injury. In this case, I guess, to see if there were any blisters—maybe to see if some hide peeled off.

The cook came to my rescue with a folded flour sack for a potholder. I told him I just wanted half a cup so it would cool faster. He went ahead and filled it to the brim anyhow. This hot coffee heated up the cup so it burned my hands. Cowboy etiquette forbade setting it down even if I coulda found a place.

I looked around for somewhere to hunker down on my haunches to be out of the cook's way and where the wind didn't blow campfire smoke and ashes in my face. I spotted a likely place and squatted down. The smoke followed. I started to move, but the old bum leg just didn't want to function so I settled down, thinking maybe somebody would come along and "tail me up" like an old poor cow.

I gingerly balanced that hot tin cup and shifted it from one hand to the other. I slowly brought it up to my lips which got burned. I backed off, licked my lips and blew in the cup awhile and tried it again. Same results. By this time, the coffee was getting cold, but the cup was still hot. I approached it carefully, stretching my neck way out like that was going to help—it didn't. I slurped a little coffee, just barely touching the cup with my lips. This is an art form that is mastered only after nursing blistered lips a number of times. This was a skill I had not yet accomplished. Fact is, I never did. The cup finally cooled and by that time the coffee was cold, and I just gulped it.

The cook had poured cold water in the coffee to settle the grounds after it had boiled. There's always hot and cold water in a camp — it's hot in the summer and cold in the winter. The cold water works pretty well, except then the pot was put on coals to keep it hot. This kinda stirred up the grounds a little so that the last of the coffee in the cup had a few grounds. Some got stuck in my teeth which was a little aggravating, but when stuck on a tonsil I gagged and coughed and made all kinds of peculiar noises. When it finally dislodged, I tried to figure if another cup was worth all the bother.

While I thought on this, I studied the cook as he went about his chores. He was an old crippled-up, worn-out cowboy. He had on an old sweat-stained, slouch hat. I imagine that at one time it was his Saturday night, honky-tonk Stetson or maybe for Sunday-go-to-meeting. A flour sack apron was tucked in his belt. His run-over boots showed the faint signs of some fancy stitching.

The west wind was blowing a gale, but he kept on working his fire, shoveling coals to one side, placing a dutch oven on them and putting some more on the lid. He mixed and worked camp bread, chopped up meat, potatoes, onions, and chili for stew. He mixed vermicelli, onions, and canned tomatoes. Then he picked beans while he rested, sitting on a five pound lard can. He worked as if it were a perfect day, seemingly oblivious to the wind. This wasn't a really genuine West Texas dust storm because the good stand of grass kept the real estate from blowing around.

I asked him how long a fellow had to live in the area to get used to the wind. He stuck his thumb over his shoulder, pointing towards Gomez Peak, then turned and squinted up at it. I guess to be sure that high mountain was still there and said, "When I come to this country that ole mountain was jest a little hill. Ever summer has been the hottest, ever winter the coldest, and ever spring the windiest." Then he went back to his rat killing and left me to ponder his remarks.

Bob Sproul's Ranch

Bob and Dude Sproul were brothers and opposites. They operated separately because their philosophies and animal husbandry practices were not compatible. Dude was kinda tall and lean. He was always neat and clean. Bob was relatively short and stocky. His clothes were always wrinkled, and I think he got them dirty walking out the front door. He kind of embarrassed me at times, doing all the dirty work of roping, tying, pulling, lifting, and carrying. When I first met him he had a baby bear in a cage that he had recently caught, being one of the last bear that I know of to be caught in the Davis Mountains. Part of his ranch was in some high rough piñon and ponderosa pine with a fair amount of juniper and oak trees. His fence posts were all juniper, cut on the ranch. The gate posts and corner posts were enormous, ten to fourteen inches in diameter. I went up on top (high in the mountains) to see a downer cow with a uterine prolapse. She was in a pole pen, a pen that is made completely of upright posts, solid wired together. She was at the far side. I wanted my vehicle close so I wouldn't have to carry my things so far and decided to drive inside. I inquired whether those big old posts were far enough apart. "Oh, sure, Doc!" He got in front and lined me up perfectly and I began to ease through. He yelled, "Hit her hard, Doc. She's narrow!" He was a doer, up to his elbows in everything.

Fortunately, he calved his heifers in a small trap (a little pasture) out on the flat, and I didn't have to go up in the high roughs often. There was a steep, little hill with a narrow, rocky road that was exciting to negotiate on the way to his ranch. I always hit high center on those big rocks, but the high rock bank on one side and a deep steep drop-off on the other side with such a narrow road didn't give me much room to maneuver. The last time I went up this road it was disgusting — all the challenge was gone. Several big houses had been constructed at the top of this hill, and a fancy, wide, smooth road had been built.

Many of his heifers were so small they couldn't be delivered, yet Bob would call early enough that the calf would still be alive. This was in contrast to many that called only after the calf was dead, and some that called me as a last resort. Because of the situation I performed a higher percentage of caesarean sections here than almost any place. There was a narrow, shallow little wash down the middle of this trap that the heifer invariably lay down in. It was very difficult to pull a calf here, but excellent to prop the heifer on her back for a ventral midline incision, which was the type operation I used until the flank site was developed.

Bob seemed always to have a Mexican hollowing out a ponderosa pine log to make a trough. I thought these were colorful and picturesque and wanted one, but they were too big to carry in my pickup, and I was too poor to hire a truck to haul it.

The Proposal

Along about February of 1950, many of the delinquent accounts had been paid up as Dr. Gearhart had predicted and I began to see daylight. A little money had accumulated in the hospital bank account and we were beginning to take some draw as income.

The calving season was in full swing with all the problems that went with it. Foremost were the difficult births, but prolapses were a close second if you counted both the vaginal preparturient plus the postparturient complete uterine. Retained afterbirths were common and there were a good many cases of metritis. Mastitis was seen, mostly in older cows. I think most of the cases of mastitis were the unclean methods used in milking a chichona[*]. Often a hollow chicken feather was used as a milking tube; others used a metal milking tube carried in the shirt pocket. Actually, a freshly plucked chicken feather was the cleaner of the two.

Lumpy jaw[†] in the cows was common. Much of it was caused by *Actino,* which necessitated sodium iodide intravenously after the abscess was lanced and packed with iodine soaked gauze.

Because many of the first calf heifers were calved in the pen, there was a problem in some of the baby calves with scours and pneumonia. These problems were almost non-existent in the calves born in the pasture.

The inventory was in fair shape and things looked so promising I felt safe in proposing to JoAnn Tyler. We were married April 12, 1950.

The Wedding

The wedding of JoAnn and me was a memorable event made especially so by Mary Martha and Ben Gearhart, and Georgia Lee and Fritz Kahl. The wedding ceremony and reception went very well, I think. I was in somewhat of a daze. I would have been able to cope with the situation better if I had realized that the bride is the main attraction, the groom, just a necessary supporting cast. My best man, my cousin, F.O. "Buster" Edwards, was my strength. The groomsmen walking down the aisle with the sly, mischievous grins were unnerving.

The excitement started after the reception. Harry Langland and D.O. Atkinson were reserved and dignified. I don't think they had any part of my troubles. Ben and Fritz aided and abet-

---

[*] Cow with a large teat which the calf is unable to nurse.
[†] Abscess.

ted by Stuart "Button" Jones were the instigators and perpetrators of my initial harassment, I suspect. My car was locked in the Tyler garage. My friends would cut the lock, replace it with one of their own, then Buster would cut that one and replace his own. I understand this occurred several times until Buster gave up and parked the car in front of the house. After the reception, I went upstairs in the Crews Hotel and after changing clothes, I couldn't open the door. I thought at first it was only jammed but after repeated jerking and hearing laughter in the hallway, I realized it was locked. I crawled through the transom. You say, no big deal? Believe me, it was a big deal.

Buster drove JoAnn and me to my car. Cars were parked in front and back of mine. Just enough room that I thought I could get out by going back and forth, turning and twisting. At the point of my exasperation, the front car moved and let me out. I sighed with relief that I had finally escaped and we were on our way. We had gone a few blocks when a noise in the back seat attracted my attention. Lo and behold! there sat Mary Martha and Georgia Lee giggling. I cannot express my feelings of shock, anger, despair, and panic. I have been accused of using an expletive, being an ex-Marine, I feel sure that I did not. I floor-boarded the gas pedal, only about 25 miles per hour. I didn't quite make it to the top of the hill east of the Alamito Creek bridge. They had disconnected some of the spark plug wires, and in my frustration I had not realized the engine was missing. When we were on our way again, I could not relax, waiting for something else to happen. The next morning at the Antelope Lodge in Alpine, I got out bright and early before the other travelers were up to wash off the graffiti from the car. I thought I was being real quiet, but soon heads appeared at all the doors and windows with a little giggling and snickering here and there.

Later at Del Rio when the oil was checked, a group gathered looking under the hood. I looked to see what the problem was, and they all burst out laughing. Written on the underside of the hood was Just Married. We never did get all the rice out of our clothes and suitcases. Isn't there a saying, With friends like this, who needs enemies?

There was a good rain the day of the wedding, and everyone was elated except JoAnn's maternal grandmother, Mrs. R.N. Settle, who said that this was a bad omen. If it rained on a wedding day, the marriage would be a sad one and the bride would cry a lot.

Rev. Nelson Wurgler, the Methodist minister, performed the wedding ceremony, and he tied a good knot. It has lasted 50 years so far and doesn't show any signs of weakening.

A Strong Back and Weak Mind?

The spring of 1950 shortly after my honeymoon, I was at Kerr Mitchell's ranch delivering a calf from a two-year-old, first calf heifer. She had been put in a crowd chute and her head tied. This was before the calf puller apparatus had been developed. After the calf had been straightened often only traction was needed. A little sorry rope block and tackle was helpful and certainly better than nothing on a particularly tight squeeze, but still there involved much main strength and awkwardness. This was the reason that most large animal veterinarians had the reputation of needing a strong back and a weak mind. The weak mind was especially valuable to go anywhere and do anything in all kinds of weather, day or night, and to continue working long after exhaustion.

I do not recall whether this was a particularly large calf or an especially small heifer. I don't guess it matters which, size being relative. The calf had his head and one leg out and was still alive, wrinkling his nose and blinking his eyes, and because of this no thought was given to an embryotomy. A generous amount of soap and water removed much of the manure. With some difficulty, I inserted my hand and arm beside the calf's head and neck and grasped the hidden leg of the calf. With my fist around the leg, it caused too much bulk to come out. I withdrew my hand and carried in a cable to snare the foot and withdraw it. A chain was put on both feet and O.B. handles hooked on and I gave it everything I had, but the shoulders and chest wouldn't come. I rigged up the block and tackle and the calf began to come. Just as I was becoming confident of a delivery, a hip lock occurred. This is really awkward, especially in a chute. I pushed down on the block and tackle, twisted and turned the calf, and performed all sorts of contortions. At the point of exhaustion, the calf came and my back went out. I couldn't get up. Kerr dragged me out of the chute and loaded me in my car, drove me to town, and half carried me upstairs to my apartment. JoAnn and I lived in Mrs. McCracken's apartments over Johnny McDonald's saddle shop. Kerr kidded me a long time about my back trouble as a new bridegroom.

Rings

I wore my senior ring from Texas A&M constantly and rarely removed it. It had taken lots of studying. I was proud of my school; besides, the ring was attractive and expensive. At least it had cost a lot for the size of my pocketbook.

One of my early obstetrical cases was a cow with one leg of the calf showing. The cowboy insisted the calving process had just started and urged me to hurry before the calf died. I failed to remove the ring and in the process of manipulating the fetus for a normal calving position, the ring came off while my hand was inside the cow. I was unable to locate it quickly, so I proceeded to deliver the calf. I searched through the blood and fluids on the ground that had come out with the calf. No luck. I then began searching inside the cow in the afterbirth. A diligent search was unsuccessful.

I was hoping that I could find it when she passed her afterbirth, so I gave an injection of posterior pituitary extract and crossed my fingers. I continued to feel in the uterus and attempted to unbutton the placental attachments. This relationship is close and complicated. The placenta of horses, dogs, and cats is not so complicated and is usually expelled within a matter of minutes. Many cows pass theirs fairly soon, but it is not uncommon for individuals in the range cows of this area to take two or three days, sometimes longer. It looked like this was going to take more time. I repeated the pituitary every thirty minutes or so while I searched. I gave intravenous calcium gluconate, hoping to hurry the process.

The afterbirth has numerous folds and wrinkles. I felt the ring once through some of the tissue, but it was so slippery, it got away from me before I could get a good grip.

The ranchhand helping was restless and began to give me a bad time, so I ran him off. He needed to get about his work and wasn't helping me with his complaining.

I was getting a little panicky after a couple of hours and even considered killing the cow and opening her up and may have if I could have afforded to buy her. I finally located the ring. I never wore it again, until I retired. My joints had gotten bigger by that time, so I had the ring enlarged so I could get it on.

*   *   *   *   *

When we married, JoAnn insisted that I wear a wedding band. I objected but to no avail. I finally decided to wear it at least a little while. A little while proved to be too long. Another OB case and another disaster. I had managed to get the ring finger in a bad place that caused it to swell—but that's another story. I couldn't remove the ring over the swollen finger, but figured that if I couldn't pull it off, it wouldn't come off accidentally.

I was straightening the calf's head and easing it into the pelvis with my left hand when the cow gave a sudden violent push as she strained to have her baby. My finger with the ring became wedged between the calf's skull and the bony pelvis of the cow. Talk about smart! My goodness, that hurt! I couldn't get my hand out, and the calf's head wouldn't move in or out. I thought I would tear my finger off.

After much moaning and groaning, with a few prayers, the ring finally came off, peeling a little hide off with it. The ring, of course, fell back in the cow. After I delivered the calf, I began searching for the ring. I about half hoped that I wouldn't find it so I would have a good excuse not to wear it again. I soon gave up and decided to give it to the cow, but the Mexican ranchhand helping me proceeded to take off his shirt to go looking for it. His hand and arm were so cruddy I tried to get him to wash up, but he said he had already been in her without washing. I went back to searching, 'cause I sure didn't want him in where I had been so careful. I finally found it and put both rings in my wife's jewelry box.

W.W. "Walter" McElroy Sr.

One of my early calls was to W.W. "Walter" McElroy Sr. The ranch was located west of Balmorhea and Toyahvale. The route was down old Highway 290 about ten miles, then turn off west toward the Davis Mountains. The graded road was a good one for that time, but I was driving a Plymouth station wagon with highway tires, so the trip was slow in order to prevent flats and blowouts. After crossing Cherry Creek and climbing into the mountains, the road was rougher and rockier. I think the place was called Fox Canyon. I crossed a nice little running creek near the ranch house, nestled in a grove of oak trees. Mrs. McElroy answered my knock and told me Mr. McElroy was in the pens.

I began walking along a path in the general direction she had pointed, looking for a way to drive my car to the pens. I walked around a shed and received quite a shock. An enormous black bear towered over me with outstretched arms and open mouth. It seemed like I stood there a long time, frozen to the spot. I suppose I stood still thinking he would not attack if I didn't move, but more likely, it was because I was surprised and frightened. It seemed like a long time, but probably it wasn't more than a few seconds until I realized that he was standing atop a three-foot high tree stump with a big leather collar on his neck and a heavy chain fastened to the tree stump. Also, he was at least ten feet away, and I am sure that I could not feel his hot breath on my face as I first thought.

Walter apologized, but he had no way of knowing that I would wander around behind that shed. The path I had followed was one used to feed the bear.

There were still some black bear and lions in the Davis Mountains in 1949. Both were soon controlled. The lions came back more numerous than ever, but not the bear, as of 1998. Walter had found one of his animals, a sheep if I remember correctly, that had been killed and partially eaten. He had returned to the house for his pack of dogs. The momma bear had not gone far because of the small cub she had with her. She was caught and killed. Walter took the little cub home and raised it.

The cow that Walter had called about was a very nice looking Jersey milk cow with a retained placenta (afterbirth). I tied her tail to her neck with a small rope, scrubbed my arms and her rear end, and proceeded to unbutton the placenta which in the cow has caruncles that engulf the corresponding structures of the uterus called cotyledons. The caruncles have small villi which are finger-like projections that fit into the crypts in the cotyledons. These are where oxygen and nutrients pass from the cow's blood to that of the developing calf. Mr. McElroy had not called me prematurely. It was ripe, the fact is, a little overripe. You might even say rank. It didn't seem quite so bad until I began to expel fluids. Walter suddenly thought of something he needed to do somewhere else. I wanted to go with him. However, these chores are just a part of veterinary practice. The afterbirth finally came out and I raked out as much juice as I could. I inserted sulfanilamide powder into the uterus, then gave her an intramuscular injection of Stilbesterol, an estrogenic hormone to sensitize and activate the uterus, followed by posterior pituitary extract (oxytocin) to cause contraction of the uterus.

I scrubbed my arm with Tincture of Green soap. Debris was tangled in the hair on my arms. It wouldn't wash off so I had to pull out the knotted hair. My arms were stinging from the irritant secretions, and the odor caused my eyes to water. I eventually decided I had cleaned as well as possible and rinsed with Quseptic solution, a disinfectant. Before plastic gloves, I worked with bare hands and arms.

My attention was called to examine her calf. It was a small, thin, weak heifer. I told Walter that I was suspicious of brucellosis and asked permission to take a blood sample from the cow for testing purposes. The family had been drinking the milk so I asked if any family members had symptoms of undulant fever. Walter said he had been sick with some disease he must have contracted in Mexico. His doctor in Pecos had not diagnosed the condition or successfully treated it, although he suspected malaria or some other tropical disease. The cow tested positive for brucellosis. Walter was then tested for the same and also proved to be positive. I was concerned that I might contract undulant fever by my contact with this cow but I did not.

Walter was well-known among the ranchers and the news spread rapidly, resulting in many ranch milk cows being tested. It was a good stimulant to the practice, but one bad aspect was that I was reluctant to drink fresh ranch milk, eat butter, cottage cheese, or acederos. (Acederos is a flat, tortilla-shaped, home-made cheese in which the milk curds have been solidified with trompillo berries. This is properly silver leaf nightshade, a toxic plant that takes a knowledgeable person to use.)

Mr. McElroy was a big man and he lost a great deal of weight from the disease and died not long afterwards from a heart attack.

The little scrawny calf died. We were sad because we thought she would have made a good replacement milk cow for her mother who was sent to slaughter. At that time we thought that a calf could be raised on an infected cow, and if it was removed before the beginning of puberty it would not contract the disease. It was later determined that this was not the case. The disease organism could become established before birth in lymph nodes and stay dormant until she calved the first time, when the bacteria emerged and spread. There was no way to test during this dormant phase, so it became a required policy to dispose of the calf. If it were a male, castrate it, if a female, either spay or send to slaughter.

Brucellosis

Brucellosis was also called Bang's disease, and when humans contract it from goats, it is known as Malta fever. When it is contracted from cows, it is called undulant fever. The symptoms can be mild with only chronic fatigue, but it is more likely to be in the form of aches and pains, chills, and fever, even life threatening before antibiotics. Most people got it from drinking raw milk from an infected animal. One of the principle reasons for the early popularity of pasteurization was because the procedure killed the bug. Many livestock people, including veterinarians, caught it by assisting in births, care of newborns, and extracting afterbirths without protective gloves. I did all the wrong things including drinking milk and eating milk products, from unknown sources, also vaccinating heifer calves with live Strain 19 brucellosis vaccine and inadvertently vaccinating myself.

I ran out of gas (chronic fatigue). I went to Dr. Walter Stover asking him to test me for brucellosis. He looked me over, poked and prodded, and started asking me questions after first sticking a thermometer in my mouth so I couldn't answer. Finally, he said, "Charlie, you're all right. You're supposed to get tired when you work 24 hours a day, 7 days a week."

I've been asked how I was able to keep going sometimes. Well, I drank a lot of coffee and smoked a lot of cigarettes. I carried a big thermos, filled with coffee and drank it all day or as long as it lasted, sometimes stopping in some cafe to have it filled up again.

Frank Warren at the Allison Ranch in the Glass Mountains

The first time I met Frank was in the summer of 1950. He had phoned me saying that he had heard of a Toyahvale area rancher who contracted undulant fever from a milk cow with brucellosis. I told him that was true. He said his milk cows had never been tested and wanted me to come by his place the following Saturday when his neighbors were having their cows tested. I told him I didn't think I would have time as I had probably made too many appointments already. There were not a large number of cows, but they were widely scattered on various ranches, except for the first which was a dairy in the old farming district irrigated by water from Comanche Springs at Fort Stockton. Frank's closest neighbors were ten to twenty miles away. He asked me to stop by, that it wouldn't matter how late it was, and that he would leave the cows in the pen.

I had been going fast and furious, so JoAnn was driving me as she often did when I was so busy and tired. It was late at night when I arrived. Frank and the ranch hands had gone to bed, and all was dark. I beat on the door and hollered, "Hello, the house!" several times before Frank finally opened the door. There was no porch, only a wide cement slab about two feet high. He had on only a pair of pants and was towering over me with his bare, hairy chest asking in a loud deep voice, "Who is it? What do you want?" JoAnn told me later that she was scared to death, that Frank looked like a monster. I told him who I was and why I came. He put on a pair of boots and we walked by the bunk house. His one call was all that was needed to bring a crew of men.

There were several cows in the pen which were roped, one by one. Frank mugged them (held around the horns by one arm and his fingers of the other hand inserted in the cow's nostrils and grasped to stabilize the head). I drew blood from the jugular vein and put metal ear tags in the ears for identification. The cows bawled and bucked, but Frank held on, having little trouble controlling them. His uproarious laughter at their struggles was enough to paralyze an ordinary cow. Frank said he bet those cows would give clabber in the morning.

I called Frank a few days later to tell him the tests were all clean and to apologize for coming so late. He said the cows didn't give much milk the next morning, but he personally had a good time. We became good friends.

He was a big man, probably six feet-five inches and weighing perhaps 250 pounds. His wife, Bess, was a little thing maybe five feet in height. I don't know if she really ruled the roost, but Frank always acted as if she did. She would just smile and say, "Oh, Frank!"

He was the manager of the Allison Ranch in the Glass Mountains between Fort Stockton and Marathon. The ranch was a big one, raising cattle and sheep. It was an excellent ranch, not much rough country but lots of cedar trees so that it was necessary to ride horseback a great deal to see the animals, especially the wormies in the warm months. Because of the need for horses, a large horse herd was maintained, the horses being raised here for this ranch and for another near Sonora.

Frank was a good-natured, congenial man, and because of his size no one was foolish enough to ruffle his feathers. I always enjoyed my calls to this ranch although they were somewhat infrequent because of the distance of about 90 miles.

One of the ranch cows developed an intussusception, a telescoping of one section of intestine inside another. Adhesions and strangulation of the gut usually had occurred before a cow was discovered to be sick. This condition necessitates a resection, the surgical removal of the affected portion. This is not easily accomplished in the cow because of the anatomy and toxemia, so she usually dies. I explained this to Frank and he replied, "Go ahead, Doc. If she dies, at least she'll die scientific."

Murphy Bennett and King Hines

Shortly after I began practice, probably 1949 or 1950, Murphy Bennett had a good stud horse. He was an all around horse being used for breeding as most stallions are restricted to because they are too ornery around other horses. This horse of Murphy's was an exception. He acted a gentleman and could be used on roundups and other cow work. He was especially good as a cutting horse. The legs of a cutting horse are subjected to tremendous stress because of the maneuvers necessary. Of course, it takes a good rider to stay with them when they are working. The rider has to anticipate the movements the horse is going to make or he'll be left high and dry, clutching a handful of air as the horse turns out from under him.

Murphy was at a cutting horse contest at Jim Espy's in Fort

Davis working a yearling when he heard what sounded like a pistol shot followed by his horse pulling up, three-legged lame, carrying a leg. Dr. Searls, a physician, took an x-ray of the leg on the sidewalk in front of his office. I didn't have an x-ray machine at that time — few veterinarians did. In fact, I had not taken an x-ray in college nor developed a film. We learned to diagnose and set broken bones by feel. I purchased my first x-ray from Dr. George Hoffman, a M.D. in Fort Stockton, in the late 1950s. He was the son of Dr. A.J. Hoffman, the veterinarian in Marfa who operated the O.M. Franklin Serum Co. store where I bought many of my vaccines and supplies. This was a Model-T type and was simple to use as compared to newer models, as it had few settings. It had been a used machine when Dr. George obtained it. I wish that I had kept it. It would now have been antique. Actually, it was when I used it. In the mid-sixties, I sent the machine in for repairs and received a letter that it was past repairing.

Murphy's horse stood perfectly still while the x-ray was being taken. This took much longer than with present day machines. The timer emitted a loud buzz not unlike that of a rattlesnake and should have caused a reaction in the horse. Later timers of mine were much quieter, but I still had many problems with animals moving, causing the x-ray film to be blurred. Murphy was talking to him, and the reassuring hand had the magic results. The x-ray revealed the suspected fracture of the second phalanx, commonly referred to as the short pastern. I applied a plaster of paris cast. He was a perfect patient, not moving while I put it on nor while it dried. Often the first few steps after the application results in some horses having a rather violent reaction of rearing and plunging and a few stomping that foot trying to get rid of the weight and pressure. The horse didn't even attempt to walk on it then or while the bone was healing. Casts were usually left on for a minimum length of time because cast sores were so common. He didn't use the leg even after the cast was removed, giving the fracture additional time to mend. However, after the horse failed to use the leg after a lengthy convalescence, I thought he was ruined. The fracture was comminuted (multiple pieces) and had extended into both joints, the one above and the one below.

Murphy had faith or perhaps it was hope; either way he refused to give up. I was amazed when a complete recovery resulted. He continued to breed mares, and Murphy said he could be ridden all day without going lame, although I don't remember him ever being subjected to the stress of a cutting horse contest again. I had several other horses with broken legs in the pastern area to heal sufficiently to be broodmares or breeding stallions, a few roping horses that were good for the short distances required, and at least one barrel horse that could run like the wind in spite of a club foot and a slight limp. Actually, the limp of that horse was pretty significant. Word was that the owner of the horse would be chided by other men when his daughter ran this horse in a race. He would defend his action by offering to bet on the outcome. It was said he took them to a cleaning. All healed-fracture horses would start limping after being ridden a mile or two making them unsatisfactory for usual ranch work, because there are few things more aggravating than riding a limping horse, although the horse may not be in pain.

I was called to the Bandera Ranch a few years later to see this horse. His leg was broken about halfway between the carpus and the fetlock, the area called the mid cannon. It was a compound fracture with both ends of the bone protruding through the wound into which dirt and old dry manure was packed including the bone marrow. The lower part of the leg was flopping around and the horse was sweating profusely from pain. Amputation of a limb in a horse was completely out of the question and not considered an option. This was a completely hopeless situation; we had to put him down.

I took it pretty hard and left as soon as euthanasia had been performed. I have had to do this many times in my years of practice. Other times have been traumatic, but I believe this was one of the worst. I left without looking at Murphy, only a pat on his shoulder for he was suffering also.

Murphy's wife, Lee, told me this was King Hines, double grandson of the original, King. She said he was all that I had written and more. She said the horse was used again as a cutting horse at least one time after the fracture.

One year the Marfa Rodeo planners wanted to have a youth cutting horse contest. They asked Murphy if his son would like to compete on King. Murphy went to the ranch and pulled King off his mares. He had been unridden for many months, maybe a year. Murphy rode him around a little, put Billy Clay, who was about eleven, on King, and he was the capable, gentle horse that I had described. They won first! Though he was called Billy Clay in his youth, as an adult he is called B.C.

An Injured Colt

I was called to Mr. A.R. Eppenauer's office at the pens behind his house on the outskirts of Marfa. It began to hail just as I arrived. The tin roof with little or no insulation caused a loud roar. I was a little apprehensive as this was a new experience. I later became accustomed to it and rather enjoyed the noise. Mr. Eppenauer related that in his wildcatting days in the oil business, he would often go broke because of a dry hole called a *duster*. He would then accumulate a stake, enough money to go back to drilling, by hauling nitroglycerine and blowing wells. One day near Crane, he was crossing a greasewood flat driving a World War I army truck containing the nitro. The cab was covered with canvas — no doors, and the back was open with no covering. It began to hail, and he piled out and started running away from the truck. Large hailstones were hitting him, and one actually knocked him down. Greasewood bushes don't offer any protection, so he returned to the truck and crawled under it. He thought he would rather die suddenly by being blown up than gradually beat to death by the hail.

When the hail and rain stopped we went outside to look at the reason for my call.

A young, unbroken two-year-old colt had a laceration on his shoulder. He kept running around the pen so that I could not see it to determine if it needed sutures. The pen was made with large upright pipe post with holes through which some heavy one-inch cables were strung. This was a good idea, we thought, because there was no wood to break or splinter. However, it didn't cause the colt to shy off and he hit it going full speed when we tried to rope him. Of course he may have slipped in the mud, but either way, he sure had a wreck. The skin on his head was torn from between his ears, down the front of his face to his nose, covering one eye and half blinded him. He was also dazed from the blow because we walked up and put a hackamore on him. The question of whether sutures were needed was settled, although the shoulder injury was not bad — just a lot of blood. But, the head looked like a hopeless disaster. I had never seen anything like this, and I saw many bad head wounds after that, but few were any worse. I cleaned it and sutured it, expecting the skin to slough. It healed with barely a scar. It made a good client of Mr. Ep and was great for my ego and self-confidence.

Screwworms

The screwworm problem was secondary only to drouth and the depressed livestock prices that always accompany a drouth as the greatest cause of financial loss in the area when I first entered practice. The poison plant problem wasn't far behind some years in some places. I am sure that it caused more illness and death loss than all other conditions combined. The death loss was not significant in cattle because they were usually found and treated before their problem became critical, but often, sheep and goats were not found in a timely manner because they were usually pastured in rough country. The loss of flesh of affected animals and the expense of locating and treating were the major cost. The expense of additional employees and extra horses needed was considerable.

The screwworm problem caused constant horseback riding to find these cases, many of which would not be obvious to the untrained eye, but experienced men could often tell a wormie as far as he could see it. A few had dogs that went with them to smell and locate cases, as they had a distinctive foul odor. These dogs were especially valuable in brushy or rough country because it was common for affected animals to hide out.

A small pasture called a wormie trap was fenced and saved to keep wormies while they healed. Usually extra feed had to be bought for them and for the horses that were heavily ridden. The cost of the worm medicine was actually minor compared to the cost of crippled horses as well as the wear and tear on pens, chutes and other equipment.

The big, metallic-bluish-green fly would lay a cluster of white eggs on the wound margin. These eggs hatched in a few hours and the larvae burrowed into and consumed live flesh. They reached a size of about ½-¾ inch in length and were somewhat larger in diameter than a kitchen match, and were a creamy white in color.

This was a warm weather problem, as the fly was particularly vulnerable to the cold. It did not winter over in this area but would migrate in from the south as the temperature warmed. All plans were made to minimize wounds during this season. All elective surgery was planned so that healing would take place before warm weather. The cows bred accordingly.

Legend has it that buffalo would wallow in mud holes to cake wounds to prevent screwworm infestation and perhaps to smother the worms. I have seen animals that wets and other Mexicans in the southern part of Presidio County near the Rio Grande treated with mud packs using the clay-like, adobe soil. I have seen dried horse manure used to pack wounds of cattle. The most common remedy was salt, preferably the coarse, ice cream salt. I frowned on the manure, but I could not condemn the use of good clean mud in certain circumstances when nothing else was available. I can definitely vouch for the salt. I have used the coarse salt to pack the scrotum of freshly castrated hogs that were being raised in the unsanitary mud wallow environment that was typical of the day. These were the larger boar hogs that I was called on to castrate.

The commercial screwworm remedy in common use at this time was Smear 62 composed of the killing agent benzol with diphenylamine to protect against reinfestation. It also contained a turkey-red oil and lampblack. This had the consistency of paint and was applied with a brush but more often with a homemade swab. It dried with a hard crust. One treatment was usually sufficient for small wounds and minor infestations.

Smear 62 had some disadvantages. One was that the worms were killed and trapped within the wound which delayed healing. Another was the necessity of dipping the applicator repeatedly into the container, thereby contaminating it badly — as screwworm cases often had bacterial infections. This caused infections in otherwise non-infected wounds. This was not usually a major problem in adult cattle but a very serious problem in horses and especially in newborn calves whose navels had to be doped until they dried up. The term *dope* was commonly used when referring to the application of external medication to animals.

The bacteria introduced into the navel often entered the bloodstream and settled in the vicinity of joints, especially the knee and hock. Thus it was accused of causing big joint. It was also said to be poison to horses, although I think for the same reason because horses are much more susceptible to infections and more sensitive to irritants than cattle.

Some of the ranchers still used the older methods. Benzol or chloroform was used to kill the worms, then they would be raked out with a twig or sometimes a pair of tweezers was used to pick them out. This was followed by the use of a homemade smear called, *tecole*. Each made this according to his own recipe which usually consisted of the black heavy pine tar oil, stinking bone oil, tincture of iodine, and saponated solution of cresol. This was a black, tenacious, foul-smelling product that no self-respecting fly should come close to.

When the insecticide Lindane was developed, it was incorporated into a clear pine oil with some agent to cause it to have a jelly-like consistency and was called E.Q. 335. This was more effective and cleaner than the Smear 62. It was often colored with gentian violet so the treated animal could be identified. It had some disinfectant property but was not altogether without problems of infections. A really great advancement was the development of 1038, a combination of DDT and Lindane in a petroleum solvent manufactured by Ortho. This was a thin liquid which could be poured or squirted into the wound. Two distinct advantages were that it caused the worms to crawl out and there was no applicator needed so that cross-contamination was not a problem.

Many of the wounds in horses were on the lower extremities which could have been bandaged, but the low grade infections would itch and the horse would chew off the bandages. Therefore, I had three screened stalls to keep out the screwworm fly. They stayed full in the summertime, but the poor horses in these close quarters suffered from the heat.

The development of 1038 and the economic availability of penicillin greatly helped in the treatment of wounds in horses. These two products also almost completely eliminated the exuberant granulation or "proud flesh" as horsemen called it.

About the same time that 1038 was made available another insecticide, CoRal, was developed. This was marketed as a soluble powder. It could be mixed with water and sprayed on animals to prevent the infestation of susceptible cattle especially ones recently castrated, dehorned, or branded. Used in this manner it was a systemic product. That is, it was absorbed through the skin into the blood and distributed throughout the body, lasting about three weeks. The powder could be applied directly to and around the wound to treat and prevent infestation.

The eradication of this pest was a cooperative effort by livestock organizations, the state and the federal government. It was the biggest boon to the livestock industry of any program, development, or advancement and probably the most successful.

The original test program was conducted on an island in the Caribbean. When it proved successful the program was initiated in the United States in February, 1962. The flies were raised in a carefully controlled environment near Mission, Texas. They were irradiated with a radioactive isotope to sterilize them. These infertile flies were boxed and distributed by airplane in a predetermined plan. The infertile flies would mate with wild native flies and break the cycle. I have to admit, I had my doubts initially, but it was very successful.

The flies were released at first in the southern part of the state where the fly winters and then gradually shifted north as the weather warmed.

Mailing cartons were distributed to all in the livestock industry with a pre-addressed label to Mission, Texas for identification. The carton contained a test tube with isopropyl alcohol for preservative into which the specimens were placed. It also contained a questionnaire to identify the origin.

The laboratory placed the unknown side by side with a known screwworm and compared them under a microscope. Previous to this time I thought I could identify a screwworm from a maggot, but I soon learned that I could not. They are very similar in appearance. The screwworm burrows into live flesh and is somewhat difficult to remove from where it is embedded. They will often become very extensive and even cause death if untreated. The maggot lives on the surface feeding on blood and serum and is relatively easy to wipe off. Both are a problem because of mechanical irritation and metabolic waste containing some toxic material. They both interfere with healing and facilitate the wound becoming infected and seem to bother the animal by their movements. The maggot is not often of primary importance, although I have seen some major problems, especially in animals with dehorning wounds. A type of maggot called a fleece worm caused a problem, living and irritating under a heavy coat of wool or mohair and occasionally in long-haired dogs.

As the eradication progressed only treatments of hot spots were needed in isolated outbreaks as revealed by the survey cartons.

Auction Ring Calves

About 1950, Kenneth Smith called me one night from Midland where he had bought a couple of truckloads of calves at an auction. He told me to meet the trucks at the Crawford Mitchell Ranch (Alta Vista). They should be there about midnight, and he wanted me to begin treating them immediately as they were all sick. I was shocked because there were few drugs available at that time, and there were serious death losses from shipping fever in newly purchased calves, even those that were healthy when purchased.

I told him I was not going. You sold at an auction, you never bought at one, and certainly not sick cattle, and that he ought to know better. Good healthy animals in this area in those days were sold at the ranch or shipped to major markets such as Fort Worth or San Antonio on the railroad. The only local animals I can remember going to auction were so-called junk, that is, the unmerchantables: those suspected of being sick or cripples, cancer eyes, abscesses, and others of questionable health. Ken gave that guffaw laugh as only he could do and told me to go on out and do my best, that I was going to save those calves and make him a bunch of money because he had bought them cheap since no one else would bid on them.

I nearly worked myself to death on those calves the next few days. I don't know if they got well because of what I did or in spite of it.

Ken must have heard that the Good Lord takes care of old men and little children, and I guess that applies to old ranchers and young veterinarians. We kept the losses to a minimum, and the calves made a pocketful of money I was told.

The Breakdown

In the fall of 1950, Hayes Mitchell Sr. made an appointment for my boss, Dr. Ben Gearhart, and me to drench a bunch of sheep at the Barrel Springs Ranch. This was west of Marfa. The first twenty miles was on paved Highway 90 to the Ryan railroad section house where Mr. Felts lived and the ranch road turned off. This road was relatively smooth. I was to bring the phenothiazine sheep drench and the drench syringes. I loaded these in my relatively new Plymouth station wagon so I could leave early in the morning and be at the ranch before the sheep were penned.

As happened so many times in my practice, an emergency came up before the time of the appointment. Dan Frank called me during the night to deliver a calf. He had the Brown Ranch leased (now called the Cathedral Mountain Ranch). There were two roads to the headquarters. The road I traveled turned off Highway 90 between Marfa and Alpine at Paisano Pass and was ungraded but fairly good except where it dropped off into the Calamity Creek valley. This portion was steep and very rocky. Some of the rocks were the size of a softball and others were big. They would make the most nerve chilling sound when they hit the undercarriage of my car. However, this part was not very long, and the rest of the road was good. This was a much shorter route. I filled a five-gallon Army surplus water can with warm water and put it in the station wagon. Other supplies were already in it, as I tried to keep it well-stocked.

When I got there the calf was already dead with only the head showing. It was blocking the birth canal, so I severed it and attempted to grab a leg. The legs were so deep, I may have had more luck by putting my arm down the heifer's throat and pushing the calf. Soapy water isn't a very good obstetrical lubricant, but it is better than nothing and something was needed because she had lost her natural slickum.

There have been many times that I have wished for a longer arm, and this was such a time. I finally got one leg and was able to bring it out and cut it off with a minimum of effort. The other leg wasn't so difficult to grab hold of and straighten. Then the calf slipped part way out only to get hung up at the hips—a hip lock. No amount of twisting and turning would loosen it, so I divided the body through the flank and loins. I then inserted an O.B. wire saw between the legs and split the pelvis. The hindquarters were pulled one at a time. This sounds rather simple writing about it, but wallowing around on the ground in the mud and muck with the heifer straining when the epidural wore off was a problem. The tight place added to the discomfort. I guess the fact that it was night and dark shouldn't matter because

I couldn't see inside there anyway.

The afterbirth refused to turn loose, so I stuffed sulfanilamide powder in the uterus and gave a couple of injections to aid in the expulsion of the placenta.

It was getting late or early depending upon your viewpoint. It was getting daylight, and it was a long ways to the Barrel Springs Ranch. I drove too fast. Actually, it wasn't very fast, but it was too fast for that road with the heavy load of drench. I hit high center several times, especially on the rocky steep-hill portion.

I stopped at Gay Howard's filling station in Marfa for gas, telling him that I didn't have time for the oil to be checked because I was in a hurry. That was a mistake! I went about ten miles out of town, and the engine began to make a horrible noise and stopped. I had knocked a hole in the oil pan and lost the oil. There I was — stranded near Aragon, a siding on the S.P. Railroad.

No one came by except some travelers who speeded up as they passed me. Eventually Hayes and my boss, Dr. Gearhart, came looking for me, thinking I had overslept. Neither gave me any sympathy as we transferred drench and supplies into Hayes' pickup. Both of them had their nose out of joint all day. I wasn't very happy either, worrying about my car. It was a bad day, and it seemed the sheep were more ornery and had more thorns in their wool than usual.

When the station wagon broke down, my father-in-law, Jim Tyler, who was a mechanic and had a garage, towed it back to Marfa and determined that the engine needed an overhaul. I was afoot. We were still living in the upstairs apartment over the saddle shop. JoAnn was working in the Marfa National Bank in the same block and bought groceries at the Safeway store just around the corner, so the lack of a vehicle wasn't a major inconvenience for her.

Ben brought an old Chevrolet pickup in from the ranch for a practice vehicle. We had a metal box with wooden drawers made to mount in the bed of it. This was a tough old pickup made with good heavy metal, strong springs, and good clearance, a good ranch vehicle made for hard use, not for comfort.

The seat had deteriorated so that folded tow sacks covered the seat springs. There was no heater. The windshield wipers were the old type, air pressure or vacuum-powered, I think. They rarely worked, but it didn't make much difference because it rarely rained after the dry spell became a full-blown drouth.

When I purchased the practice in 1953, the pickup was included. Jim Tyler kept that old thing running.

Some Aspects of Early Day Practice

The practice was very informal in the early days, and almost all my clients became friends. Sometimes we had a cup of coffee before seeing the patient. Of course, an emergency was attended to first. Often, we had coffee and a snack afterward, frequently consisting of a biscuit or homemade bread with preserves or jelly.

When an early morning obstetrical case was treated, we would eat breakfast afterwards. If a work was finished near mealtime, I was invited. The noon meal was dinner, and the evening meal was supper.

The larger ranches often had camp cooks with a chuck wagon or at a cook shack, but most of the time a rancher's wife would bring us the noon meal. Or, if we were close by we went to the house. Sometimes the rancher would bring a lunch for us to eat at noon.

Many of my calls were to ranches some distance from town, and I would often take the mail and a newspaper. Sometimes they would ask me to bring a box of groceries they had ordered or some part from a hardware store. I would bring letters to be mailed back to town.

Sometimes I would be given a loaf of homemade bread, a pie or a cake, preserves or jellies, as well as fresh fruits and garden vegetables. During the hard days of the drouth of the fifties, Ralph Boone gave me steaks from a buffalo calf. Others would give or trade me items for services: beef, eggs, sausage, ham, and bacon.

After a hard day's work on the drive back, I would often worry what might be waiting for me: a calf delivery, a uterine prolapse, a wire cut horse that needed to be sutured, a horse with colic, or a cow with bloat—things that had to have immediate attention, even though I may not have an appointment the next day. My help understood that they were required to help at night when needed — part of the job. I didn't call them unless it was absolutely necessary, often utilizing the rancher or his hand and many times performing surgery or treatments unassisted.

I had some very good men helping over the years. Those that couldn't handle it would soon quit. Most that quit didn't give me notice of any kind. They just didn't show up and wouldn't talk to me either on the phone or when I went to their house. At first this infuriated me, especially when I only had the one employee and things were planned. Later, I would accept this as a fact of life.

The solo surgery, although inconvenient, was not as bad as it may seem because the procedures used at that early time were hardly aseptic—no gloves, no gowns, no masks, or surgical drapes. Instruments were scrubbed in soap and water and disinfected in a solution in which they were kept during surgery. If they had become grossly contaminated, they would be sterilized by boiling. The glass syringes were boiled in distilled water so that mineral deposits would not form and interfere with the fit, as barrels and plungers were ground for an exact fit. Needles would be boiled and stored in alcohol until used. Most of the needles were brass with chrome plating. Later, they were stainless steel, then still later, I used disposable aluminum needles and plastic syringes that were used once and discarded. I was never comfortable with this as it seemed so wasteful, as did the disposable surgical gloves and other disposables.

I often operated on dogs and cats on a kitchen table and sometimes on the tailgate of a pickup.

Squeeze chutes were scarce at first and most of my work on cattle was in a crowd chute. A few cedar posts were used to block the front and another post called a scotch bar was put behind to prevent backing up. If the head was to be examined or treated, a rope was put on the horns and the head snubbed close to a post. Then a nose lead was inserted in the nostrils and a wrap taken around a post to further stabilize the head.

Sometimes not even a crowd chute was available, so the animal was roped and stretched out on the ground by heading and heeling. If eye work was needed, a large post, preferably a railroad crosstie was placed on the neck and the head bent around. Usually a nose lead was inserted and its rope tied to the upper hind leg.

Cattle vaccinations were given with a heavy duty metal syringe with a glass barrel. The plunger had a rubber packing which was adjustable. This syringe could be completely disassembled for cleaning.

Although these procedures may seem sloppy and haphazard, actually, infections were rare. General anesthesia was my worst problem, especially when unassisted. I would clip the hair on a leg to expose the vein, then hold the dog or cat and give ether with a cone until they relaxed, then insert a needle and syringe loaded with pentobarbital which was slowly injected. A toe pinch reflex was used to determine when the anesthesia was sufficient enough to perform surgery. The syringe was taped to the leg, and additional was given as needed during the operation.

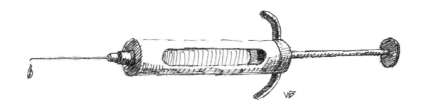

Metal ranch syringe.

Horses were anesthetized with intravenous chloral hydrate and magnesium sulfate. Later pentobarbital was added to this solution. Cows were rarely given a general anesthetic, only a local infiltration, nerve blocks or spinals.

The general anesthesia used on dogs, cats and horses was neither simple nor safe. I had some anesthetic accidents, but even though the percentage was low and the client-owners were understanding, it depressed me greatly. Of all the advances in medicine over the years, I appreciated that made in anesthesia as much as anything. Well, maybe not as much as antibiotics.

I did not have a receptionist or bookkeeper until Mrs. Lorene Tyler, my mother-in-law, came in 1960. Before that when things were busy, I often stayed up late at night doing bookwork, especially at statement time. Rarely were they sent on time at the end of the month. Many clients told me they knew when all their bills were in when they saw mine. After the hospital-residence was purchased and we moved, JoAnn helped with the bookwork and answered the telephone at times because both places had the same number.

Kerr Mitchell's Calving Shed

Kerr Mitchell had some of the prettiest, gentle, Hereford cattle in the area, and they were a pleasure to work with, except that the first-calf heifers had trouble calving, which was typical of the conformation that was desirable at that time. He had some of the best facilities when I came to the area, probably because they were relatively new, having been built in 1940, only nine years before. There was a nice saddle and feed room adjacent to a hay barn with a feed trough attached.

His only disreputable outfit was the calving shed. Now, some might call it quaint. It had been a chicken coop that had been tacked on the south side of the saddle room. It was a little lean-to shed with a west wall and roof made of old, beat up, rusty tin that had been scrounged from some abandoned building. The east and south sides were enclosed with chicken wire. It was very small. The door was a sagging wooden affair with leather hinges and fastened with baling wire, wound around a nail. In spite of its condition, it was great in inclement weather.

How he managed to put a heifer in it could only be explained by his being an excellent cowman, as the door was in the middle of it without benefit of a "blind" or "wing." He would have the heifer snubbed in a corner for me when I arrived so that her side to side movements were somewhat restricted. Although her head was tied close, there was still an amazing amount of forward and backward movement. The neck can be extended and contracted or kinked to a most remarkable degree.

It seems that when I was in up to my armpit, the ballet began. A quick twist of her rear end would soon be followed by another to the other side while squirming and tippy toeing. I was fairly agile in my youth, but some of the heifers really put me to the test as they danced about. Most of them didn't show favorites as they would step on first one of my feet and then the other. When I was exploring deeply or attempting to straighten a nose or foot, my chin would be resting on her rump and she would give a little hippy-hop and pop my neck. I think this is called whiplash. A quick drop downward would almost tear my arm off at the shoulder. Sometimes a quick twist with my arm halfway in would cause my elbow to bend backwards. If I had been a football quarterback, it would have been called hyperextended elbow. I would have been able to sit out a few downs with a trainer fussing over me, maybe even be put on injured reserve. As it was, I didn't even get any sympathy. Kerr was very compassionate towards his cows but not to his veterinarian.

I arrived on a call one day to find him sitting on a sack of feed looking very dejected. He had managed to get a wild heifer in the delivery room, but she didn't respect the flimsy nature of the structure and had demolished it. By his attitude, one would think the heifer had destroyed a work of art. Kerr rebuilt it with better material, but it just didn't have the same atmosphere as before.

The Over Zealous Ranch Hand

This ranch hand was very conscientious taking care of the boss' cattle. He either fed and pampered them too much, or the genetics were faulty as far as ease of calving was concerned. He had more trouble calving than I was seeing in other herds, even though he had the reputation of being very adept at calf delivery.

In retrospect, I wonder if I may have caused some of my problems there by delivering the first calf so quickly and easily. I was a young button, fresh out of school and new to the area. I was anxious to make a good impression as to my ability. I straightened a leg and slipped that little booger out, rubbed it down until it was breathing good, and left.

After that, when I arrived, the guy would still be working trying to get the calf. He wouldn't let me at her. This happened several times, mostly at night. I strongly suspect that I hadn't been called until late, and he was determined to deliver it himself. Perhaps he was trying to impress me that he was really trying before I was called and not just loafing on the job.

This was certainly aggravating to me, as nothing ever bugged me so bad as waiting. I nearly froze on a cold, windy night with my shirt off, ready to work, just standing around doing nothing. I'm not sure that I ever timed how long I was kept waiting, but one particular cold, drizzly night I had waited what seemed like a long time. I finally got in my car and left. I took the telephone off the hook and went to bed. The next morning, the rancher, who lived in town, called, and I explained what had been happening. He said there would be no more of that, and there wasn't. The heifer had died, and I guess he got somebody's attention. I thought the ranch hand would be angry with me, but on the contrary, he would be waiting with a smile and we became friends.

Frances and S.S. "Ted" Harper

Ted and Frances Harper had a little place west of Marfa that straddled Highway 90. This place was primarily a place for Frances and the two girls, Tana and Amy, to live while they were in school. Years before, Casa Piedra had a school when it was a bustling community, but now few people lived there and the town pretty much consisted of a rock house residence with a combination post office and store with a gas pump. The closest school was in Marfa.

At Marfa there were a couple of little pastures where cattle and horses were kept that Ted brought from the ranch when they needed special attention. They were hauled between here and the ranch in a rack on the back of a pickup or in a two-horse trailer that was also used for transporting the girls' barrel horses to rodeos. Those two pretty little girls riding the barrels was a thing of beauty. Ted was a good roper and often entered the roping contests.

Frances and the girls went to the ranch on weekends to help with the ranch work, and most of the summertime was spent there.

I had been called to see a milk cow with a spoiled bag, but she had been turned out. Frances said she would have her back in short order and put a bridle on a horse, then mounted bareback with a graceful motion. She trotted down to where the cow was grazing and started her back to the house. The cow had already been milked and fed this morning, and it wasn't time for the evening milking, so the cow realized something was out of the ordinary and didn't want any part of it. She was reluctant to go through the gate into the pen. Of course, she may have seen me peeking around the corner of a shed and got boogered at seeing a stranger.

The horse put on a pretty good show as he worked that cow back and forth until she gave up and went in. How Frances was able to ride that horse bareback was quite a feat.

A few years later I was at Cienaga, the Hart and Amy Greenwood ranch, that had been one of Milton Faver's part-time residences and a full-time fort in the Indian days. I had just finished replacing and treating a particularly difficult vaginal prolapse. The cow had hid out in the brush where Mr. Greenwood had trouble finding her, resulting in the prolapse being swollen and hard. The Mexican ranch hand that had been watching the proceedings, continually shook his head and muttered, "*El no puede, Señor Corazon.*" ("He can't do it, Mr. Hart.") I sat down on the old rock fence and smoked a cigarette. This ritual gave me time to rest and recuperate from the ordeal without it being too obvious. I told him how impressed I was with Frances' horsemanship. The Greenwoods were her parents.

Hart said that Frances had ridden all her life, besides having come by it naturally because Amy, her mother, was as good as they come. He related that not long after he and Amy married, they were in on a big roundup. The cattle hadn't been bred up like they are now, still being mostly Longhorn and none too gentle. Hart said he and another cowboy had been working some hills, and each had picked up a few head and drifted them to a point where they came together. About the time they met, there was an awful racket down in the bottom of the draw ahead of them. Hooves were cracking, rocks were rolling, and the brush was popping. Every once in a while they could get a glimpse of cattle running full speed with a cowboy in hot pursuit, leaning low in the saddle and seemingly oblivious to the limbs that clawed at him. The man with Mr. Greenwood exclaimed, "That's the wildest, craziest cowboy down there I ever saw!" Hart told me he had been watching closely and said kinda matter-of-factly, "That's my wife, Amy."

Calf Meningitis

A rancher brought in a steer calf about one month old, lying on its side and periodically suffering convulsions. I tapped its back and it stiffened into a typical strychnine poisoning convulsion. The rancher assured me there was no way the calf could have gotten a-hold of strychnine. There were still many sheep and goats in the area and strychnine baits were commonly put out to control predators. I tried to convince the rancher that was the problem, but he wasn't buying that diagnosis. The rectal temperature was 106° which was unusual for strychnine.

The calf had recently been castrated, branded, and dehorned so I tried to call it tetanus. Again, the rancher wouldn't go along. I finally questioned the dehorning process. He said they had recently changed the method. In the past, they had used a spoon. This was a homemade device sharpened to cut off the horn bud. His buyer was complaining about the scurs[*], so he asked a neighbor who suggested a tube dehorner. This is a small steel tube sharpened all around on the business end and a large wooden knob on the other. It is placed down on the small horn using a size that completely encircles the horn plus a little of the adjacent skin. Then it is pushed down and twisted to cut through the skin which is then scooped out. He was also advised to use a blunt rounded hot iron to sear it. He had chosen a big husky young cowboy to do the work and instructed him to be sure and get the roots. Well, the kid did as he was told. He went too deep with either or both instruments, resulting in cerebral meningitis.

I was really proud of myself for finally diagnosing the problem. The rancher left it for me to treat. Kenneth Smith, a local rancher, came by soon after, and I took him back to the pens asking him if he knew what was wrong. He just glanced at the calf, clapped his hands loudly, and when the calf jerked, Ken calmly said it was meningitis. I was really subdued. He had diagnosed it in a minute, and I had poked and prodded an hour or more.

W. E. "Bill" Bunton

W. E. "Bill" Bunton ranched at Bunton Flat, an area about 30 miles south of Marfa. He came to Marfa most nights and left early the next morning to be at the ranch at daylight. Occasionally, he would need some vaccine or medicine before he left town and would phone me with the greeting, "Get up and listen to the birdies sing."

I have never been very good about remembering names. It was the major cause of my being disciplined when a freshman at Texas A&M, where great importance was placed on knowing as many as possible. I had met Bill on more than one occasion soon after coming to the area and should have remembered his name, but I

---

[*] Distorted regrowth of horn.

didn't. When I asked to whom I should charge an item that he purchased, he answered, "Oh, just anyone you think you can get your money from," and walked out. You can be sure that I remembered him after that.

On another occasion he asked for a check to pay for a service. This was at the time when a person could use counter (or generic) checks to access their money at a specific bank and the bank would verify and pay by name and not by account number. I asked him which bank, to which he replied, "Oh, any bank should have $5.00 in it, shouldn't they?" Then to add to my confusion he finally decided on the Bank of Casa Piedra. Dr. Ben Gearhart, my boss, had obtained counter checks from both the Marfa banks and all the banks in adjacent towns. I had quite a stack that I frantically looked through. Finally, he laughed and named a local bank. I found that Casa Piedra was only a post office and a small grocery operated in Mr. Vasquez's house with a single gasoline pump in front.

I was repairing a prolapse at the Bill Bunton Ranch. Pete Chavez, his ranch hand, was helping me. I commented to him that I was never called to that ranch to deliver calves and asked if they ever had trouble. Pete answered, "Very little," that the heifers were out in the roughs with the rest of the cows. They were not watched and not helped. This really disturbed me because most ranchers brought their heifers close to the house, put them in a small open trap, and fed them on 41% cottonseed meal cake. When parturition seemed imminent, they were put in a pen, fed alfalfa and cake, and watched day and night. A peculiar thing about man and beast is that most are born at night. I have wondered if this may be a built-in safety device because both mother and baby are particularly vulnerable during this time, and darkness is a protection. However, this made it pretty hard on ranch hands and veterinarians.

When I got to know Bill a little better, I questioned his handling of the heifers. His explanation was that pampering the heifers and helping them was propagating problems. The ones having trouble calving would be eliminated—the hard way, I might add. Bill continued to explain that he had done this many years and had very little trouble. Also, the feed and labor saved offset the losses. I thought also, out of sight, out of mind. A heifer out in the pasture wasn't observed in trouble, therefore, her problems could be ignored. Most ranchers are very compassionate and, if a cow was seen to be in trouble, they could not stand by and allow her to go unaided.

This bothered me, and I began to speculate that perhaps his reduced problems might be due to other factors. I had heard that Chinese women continue working in the fields until immediately before childbirth with very little difficulty. Physicians had begun to stress to women that they exercise while pregnant and restrict their diet to prevent weight gain. Perhaps the customary way of handling heifers was compounding a problem that was being blamed entirely on the new genetics in cattle. That is, the short, broad head, short legs, and heavy shoulders.

Chow Dogs

There were few dogs that I did not like and enjoy. Some of the dogs that had a bad reputation would cause me the least trouble, such as pit bulls, Dobermans, and German shepherds. There was one breed that I had a healthy respect for. No, that is not the way to describe it—an unhealthy fear is more accurate. That was the chow or more properly called the chow chow. I never did understand why the name had to be repeated unless it was to warn the unwary to be sure they understood.

I didn't vaccinate many chow dogs and treated even fewer. A good example of the reason I didn't was an incidence stemming from a request from my plumber, Henry Magallanez. Henry was at my hospital cleaning out a sewer line that was stopped up with dog hair because my help had been bathing long-haired dogs. He had always come when I needed him and was reasonable in his charges. He asked me to come to his house to vaccinate his dog because it didn't like to ride in his truck, and his wife didn't like for the dog to ride in her car. I was glad to accommodate him. I followed him home, and he took me around behind his house. Inside a high chain link fence was the most ferocious beast I had ever seen. I don't know if that chow was as big as he seemed. It may have been the way he was barking, jumping, and biting at the fence. I kept waiting for Henry to make a move, or maybe I was hypnotized. Henry finally said, "There he is, doctor." I had to agree, he <u>really</u> was! I asked how we were going to vaccinate him, to which he answered, "I don't know. You're the doctor." I asked if he or his wife could hold him. He answered no, that one of them would entice him to one side of the pen while the other opened the gate a crack to put in feed and water. I tried not to show my fear while I studied the situation. Finally, I told him that there was no way an animal could get to the dog to give him rabies; and if by some strange circumstance he did contract rabies, there was no way he could spread it. So there was no need to be out the expense of vaccination. Henry thanked me, and I bowed out gracefully.

*   *   *   *   *

Bennie Durrill had a big red chow dog that eyed me, and I eyed her. I would step gingerly around, glancing out of the corner of my eyes and kinda side-stepping. She didn't act too aggressive, but my instincts were to beware. She would approach me, and I would shy away. Bennie tried to assure me that she was very gentle and wouldn't bite. I had heard that song and dance before. I wasn't buying it. One day, I was lying down behind a cow feeling for an elusive calf's foot. The dog kinda eased up on her belly beside me and put her head on my shoulder. I lost all my fear of her, and I would bring her a tidbit when I came to the ranch. She would stay right by my side. I learned to love her, and it was a sad day when I had to put her down.

The Bashful Bull

Guy Garren ranched in some hills between the Wiley Mountains and the Chispa Mountains about 15 miles southeast of Van Horn in Culberson County. He was a slender, dried-up, weather-beaten, old man. I guess his brother, Fatty, had hogged all the groceries. He looked all the more distinguished by his having only one eye — the missing one was a sunken socket with no glass eye.

Guy had called me to come see his herd bull which was not showing any interest in the cows. Frank Newsom, the county agent in Alpine, went with me to look for club calves. Guy had one of the better registered Hereford herds and Frank's 4-H Club feeders had been very successful in showing these calves. Guy complained about Frank castrating his good registered bulls, to make club steers. Frank argued that Guy was getting invaluable advertisement for his cattle by Frank's skillful guidance of his club kids. I was caught in the middle of these disagreements. I finally had to quit those two banty roosters. This really wasn't a good way to describe them. Guy was a smaller man, okay, but Frank was a long, tall, lanky guy.

Dr. Ben Gearhart was at a stock show when a man approached him, wanting to know if someone could point out Frank Newsom for him. Ben told him that wasn't necessary, to just walk around and if he saw a fellow that looked kinda like a sandhill crane, that would be Frank. Sure enough, the man didn't have any trouble finding Frank because the description fit him so well.

I collared the Mexican ranch hand to help me examine the bashful bull. He was a gentle bull and allowed me to take his temperature, listen to his heart and lungs, feel the texture of the skin and hair, and look at his eyes and in his ears. He even allowed me to nick an ear for blood to test. This was examined very scientifically by rubbing it between thumb and forefinger, smearing it on the palm of my hand to observe its density, clotting time, and length of time that it took to absorb oxygen by turning from dark blood to bright red. Everything seemed normal, so I hunkered down under him to examine the underside. The bull didn't object as the Mexican scratched his back. They had finished their discussion and had come to give me helpful advice and suggested numerous diagnoses and treatments. I caught a urine specimen in a tin cup. I placed a small amount in a glass Bangs (brucellosis) test tube, looking for blood or the deep golden color of yellow jaundice (icterus). I then heated it with a match. It smelled just like hot urine, no acetone odor. There was no cloudy formation of precipitated protein. The feces made a nice mashed potato patty with no visible blood or mucus. The texture was normal for well chewed and digested feed and had a normal odor. I put a little in a tin can to test later for the microscopic size eggs of internal parasites, commonly called worms, with Guy assuring me his cattle were not wormy, as if this was a reflection on his morals. Because I could find nothing physically wrong, I dispensed an aphrodisiac, "Elixir of Yohimbine," which contained tincture of yohimbine, tincture of cantharides (better known as blister beetle and the historical nickname of Spanish Fly), with a little strychnine in a syrup base. I had excellent results with this in buck sheep (rams) as well as bulls and carried a gallon jug to dispense in four-ounce bottles for sheep and pints for bulls. I put a label on it for directions. At that time a client wasn't told what a medicine contained and rarely cautioned on its use. (Give it like I say and don't ask any questions.)

I asked him to report to me in a few days, which he did, saying the bull had gone right to work. I later learned in a coffee shop in Van Horn that he had told someone how good that medicine, that "ole Doc Ederds" had given him, worked on that bull. The person asked what was in it, and Guy answered, "I don't know but it taste kinda like molasses." I got lots of mileage from that story. It was told far and wide for years. I sometimes hear it now, the participants having been forgotten or substituted. It is told as a joke not realizing that it actually happened.

The FDA (Federal Drug Administration) in all its wisdom soon had the product taken off the market, claiming it wasn't any good. I'm glad my bucks and bulls didn't know that.

Castration Infection in Calves

A local man was a prominent rancher in the Marfa area. He owned one large ranch southeast of town and leased another near Paisano Pass where he raised both registered and commercial Hereford cattle. He was manager of a good size ranch for a woman after the death of her husband and also a very large ranch for another widow.

He was in a business partnership with his brother. They bought and sold cattle, mostly for others, on a commission basis. A large number of the calves raised in the area and shipped to the Midwest corn belt were handled by them.

He was spread pretty thin, having so many irons in the fire, but he had a good crew of Mexican ranch hands who had worked on his ranches for years, especially the *corporal* (foreman). Therefore, he felt safe in letting them do the branding work without close supervision. This term was used for the process of working baby calves. They were branded, ear marked (a piece of the ear was cut for identification), and vaccinated for blackleg. The bull calves were castrated and dehorned also.

He had gone to the ranch to check on the work and found several dead and sick calves at one of the first waterings he came to upon entering the ranch. He went no farther, but returned to

Marfa and called me to look into the problem.

The ranch was southwest of Marfa down the Ruidosa Road which was a graded county road. It was later paved, but at this time it was dirt and kept in fairly good shape most of the time when the county road crew could get to it. This precinct had only one maintainer (grader) and lots of dirt roads, so it was spread pretty thin. The ranch road that turned off this county road was a different story, especially after a rain. A couple of miles down this road was a water trough with several dead calves nearby.

I performed a postmortem examination, also called a necropsy, on one that revealed a massive abscess in the scrotal region that extended up the inguinal canal and involved the abdominal cavity with peritonitis resulting. I opened a couple more with the same findings, then looked around and realized that all the dead calves and a few humped up sick ones hanging on the water were freshly castrated steer calves.

I had been told where the branding crew was working, so I drove there to observe their procedure to see if I could discover the cause of the problem. I found them, stopped and climbed up on a fence to watch the Mexican crew working. They seemed to be very skillful, heeling the calves, dragging them to the branding fire and flanking them. I could see nothing amiss from my vantage point, so I climbed down and moved closer so I could observe more carefully. The castration procedure was typical. The man castrating grasped the end of the bag and cut about half off then stripped the testicles out and cut the cords. There was one major exception. A small Mexican boy was carrying a bucket in each hand. The testicles were dropped in one, and then the man reached in the other bucket removing two horse apples (the formed fecal balls from a horse) which he then inserted inside the scrotum.

I asked him why he was doing it, and he said the first few calves they had worked on this roundup had bled so, they had begun doing this to stop the blood. I was able to control my anger and asked that they not do that any more and had him wash his hands and knife with my soap and disinfectant water. He obliged, not seeming to resent my interference. I watched a good while to be sure he didn't revert to his old practice. I had experienced a few instances previously where I corrected some procedures to which the men seemed to understand and agree to, but as soon as

I got out of the way, they went back to doing as they pleased. The fact that these calves weren't bleeding may have been the reason he complied.

I went to the boss man's office and reported. His face went pale, then red. I doubt seriously if those Mexicans ever used that method to control bleeding again.

It was quite a job cleaning up that wreck, but the losses weren't nearly as bad as I expected.

Fayette Yates' Poodle

Fayette Yates called me one day and asked if he could bring in a dog after-hours when the help had left. I was curious because this was a very unusual request, but I agreed to the arrangement.

He showed up with a French poodle. In the 1950s they weren't just called a poodle, they were French poodles. This one had a classic poodle trim — a top knot, feathers on the ears, clipped face and feet, rings around the legs, and fluffy bush on the end of the tail. This was the first live one that I had ever seen.

Fayette said it had whooping cough. It may have been kennel cough, but I diagnosed tonsillitis. I gave a penicillin injection and dispensed some triple sulfa tablets with instructions to give a little honey several times a day to soothe the throat.

He swore me to secrecy, not to tell anyone about this dog. He, his wife, and daughter had been to New York City where his daughter had fallen in love with this dog. He didn't want anyone to know he had it, because he claimed the only people that had them were pimps and prostitutes. I asked him how he knew that, and he just gave me a dirty look.

Cancer Eye - Pinkeye Seminar

The Highland Hereford Breeders' Association held a cancer eye - pinkeye seminar in Marfa, Texas, in 1951. David Combs was a prominent rancher in the Marathon area. He not only had his own ranch, but he also managed family ranches that operated as the Combs Cattle Company. He caused his brother-in-law, one of the owners, Dr. Matthews, a physician in San Antonio to become interested in the idea. The Combs Cattle Company was experiencing a large number of both types of cases, as were all the ranches in the Big Bend area. These were my main cases at that time, being in excess of fifty percent of my practice.

Dr. Matthews was well-known in the human medical community and was instrumental in getting many to cooperate and attend. Dr. Maxwell who had a private, cancer clinic in Dallas and Dr. Queen, together with several of his associates from the M.D. Anderson Cancer Hospital in Houston, were some that I recall attending. There were representatives of the veterinary profession, including some from Texas A&M and the State Extension Service as well as private practitioners. A large number of local, prominent, and knowledgeable ranchers as well as some from throughout the state and a few from New Mexico attended.

I presented a paper and gave a demonstration on cancer eye surgery on several cattle at Joe Mitchell's ranch near Marfa. Most of the people were particularly interested in the so-called trim of the relatively small growths on the surface of the eye. An 18-gauge, 4½-inch needle was inserted in the temple and angled towards the nerves to the muscles of the eye as they emerged from the skull. A local anesthetic was injected to deaden these nerves and relax the muscles. This allowed the eye to be popped from the socket for easy access to shave the growth off with a scalpel. The site was then cauterized with silver nitrate. I would later use Dr. Maxwell's Hyfrecator to cauterize, which improved my success rate. The length of the needle and the direction of insertion produced a few gasps. It looked like it was going into the brain.

Dr. Maxwell showed us his Hyfrecator. This was a high frequency electrical applicator that basically emitted a spark which caused tissue coagulation. He stated that he had remarkable success treating superficial skin lesions. He gave me his unit and encouraged me to experiment with its use on eye lesions.

I read the accompanying bulletin which described the painless removal of unwanted hair and its use in the removal of warts. I had developed a wart on my finger after I had surgically removed numerous warts from a show steer. This was done without the use of surgical gloves. Humans cannot contract warts from cattle. I guess that must say something about me. I decided this would be a good way to try out the instrument.

I set the dial good and strong to give it every chance for success. I stepped on the foot switch and touched the wart with the needlepoint. A blue spark shot out, and I smelled burning flesh. I threw the Hyfrecator across the room and made derogatory remarks about the person who had written the bulletin, his ancestry, his offspring, and all future generations. It got rid of the wart okay, but it sure wasn't painless by a long sight.

I reread the directions more thoroughly and completely. I always used a generous amount of anesthesia when I used it on animals.

I initially practiced on some eyes that I enucleated, then gradually on other eyes with fear and trembling. It eventually became one of my most valued instruments.

A great deal of interest was generated by this seminar. Dr. Burns, a Presbyterian minister, made a home movie showing Dr. Ben Gearhart and me demonstrating the lesions, treatments and surgery of various subjects.

Subsequently, I presented a paper and showed the movie to several organizations including the Pre-vet Club, the student chapter of the American Veterinary Medical Association at Texas A&M and also at a rather large seminar at Victoria, Texas.

I enjoyed these meetings and the experiences I shared with others, but I was unable to continue to accept their invitations to speak because of the distance and expense. The drouth had caused me to suffer financial hardship. This was in the days before honorariums were customary, and all expenses were borne by the speaker. It was considered the duty and obligation of a professional man to contribute to the advancement of the profession by the dissemination of knowledge and skills.

Dr. Queen and his associates from M.D. Anderson began making periodic trips to the area. They had been particularly intrigued by my surgical technique whereby I shaved growths from the eyes of cattle without contaminating or damaging the lesion. I would make the preliminary arrangements with various ranchers to study cases. We examined and treated eyes. A detailed description of the lesion, treatment, and animal was kept, with the animal identified by eartag. Specimens were collected to be taken back for histological study.

At first two or three came, then only one, Dr. John Sykes. He had immigrated from Scotland by way of Canada. He had spent the war years in India and Burma. I always introduced him as a

Scotchman and he would promptly correct me saying that a man from Scotland was a Scotsman, that a Scotchman was one that drank Scotch whiskey. He admitted that the two often went together.

John came out several times a year and we made some interesting observations. I was able to learn to make some very accurate eyeball diagnoses and prognoses. I was able to perfect my surgical techniques so that I obtained a high degree of success.

M.D. Anderson hired their own veterinarian, Dr. Jardine, to care for their laboratory animals, and he began to do the eye work on cattle in the Houston area. John went to California to do research and I lost touch with him. He was a hard man to convince that he should wear a hat in this country to keep his bald head from getting blistered.

Punkin

Punkin was Mrs. Em Mallon's dog, or perhaps I should say Mrs. Mallon was Punkin's owner. Mrs. Mallon owned and operated the Paisano Hotel in Marfa.

The dog was a honey-colored, male cocker spaniel. He was very well behaved, spending most of his time in the hotel lobby, discreetly greeting the guests. The doors to both the coffee shop and the dining room were almost always open, yet I never saw him in either place.

I don't remember Mrs. Mallon ever bringing him to my hospital. He would come on his own accord. Most times it was only a visit. Other times he would lick his lips and stretch his neck to show he had a sore throat. He would tilt his head and gently rub an ear with a paw when a tick or grass awn needed to be removed. At times he would sit by the office door until someone let him in, or he might sneak in at an opportune time. After he said his howdys or when the treatment was finished, he would lie quietly out of the way until someone took him back to the hotel. He would hop out of the vehicle and look back as if to say, "Thank you, see you later," then trot to the hotel door.

Clay Espy's Horse Guante

Along about 1951 or 1952, Clay Espy was shipping calves in the Marfa railroad stockpens. He had hauled a young horse he was training to town. Guante was from an exceptional bloodline that Clay was breeding, and he was particularly proud of this colt. I don't remember the reason he was brought to town, perhaps to show him off.

The stockpens were busy, so Clay had tied the horse to a post on the railroad right-of-way fence. A train came by and whistled. The colt was frightened and jumped the fence, or rather attempted to do so, and landed on the post which was about three inches in diameter.

When I arrived, the horse was walking slowly down a gravel road with about ten feet of intestines dragging on the ground. He was kinda side stepping along as if he was trying to keep from getting tangled up in them. Clay had ahold of the bridle trying to calm him and slow him down. The guts were bloody and dirty. I took one look and knew it was hopeless, so I recommended that he be put down. Clay refused and insisted that I try. Well, I was young and thought I could walk on water. I was secretly glad of the opportunity, so I didn't put up much argument.

Dan Perry, a Negro cowboy and horse trainer, was my assistant at the time. He took ahold of the colt's ear, twisted it and began talking to him which caused him to quieten down and stand still, while I administered a chloral hydrate and magnesium sulfate intravenous anesthetic.

The horse laid down smoothly. Men put ropes on all four legs and rolled him on his back. Dan held the bottle of anesthetic, allowing it to drip slowly while watching and checking the eye reflexes.

The wound in the abdomen was about six inches behind the ribs and to one side of the midline, a ragged, shredded wound. I trimmed off the badly damaged tissue and cleaned up the area. I began to wash a little of the gut and patch small holes caused by dragging in the gravel. I gently milked the intestinal contents into the part still in the abdomen, applied an antibacterial solution, Disulfalac, then coated it with finely powdered sulfathiazole as I gently worked it into the abdomen, ligating bleeders as I went along. This was a very slow, tedious task.

I would stop occasionally to rig up a fresh bottle of anesthetic for Dan. I think his stroking and talking soothingly to the colt had much to do with his lying quietly. The gravel on the road ate into my bony knees. I may have made some emphatic comments about the discomfort because someone placed a folded saddle blanket down for me.

There for a while, it didn't look like it would all go in. I was reminded of an expression, "trying to thread a needle with a wet noodle." I had an immense sense of relief and satisfaction when the last went in. Now I was faced with another dilemma: how to close the hole in the abdominal wall. The shredded tissue had left a gap that I could not close by pulling on the muscles. The peritoneum was sutured fairly easily, then each succeeding layer of muscle was patched by weaving catgut. Fortunately, there was some overlapping of muscle layers. I was able to stretch the skin to close it using one-eighth inch umbilical tape for suture, hoping that this was wide enough to keep it from cutting through the skin. I thought I would get some comments from the many onlookers because of this sloppy suturing but nary a word. I really wouldn't have cared if they had — I was so glad to finish.

I gave twelve 1000cc of lactated ringer's and 250cc of calcium gluconate. We give a solution nowadays measured as a liter and a milliliter, but we gave it as a *cc* then, and it seemed to work just as well.

The horse began to awaken soon after the anesthetic was discontinued, but Dan's gentle hands and voice caused him to lie quietly while I finished the intravenous therapy and he had time to recover. With gentle urging the horse made an effort to rise with all of us assisting him anyway we could and continuing to support him as he swayed, becoming accustomed to standing. We fitted a corset-type rigging around the body. Gauze was placed on the wound, then a thick pad of Belleview surgical wadding held in place by two girths, one under the belly and the other over the back, padded with a tow sack. This acted as a wound covering but more importantly as a support for the weak, damaged abdominal wall.

There were no trailers available as they were not yet common. Guante had been brought to town in a pickup rack. Dan began leading him slowly towards my hospital, taking a shortcut by letting down a couple of fences for him to walk over. Dan had some help with this and gave the horse support during frequent stops to rest. There were lots of men pulling for the game horse as he fought to live. I met him about halfway with tetanus antitoxin and intravenous sodium penicillin. Also I gave him what I thought was a massive dose of penicillin in oil intramuscularly.

Dan arrived with him late in the afternoon and gave him a few swallows of water off and on. He tried to feed him a hot bran mash, but it was refused. The next few days Dan hand watered and kinda force fed him by putting feed in his mouth and holding it closed. I kept him on penicillin in oil in the muscle and Disulfalac intravenously. He began to eat of his own accord but was fed cautiously to prevent abdominal distention. Between his poor appetite and our restricting his intake he got pretty slim of gut.

He made an uneventful recovery that truly amazed me. He had only a small indented defect and lived a long, useful life.

A Very Late Night

Bennie Durrill ranched north of Van Horn, the house being about ten miles from town. He called me one night in the fall of 1951 with a calving problem in a heifer. It was almost midnight when I began a complicated delivery, and it took most of the night to accomplish it with the use of a flashlight whose batteries gradually faded out. By the time we finished, Bennie, his ranch hand, and I were cold and exhausted. Bennie tried to get me to come in the house to drink some coffee and warm up, but because it was so late I thought I should go on home some 85 miles away. Bennie promised to call my wife and let her know I was on my way. As luck would have it, his phone was out of order. I don't remember it being a windy, stormy night which was usually the cause of those ranch telephone lines going out, but actually, much of the time, they didn't need an excuse.

JoAnn awoke, or perhaps she hadn't been able to sleep between baby Nancy and my not arriving home yet. She became concerned, then began worrying, and finally bundled up the baby and called her father who she prevailed upon to take her to look for me. I was in our only vehicle, and it was a worn-out ranch pickup that my boss, Dr. Ben Gearhart, furnished when my station wagon had engine trouble. The old beat-up pickup may have been partially the cause of her anxiety, with good reason. I was afraid to drive it fast.

I got back to Marfa just as they were leaving, meeting them in the middle of town. In retrospect it probably was a good thing we met instead of missing each other. However, in a little town it is easier to meet than miss. I was furious that she had gone to all that trouble, not knowing that she had not received the phone call. I wouldn't talk to her, only pouting like a little kid.

I have regretted very few things that I have done as much as the bad way I acted that night responding to JoAnn's anxiety.

The Holstein Bull at Lobo

About 1952 I was brucellosis testing at the Lobo Dairy of Holstein cows. I had finished the cows and a young bull when I was directed to a pen with the biggest Holstein bull I had ever seen. He was bellowing and pawing. I didn't want anything to do with that bull, especially because there was no working chute of any kind. We had been mugging the cows and young bulls. "Mugging" is a type of manual restraint of the head of cattle. In this case the opposite ear was grasped with one hand and a nose lead was inserted in the nostrils with the other and the neck bent or bowed to give access to the jugular vein for taking a blood sample. Later, a technique was developed to bleed (take a blood sample) from the tail, which was an easier and faster method.

The bull had a brass ring in his nose and had been dehorned. I had often jokingly chided some cowboy for climbing a fence to escape a wild, fighting, muley cow, telling him the cow couldn't hurt him with no horns, and he would spoil that cow by running from her. Now it was my turn to see if I had good red blood. I really didn't want to see it bad enough to look at it scattered all over that bullpen. One of the men had a long pole with a hook on the end. It was long, slender and lightweight, probably made from a cypress sucker rod[*]. The bull didn't want that hook in his nose ring. Secretly I was hoping they wouldn't be able to hook him, and I wouldn't have to test him. The bull couldn't tolerate being teased and kept butting the fence. The nose ring was eventually hooked, and the bull settled down a little. The fellow with the pole said, "There he is, Doc." I had to agree, he really was! But I made no move. The man added, "He's all yours, go get

---

[*] Part from a windmill, nowadays made of fiberglass.

him." The other gents watching the goings on looked at me. When I hesitated, I was prompted with, "Hurry, Doc. I can't hold him all day!" I really hated to climb down in that pen with that bellowing beast. The restraint was less than ideal, but I finally got up enough courage to crawl off the fence and ease up beside him and jab a needle in his neck aiming for the jugular. He came unwound and threw a wall-eyed fit. I went down in a pile of manure with him on top of me, kicking and pawing. When he settled down and the dust cleared, I was able to stand up, much to my surprise. There was blood coming from the needle, and I caught some in the test tube that had survived, unbroken. I started for the fence, but I didn't make it. My legs gave way. A big, stout Mexican grabbed me and literally threw me over the fence. It was several minutes until I could stand. There was blood on my clothes and by the aches and pains, I knew it was mine. I could feel it running down my leg and into my boot. When I got home, I looked sorta like some roadkill the dogs had drug up, hobbling and bent over. JoAnn was concerned as I eased off my boots and pants. No blood, no abrasions, no swellings, not a mark, nothing to show for my pains. What I felt running down my leg wasn't blood! JoAnn looked at me questioningly but made no comment, only a sympathetic pat. The blood on my clothes had come from the needle in the bull's neck. How disgusting!

JoAnn fixed me a tub of hot water, and I climbed in to soak. When it got cold, I filled it again with hot water and soaked some more. This was kinda routine after hard work, and occasionally I would fall asleep in the tub.

The Calf Puller

I had seen commercial advertisements promoting a new calf puller. Among the many claims was that a twelve-year-old boy could deliver the most difficult case. The mechanics were entirely too simple. It couldn't be any good, or it would have been thought of and used years before. I had been a sucker for several new contraptions that didn't work nearly as well as advertised, if at all. The reason I was so gullible was because of the rapid advancements being made shortly after World War II, especially in the field of pharmaceuticals but also in equipment and surgical instruments.

Kerr Mitchell was having his share of problems calving heifers and ordered one of the new fangled gadgets, disregarding my bad mouthing it, telling him it was probably made to sell, not to use. Shortly after it arrived, he began to brag to me about its value. I didn't take him seriously. In fact, I accused him of exaggerating, trying to justify his waste of money. He had arthritis in his hands and was limited in his ability to straighten a malpositioned calf. He called me and I corrected the turned-back head and one leg of the calf, attached the O.B. (obstetrical) chains to its legs, and then hooked on the calf puller. It was Dr. Frank's Fetal Extractor and we pulled the calf slick as a whistle. I was duly impressed.

I bought one immediately, and it, or one like it, was my most valued piece of equipment. I wore out several, but I was never able to find the twelve-year-old boy who could deliver the most difficult case. I still had to do many embryotomies and caesarean sections.

Late Spring Frost in 1952

Range conditions were exceptionally good in the spring of 1952. There had been wet snows in the winter, and the weather had warmed up nicely. The grass had greened up, the brush had put on leaves, and weeds had come up. These conditions are rare in the area. The soil conditions usually are very dry, and the wind is blowing in the spring. The first moisture to fall usually comes in the summer.

Brush and weeds are an important part of the diet of sheep and goats which were raised in large numbers at that time.

A hard, killing freeze occurred on April 22, 1952, after animals were accustomed to eating the green vegetation. The leaves dried up and fell off the brush. The weeds were killed and shriveled up to nothing. The grass turned brown. The only green left was on plants not sensitive to the cold. The animals kept searching for these, many of which are poisonous.

Bob Dod was the foreman of the Ray Willoughby Lobo Flat Ranch between Valentine and Van Horn. He called saying that many of the sheep were getting sick and dying. He was a man in his late forties or early fifties, raised in this area and experienced with livestock.

We caught a few weak, lethargic individuals to examine, seeing a green stain around the mouth and nose. I opened up several that had not been dead long. I found some congested lungs, a few hemorrhages on the heart and some on the lining of the true stomach. The rumen contents were green, but I could not identify any of the plant material. We looked for green plants and found only one that had been grazed. It looked like bitterweed, had a little aromatic odor when rolled between the fingers and had a bitter taste. When I could not definitely identify a plant, I often tasted it because, as a general rule, a poisonous plant has an unpleasant taste. Bob said he had been told by some men that it definitely was bitterweed like that around Ozona and Sonora, but others said it was a little different and wouldn't cause a problem.

We found sick and dead sheep around all the waterings where this plant was found and much had been grazed. Bob pointed to the next watering that he wanted to go to but said we couldn't go straight to it but would have to detour around a crack in the ground. He said this was caused by an earthquake. I was curious so he drove to it. The crevice was five or six feet across as well as I can remember. It looked to be about twenty feet deep, but Bob said it was much deeper, that you couldn't see farther because it was not completely vertical. Bob said he was told that it had been found soon after the earthquake in the early thirties that cracked adobe houses in Valentine. It must have been the one I felt in Del Rio when I was a boy.

I recommended the sheep be moved to the north end of the ranch where this weed was not present. Bob told me later that he was nearly 800 head short when he rounded up in the fall.

This was the only bitterweed poisoning I saw west of the Pecos River. It was the first time I saw such a large number of deaths.

Lechuguilla

Agave lechuguilla consists of a crown or heart that is white and grows close to the ground, without a trunk. A number of broad, fleshy, green leaves or blades ending in a sharp thorn radiate from the crown. The immature stalk and flower are palatable and nutritious to animals although somewhat difficult to graze. The plant dies once it has bloomed, similar to its close relative, the century or maguey plant.

The green part of the leaf is toxic to sheep, goats and cattle that will eat it when there is a shortage of feed, causing a poisoning. I have never heard of horses, mules or burros eating it. Deer will paw up the plant and javelinas will root it up, both eating only the white heart. It was said that Indians roasted this heart for food. The freshly roasted portion could be chewed, sucking the juice and flesh from the tough coarse fibers which were then spit out. Many of these are found in caves that had been inhabited by Indians. They have been called lechuguilla cuds, being black from the roasting and with tooth marks. The roasted portion was also ground into a flour in a mortar called a *metate* or *mortero* using a hand-held rock called a *mano*. This flour could be saved and later made into a tortilla. It was also made into small loaves, probably incorporating other ingredients.

My helper, Paul Spitzer, told me that his father-in-law, Pancho Escarcega, was raised near Coyame, Chihuahua, Mexico, west of Ojinaga. Coyame was well-known for the production of sotol, an alcoholic drink made from the plant by the same name. Pancho said that when he was a small boy, he would go into the hills and gather lechuguilla hearts, carrying them in tow sacks on a burro. They were brought to a place where men expressed the juice which was fermented to make an alcoholic drink which he said was a cheap substitute for and sold as a second class sotol. This was during prohibition in the United States and any kind of liquor was in great demand. Pancho said both lechuguilla and sotol pulp was mostly fed to hogs but also ground into flour and used as an extender for wheat flour for human food after being roasted. Probably the part used for food had not been processed by extracting the juice.

A drink was made from the sap of the century or maguey plant stalk and some said that its root bulb was roasted and made into a flour for food also. Both the drink and the flour are called mescal.

The Mescalero Apaches that inhabited the Trans-Pecos region when the white men came were called by that name because they both ate and drank mescal. It is not known if the Indians used the one word, mescal, for the food and drink made from all three plants or if the early settlers failed to make a distinction.

Pete Salas, a ranch hand who I worked with at the Paisano

Cattle Company ranch at Marathon, was raised on the border with Mexico near the Rio Grande, an area that is now in the Big Bend National Park. He told me his father would gather the growing stalk of the maguey (century plant) which he then roasted. This would be chewed, sucking out the juice and pulp that was sweet. This was very similar to chewing sugar cane.

The mountain laurel bean which is brilliant red, about the size and shape of a pinto bean, was also called a mescal bean. It was said that the bean was ground and added to the alcoholic drink, mescal, to make a hallucinogen. The bean is poisonous but like other toxic plants, the Indians knew how to prepare and use it.

Lechuguilla poisoning results in a thick tenacious discharge from the nostrils and lacrimation, a weeping from the eyes that cause stockmen to describe them as fevered. They do have the appearance somewhat of cattle with shipping fever. The secretions and visible mucus membranes are a golden yellow. This color is more easily seen in the vulva of females and the prepuce of males, especially in pigmented animals such as Suffolk sheep and Angus cattle where the color is obscured in other visible areas.

The urine is yellow in the relatively early stages and red-tinged later. When lechuguilla poisoning is present or suspected, a careful watch for the telltale, yellow urine will disclose animals in the early stages when they can be removed and fed, with a high percentage of recoveries.

Photosensitization is common, evidenced by thickening of the ears. If only small numbers are affected, keeping them in the shade is beneficial. There is weight loss, some becoming very thin if they live long enough. They are lethargic and often off by themselves or dragging along behind the group.

A distinct, golden-yellow color is seen on postmortem especially on the flesh side of the skin, the fibrous connective tissue and any fat that may still be present. The liver is a dirty yellow color and the kidneys almost black. There is a characteristic fiber ball in the paunch (the rumen), except in one unusual case that I saw.

Horses did not eat lechuguilla but suffered badly by being crippled by the thorns. This was especially true when sheep were still plentiful in the area. The plant has a tendency to grow in patches, and sheep would go in these to eat the grass because cattle and horses usually did not. They seemed to delight in getting in a big patch and balking. Hollering, waving a hat, slapping leggins with a rope and even rattling a can with rocks would sometimes be ignored, and the only way to get them out was to ride in and drive them out. If given time, most horses would pick their way if familiar with the plant, but too often a rider would be impatient and charge into the mess.

Those vicious thorns would easily penetrate a horse's skin. The hairline, coronary band, was a favorite place and very painful to the horse. However, I had more success locating and extracting the thorn here than in other places. The thorn would break off and remain in the horse. All too often the thorn would not be visible and only a small puncture wound could be seen. Most were a real challenge to find and remove.

The worst were those in the joints such as the pastern and fetlock, but those embedded in the flexor tendons were especially bad. Too often the thorn could not be located, and the horse would be permanently crippled.

The ones penetrating the pasterns could usually be located by shaving and scrubbing, then probing with mosquito forceps. Mexicans would make a poultice with a prickly pear leaf by splitting it and bandaging, in an attempt to draw out the thorn. I usually used icthammol ointment. A physician and I were visiting near McCamey, and he told me he used Ergophene ointment made by the Upjohn Company to draw out mesquite thorns in people. I liked this, not only because it didn't smell so bad and was not as messy as the black tenacious icthammol, but also because the dark colored thorn, if it came out, could be seen in the light gray Ergophene.

The thorns seemed to have an irritant on them which make them more painful than just the injury. I had a few penetrate my boot and stick in me as I was engrossed in hunting a deer and not watching where I stepped. Therefore, I can vouch for the pain. They wouldn't fester like a splinter and come out. If anything, they seemed to have a tendency to migrate deeper. I could not see them on an x-ray.

Deer killed in lechuguilla country would be found to have many of the black thorns in their legs, but they would be soft and pliable, not causing the deer any problem. Deer are native to the area and nature provided them this quality. Domestic livestock and people are intruders.

A common belief when I came to the area was that lechuguilla caused trouble because a large fiber ball would form in the rumen. Many of these fiber balls were packed so tightly that they did not deteriorate readily and could be seen in a carcass long after little else remained. I was approached a number of times requesting that I surgically remove the fiber ball.

Dr. Burns, our toxicology professor at Texas A&M, had assured us that the toxic principle was an alkaloid in the sap. Experiments had been performed by placing the plant in a cider press to extract the juices which would be fed, producing typical symptoms.

My father told me that a neighboring ranch of our family in the Comstock area had fed lechuguilla during the severe drouth of 1917-18. They had men gather the entire plant and chop it up fine in a hammer mill. It would be mixed with cottonseed meal and fed in troughs to sheep. The theory was that the very small pieces would not ball up in the rumen like the natural long fibers. A large number of sheep died with typical symptoms yet no fiber ball was present.

It was never fed intentionally during the drouth of the 1950s to my knowledge.

The late spring freeze of 1952 caused the first significant number of complaints that I had with livestock eating lechuguilla. Sheep and goat problems were numerous and some severe losses occurred — cattle less so, but they were significant.

Affected cattle were put in the shade during the day when possible, and some were given glucose intravenously. I guess it was technically dextrose, but this simple sugar was called glucose at that time. This really impressed the Mexicans. Their eyes would get big, look at each other, and nod knowingly, saying, "Ahhh, suero!" The other would answer, "Sí, suero!" *Suero* is the Spanish word for *serum* and is used anytime a volume of solution of any kind is given intravenously. I would also give water and light feed with a stomach tube and pump. Vitamin A injection from cod liver oil and B-complex vitamins were given intramuscularly. I don't remember saving many that I treated, I think because only advanced cases were presented to me. The less severe cases were treated by the owners, primarily with tender loving care.

Sheep and goats were brought only for diagnosis. I never treated any because the value of the animal versus the cost of the treatment did not permit it.

Switching pastures would sometimes cause the trouble to stop or at least slow it down temporarily, even if both pastures had lechuguilla problems. Once sheep and goats started eating lechuguilla, often they would stay out in a patch and not go to water. It is possible they were getting enough moisture from the plant to dull their thirst, but I suspect that thirst was actually killed because when placed in a corral, they frequently would not drink. We called this "the dry mouth" and much of the time drenching of water with a coke bottle would start them drinking again. This method seemed to be more successful than giving water with a stomach tube or with a drench syringe.

Dan Frank was leasing the Drake Ranch north of Kent. His sheep started eating lechuguilla, and switching pastures was moderately successful. He and his ranch hand rode the pastures horseback, picking up any sick or suspicious animals. They were placed in a pen and fed hay. He told me that almost all died that were fed alfalfa and yet few died that were fed grass hay. I have been told that alfalfa is hard on the liver and kidneys which are the two organs primarily affected by lechuguilla. Knowing Dan like I did, I imagine both men produced lots of wet saddle blankets caused by riding can 'til can't.

Lechuguilla in South Brewster County

A ranch foreman called me two or three weeks after the late spring frost that caused so much trouble in the sheep at Lobo and asked me to meet him at a water trough about a mile west of the Park boundary at Persimmon Gap. I turned off the highway onto a dirt ranch road and looking ahead, I saw the side of the hill was white. My first thought was that it looked like snow or hail, but these ideas were quickly discarded. I thought it might be the white rock such as on the scalloped hill tops a short ways south of Marathon. But it didn't look right. When I drew near, I was surprised to discover this was bare lechuguilla fibers that had bleached white. Close inspection showed that sheep had chewed the green part of the leaves and sucked out the pulp and juices, leaving the bare fibers between the crown or heart and the thorn on the end.

A number of dead and sick sheep were in the vicinity of a water trough that was in the middle of the area. I examined a few of the very sick, weak ones that I could catch afoot. They showed typical symptoms of lechuguilla poisoning. I performed a necropsy on a couple of fresh carcasses that also showed the typical postmortem lesions, except there was no fiber ball, which was always thought to be present in the rumen. This was easy to explain because the fiber was still on the plant.

The ranch foreman arrived soon and was surprised that I was already there and had completed my examinations. The ranch was about a hundred and twenty-five miles from Marfa, but I had a pretty heavy foot in my younger days. I explained the diagnosis and the reasons for it, but he had a problem accepting it.

He was an experienced rancher and had been around lechuguilla much of his life and had seen many deaths caused by it. He had always seen the fiber ball and was a firm believer that it was the cause of the problem. He wasn't ready to accept the diagnosis of the young pipsqueak of a veterinarian with his book learning. We sat down on a rock and discussed the symptoms, which he readily admitted looked like it should. I then told of my father's knowledge of the Comstock rancher who had fed chopped lechuguilla that resulted in the death of sheep without the characteristic fiber ball. We then examined the chewed plants.

What could I recommend? He knew what should be done. Take them off the plant and feed them. This wasn't so simple. The pastures were few and large. We decided that if he tied off the float on the water troughs on that side of the pasture, it would force the sheep to change their grazing habits away from this heavy thick growth of lechuguilla. Also the sheep should be driven horseback and kept out of the area for some time. I also suggested that he switch pastures with the sheep. I had been told that sheep doing poorly in adjacent pastures could be switched and both bunches would pick up and that losses would slow down or stop. I could not recommend any medication.

Mr. Matthews, Elsinore Cattle Company

Mr. Matthews was the manager of the large Elsinore Cattle Company Ranch near Fort Stockton. I considered him to be one of my best friends in the early 1950s. Therefore, it is embarrassing that I cannot remember his first name or initials. Perhaps it is because I never addressed or referred to him as any other than Mister Matthews. I always held him in awe — he was that type of person. He told me that he had been a sheriff in south Texas with a reputation. The Elsinore Ranch was owned by a group of investors who were extremely upset because there were no deer on the ranch, and there was a continual loss of cattle from rustling. The group hired Mr. Matthews to correct the situation, which he did in short order. The cattle losses stopped and the deer increased. I have forgotten almost all the stories he told me, and it is probably better that I did, as some things are best not written or repeated.

I usually left Marfa early in the morning and would drive ninety-three miles to Fort Stockton and would eat breakfast in a cafe before going to the ranch. Most of the men I talked to there swore they wouldn't set foot on that ranch, that too many men had disappeared there, and that I was a fool for going. The first time I went on a call there was in the early days, and it was still my practice to take a newspaper and a bottle of whiskey. This really impressed the old gent and made a staunch friend of him. I call him old, but I was 24 at the time and anyone with gray hair was old. His son, Peeler, was about my age.

It was a big old ranch with lots of cattle. There were hills and brush with mesquite in the flats and cedar in the hills. They raised lots of horses that were needed at that time. Many colts needed castration, and many became lame and wire cut. They ran Hereford cattle, so cancer eyes were also a problem.

When the work was finished we would go to the house and nip at the bottle. (Of course, at that time it would have been impolite not to join him.) He would tell tales of south Texas. He never shared any of the happenings at this ranch, so I never knew if the rumors had any substance. Some men's reputation and bearing are all that are needed. He died during the worse part of the drouth, and Peeler took over management.

Peeler was a good manager and a good man. He took over the ranch at a difficult time, and I was afraid the owners might hold him responsible for the poor showing the ranch made financially, but he stayed on. We were never close. He was all business and no foolishness. Eventually, veterinarians settled in Fort Stockton and I ceased to go to the ranch. An end of an era.

J.M. "Manny" Fowlkes and the Lion Dogs

J.M. Fowlkes was always called Manny. He may have signed his checks that way — I don't remember. He was known as one of the whispering Fowlkes boys. They had the most remarkable volume to their voices. A normal conversation voice in front of the Paisano Hotel could be heard a block away. I never heard him raise his voice. He didn't have to.

Manny's ranch bordered the Rio Grande River for several miles in rough, mountainous country. He ran mostly sheep which mountain lions love to kill, but seemingly not to eat, just for the pleasure. He had one of the best pack of lion dogs and was very successful in catching lions. He didn't eliminate them, just attempted to keep his losses to a minimum. This was a constant battle though, as they kept coming from Mexico where they flourished. There was little or no effort to fight them there.

A big cat, lion or panther, escaped from the zoo in Oklahoma City. There was lots of publicity, and dogs came from all over the country. Manny took his best dogs there. The cat was captured. Manny had good heavy leather collars on his dogs with brass name plates riveted on. One of his best dogs was claimed by another man who Manny suspected had removed the collar. The dog's neck showed a well-defined area where a collar had been worn. There was no doubt who the dog belonged to. The other man was a pretty salty individual, and the situation became tense. Manny came back with the dog. Rumors filtered back that this was the first time the other guy had ever been known to back down. Manny was an imposing figure of a man in stature, demeanor and voice. Quite intimidating, I'm sure, and I feel certain the man was very wise not to have pressed the issue too far. Manny brought the dog to me to have it branded. I don't recall the shape of the brand but it was a long running figure to be put across the entire left side. I gave the dog a general anesthetic and clipped the hair closely. I had branded many cattle and quite a few horses but this was my first dog. The skin resembles that of a horse, so I determined that I should not use a very hot iron and, at that, leave the iron on only a short time. It was still a mistake! The skin immediately puckered up something terrible. The brand wasn't legible as to it shape, but it was certainly legible as to its presence.

The trip was a disaster for Manny. He had raised his dogs on the ranch. He had never brought them to town, nor were they ever commingled with other dogs. Therefore, he had not taken the trouble to keep them vaccinated for distemper. Distemper is a very deadly virus disease of dogs and other members of the canine family. It is particularly vicious in that it is slow to incubate and has a high mortality rate with a prolonged period of illness with pus type gummy discharge from the eyes and nose. If the dog does live, it has an impaired sense of smell because of the long time the nose was irritated. This essentially ruins the usefulness of a dog that depends on its sense of smell. Most so-called recoveries are affected with a nervous disorder called chorea, a pitiful condition, especially the chomping or chewing gum fits, a constant chewing movement of the jaws. These eventually die. Many are affected with a rhythmical jerking of a leg or multiple legs, similar in appearance to Parkinson's in humans. This was very sad to see these exceptional dogs deteriorate. Manny took it pretty hard, not only because it wiped out his pack of good dogs but also because he was a very compassionate person, despite his rather brash manner.

Rabies

The "Mad Stone", the Rabies Epidemic, and Vaccination Clinics

A so-called old wives' tale was that a skunk, called a hydrophobia cat, was a carrier of rabies, even though apparently normal. Animals that had rabies were said to have hydrophobia, or to be mad. This notion was ridiculed for many years until research proved that a skunk, often called a polecat, (or civet cat) could have rabies and secrete the virus in the saliva for prolonged periods before showing symptoms and dying.

We thought skunks made good pets, and I de-scented several. The first was Pepe Le Peu that belonged to Mary Martha Gearhart. He was a cute little fellow, very colorful with clean body habits and a good disposition. He caused quite a reaction in people who did not realize he was de-scented, and even when told, they would give him a wide berth.

Dr. Gearhart and I operated on him in the hospital with disastrous results. We really smelled up the place. It seemed as if the odor persisted forever. After this I operated in an open air environment, wearing old clothes, that could be left outside to air out.

It was believed that skunks and raccoons were susceptible to both dog and cat diseases, so I gave rabies vaccine plus canine distemper and feline distemper (panleucopenia) vaccines to them. Later, when skunks were determined to be carriers, it was prohibited to vaccinate them, as well as raccoons. I no longer operated on or treated either, discouraging their being kept as pets.

There were several conditions that were confused with rabies. I suppose strychnine poisoning was the most frequent because of the champing of the jaws and profuse salivation. Perhaps chorea, the nervous form of distemper, may have been equally mistaken, especially the so-called chewing gum fits.

I was told there were many cases of running fits in dogs during the 1920s and 1930s. It was thought to have been caused by a preservative in light bread, as store-bought bread was called. The problem stopped when the preservative was discontinued. Most dogs were fed table scraps and leftover bread was a common ingredient.

I met a lot of resistance to rabies vaccination, not only from those who did not believe it to be a contagious disease but also because of the problems with the vaccine. It was a 5 ml suspension of caprine (goat) brain tissue. This caused an occasional sterile abscess. The body was reacting to all the foreign material as if it were infectious bacteria. This caused the clientele to think we were using dirty syringes and needles.

The mad stone was used as a preventative in cases bitten by a mad animal. The mad stone was supposed to be a calculus, technically called a trichobezoar, that is formed in the stomach of an albino deer. They were quite rare and a highly prized possession. I never saw one. In fact, I never saw a white deer, much less an albino. I never even talked to anyone that had seen either. It was either "they said," or "I was told." Sometimes the patient was taken many miles to a mad stone. If the stone stuck to the bite, it would draw out the virus, and the treatment would be successful.

I saw very few confirmed cases of rabies until a major epidemic occurred in the area. I think it was in 1952. There were twenty-nine cattle, four horses, six cats, but only two dogs that were confirmed by laboratory examination. Few dogs were tested because almost all were shot in the head, resulting in the brain being destroyed. Another reason few dogs were tested was because of the frequent delay from the time of death until testing. The test was a microscopic examination of brain tissue which could not be performed if decomposition had taken place, which occurs very quickly in delicate brain tissue.

There were numerous other cases especially in cattle, skunks, fox and coyotes that were suspicious, but were not tested, either because there was no human exposure or because the animal could not be found to kill and obtain the head.

A number of bats were found dead and others that were unable to fly. An occasional one was seen on someone's porch or alone in an open garage, apparently having become disoriented and lost its way. This led us to believe bats were the primary source of the disease because of the distances they fly to feed and when migrating, although none were tested. In recent years a technique has been developed whereby the strain of virus can be identified, revealing the animal origin.

Many people in the area took the anti-rabies prophylactic series, myself included. Rabies was so feared that many took the series even though there was no exposure, only a vague suspicion that there could have been.

*   *   *   *   *

The 1952 Rabies Epidemic was particularly serious along the border. The Lions Club in Presidio invited me to talk to them about the disease. The meeting was held in the old Oil Flyer Cafe which was a remarkable and colorful building. I wish I knew its complete history. It was a large lumber building, that in itself was unique in Presidio, as all the other buildings were adobe and a very few of red tile construction. The ground floor was divided by a partition that had a lower solid panel and a lattice upper portion. The west side was equipped with tables and chairs for eating. The east side had a long counter with stools. It looked very much like a bar, which I was told it had been. There were booths near the partition. The back was a kitchen. A wooden staircase led to a balcony which looked down on the west side. There was one large room upstairs on the south side that we met in and a series of smaller rooms on the east and west sides, that, I was told, had been sleeping rooms. I was told that the building had originally been a saloon with a ballroom on the ground floor and hotel rooms on the upper floor. I was very sad when it burned. I always ate there. I don't know if the food was especially good or if it was because of the quaint atmosphere. I wasn't much of a connoisseur of fine food then, or even now. If it was greasy, salty, and hot with chili peppers, it was good. Of course, there weren't many places to eat in Presidio at that time.

The meeting was well-attended by Anglos, Americans of Mexican descent, and Mexicans from across the river in Ojinaga, Mexico. They fed me a big thick steak with french fried potatoes and some Carta Blanca beer. We talked half the night. I've talked at various meetings, but I'm sure this was the most enjoyable. We planned a vaccination clinic that we set up a few days later across the street in a vacant area in front of the Phillips Hotel. They nearly worked me to death, many dogs being brought from Mexico.

Not many cats showed up but the few that did caused considerable excitement. There weren't any cat carrying cages, and very few got vaccinated. Some owners got scratched up pretty bad and some of their cats received some rather harsh verbal abuse in Spanish or English and some in both languages, especially when the dogs started barking, scaring the cats which scratched the owners, who turned them loose, resulting in havoc among the dogs who then decided to have a dog fight. A few owners got bit trying to separate the dogs. Very exciting time!

I didn't worry much about the cats missing the vaccinations because I was under the false impression that cats were not a menace, not likely to get rabies because they would sit on top of a fence watching a dog or wild animal and not get exposed. I was wrong, as there were more confirmed rabies cases in cats during this epidemic than in dogs. A high percentage of the people that took the shots (anti-rabies prophylactic series of vaccinations) were bitten by cats.

Some of the Lions Club members made out rabies certificates and put on tags. I vaccinated with the old caprine (goat) brain phenolized type, rarely changing needles until they got dull, and the syringes were changed only when they began to stick. Stainless steel, reusable needles and glass, reusable syringes were used, as the disposables were not yet available. I certainly wouldn't vaccinate animals that way now, but that was a different era. I guess the phenol in the vaccine and the alcohol used to wipe the needle and the skin must have been sufficient, or the Good Lord was looking over my shoulder because I did not get any reports of abscesses.

I was always concerned when I vaccinated during an epidemic because a dog may be incubating the disease. A single dose of vaccine does not abort the development, and owners may either blame the vaccine for causing the disease or not take precautions with a pet showing the symptoms. I was fortunate as I did not receive any reports of vaccinated pets developing symptoms after they had been vaccinated.

We continued to have rabies cases the next few years but with diminishing frequency. We attributed the control to aggressive vaccination programs partially, but more to the widespread use of strychnine baits to control carnivorous wildlife. Also, there were coyote drives by men horseback aided by airplanes.

Kerr Mitchell bought a fox and coyote call that imitated a crying, injured rabbit. He drove down to his Alamito Creek pasture where tracks of both fox and coyote were plentiful. He rolled the window down and stuck his gun out and began the call, peering intently into the dark. He was still and quiet, concentrating on any sound or shadow that might move, as it was a particularly dark night. Suddenly, something jumped through the window and began running around inside the cab of the pickup. It almost scared Kerr to death. He frantically grabbed for the door handle to open it and get out, letting that varmint have the pickup. He soon discovered it was his dog that had followed him the four miles or so from the house. The last time I heard, he had not used the call again.

My personal exposure to rabies was frequent, and I took many series of rabies shots. Some of the exposures were due to carelessness, but most were due to the type of practice I had. Dr. Stover, my physician, began to give me only a series of five daily injections followed by three additional, given on alternate days. This was later reduced to a daily injection for three days followed by taking a blood sample about one week later to test for antibody titre. The test results were always very good. I finally lost count of the number of series that I received, not only because there were so many, but also because the number of injections per series varied so much.

Poppy

Jim Bob Steen was the Presidio County Agent for a number of years. He told me he resigned because the paperwork had become a nightmare. I know the feeling! The last few years of practice the paperwork became a major burden. I suppose with a voice activated tape recorder, a computer, and a staff it would have been easier, but I didn't accept or understand all the new technology. I would mentally do the arithmetic to check the calculator.

Soon after he came to Marfa in 1953, he went with me on my annual rabies vaccination tour along the Rio Grande where I started in Redford, went to Presidio, then to Ruidosa, and ended up in Candelaria. I sometimes stopped in Shafter, and occasionally someone would flag me down on the highway, especially at places where ranch roads turned off. I would come back up Pinto Canyon, returning to Marfa, usually quite late. Jim Bob wanted to learn the area and meet the people. He was a great help to me, filling out rabies certificates and handing out the tags. On our way back, he commented there certainly were a lot of dogs named, Poppy. I explained they were saying "puppy," with a Mexican accent as they had never given them a name. Most cats bore the name, Kitty all their lives.

Jim White and Our Rabies Exposure

Courtney Mellard's grandson, the son of Kenneth Mellard, had a very good 4-H Club calf in the pens behind the ranch house. Little Courtney called me complaining that the calf was not eating, but was drinking all right. Jim White was at my hospital at the time and decided to go with me to the ranch. Kenneth and Courtney put the calf in the chute, and I took the temperature and listened to his chest.

Jim was cleaning out the calf's water trough with bare hands commenting that it was full of saliva. I suspected a mouth lesion or something caught in the throat so I examined the mouth, especially the teeth, gums, tongue, and throat. I was unable to find anything wrong, except a fever. The calf was a little lethargic, which is not uncommon with a fever, but showed no sign of aggressiveness or mental derangement.

The next day I was called with the report that the calf went berserk, bellowing and soon died. I opened the skull, removed the brain, and sent it to the lab. It was positive for rabies. Kenneth and Courtney started their treatments immediately, but I had finished one of my short series recently with a good report on antibody titre so did not intend to take any additional. Jim was so gun-shy of needles that he refused to take them even though Dr. Stover no longer insisted on the belly shots, and the vaccine had been improved so that I thought there was little pain. Many still complained of pain, and I suppose some were affected, but I think many just wanted sympathy or were trying to spook someone into a fear of the shots so they would be careful or to harass someone with an exposure or a suspected one. Jim finally agreed to take them if I would also.

We arranged to meet the first thing each morning and get our shots so we could get on with our work. The first morning, we were waiting in the office with our sleeves rolled up. Jim was looking at some charts on the wall. Dr. Stover came in with loaded syringes, gave me mine and started for Jim who balked and said that the agreement was that I would take mine first so that he could see how I reacted. We assured him I had taken mine already. He didn't believe it, stating that no one could take any kind of injection by just standing out in the middle of the room and not making any noise. We tried to show him the empty syringe and the little pin prick on my arm. He wasn't buying any of it and insisted that I take another with him watching. He wanted it to be the one intended for him so Walt couldn't fake it. He watched the preparation closely and I watched his face. He had his face screwed up and shut his eyes at the moment the needle went in. I wanted to tease him by hollering and flinching but thought better of it as we were having enough trouble with him. He finally took, his but I thought I was going to have to put a twitch on his nose and ear him down.

He was insisting that I go the whole twenty-one injections with him but, after a couple of weeks I had a call to Fort Stockton and would have to leave town by 5:00 in the morning. I called him and he agreed to try to take them without me that one morning. I called him that night when I got in to see if he took it. He said that he had, that Dr. Stover only had to run him around the office twice and hem him in a corner.

Jim insisted that I complete the series with him. I was afraid he was going to stop when he started complaining of nervous symptoms, which were reputed to be an adverse reaction to this nerve tissue vaccine. That was the last time I received the full twenty-one injections — two the first day and nineteen additional. I don't remember Jim ever going on another call with me.

*   *   *   *   *

When I held vaccination clinics on the border the first year, it was only at Presidio, but I made three trips there as interest was intense. When the number of rabies cases declined, interest in vaccination diminished, and I began to accomplish the task with only one trip.

At one of these vaccination clinics, a little Mexican boy about six or seven years old faced his dog with an ear in each hand and pulled his head down. I imagine he had seen his father ear down a colt this way. The dog never moved.

One year when I arrived at the store in Candelaria, run by Marian Walker and Nellie Howard, to vaccinate dogs, a most disturbing sight greeted me. There were about thirty dogs running loose. A few dog fights, but mostly sniffing noses, chasing females in season, drinking from a common water trough while the owners sat around smoking, drinking some beer and a little sotol and a few pitching washers. In general, a typical Saturday night in the city.

A large percentage of the dogs had the typical symptoms of distemper. It was highly contagious with no satisfactory treatment. There were rumors of a few rabies cases along the river, almost all of which were reported by Mexicans and none of which I saw. In retrospect, I feel these were distemper complications, chorea, instead of rabies, but at the time I decided that the distemper had already been spread and the danger of rabies was imminent, so I had nothing to lose by vaccinating.

I was wrong! A high percentage of the dogs died. My vaccine and I got the blame. After that, no dogs were presented in Candelaria, Ruidosa and Shafter, none in Redford and only a few in Presidio. I stopped making my annual trips. A few dogs and some cats were brought to Marfa for vaccinations but mainly for spay and neuter, broken legs, and illnesses. A new rabies scare, some thirty years later, prompted the Ladies' Club to organize a vaccination program, the older generation having died, forgotten or were being ignored.

* * * * *

Joe and Hayes Mitchell bought a Hereford bull at Kansas City for $5,000, which was quite a sum at the time. He became sick during the first big rabies epidemic in the fifties. He was lethargic and not eating his range cubes, so was put in the pen and I was called. He had a fever but no other symptoms, except the fact he wasn't eating. I gave Sulmet boluses and penicillin injections.

The next day, he was down and straining as if to have a bowel movement. Autointoxication from constipation was a common problem then, but it is not usually accompanied by fever. However, that was my tentative diagnosis. I passed a stomach tube, pumped in a gallon of mineral oil and gave intravenous calcium gluconate and dextrose. Later that day they reported bellowing and hooking the ground — death soon followed. I removed the brain and the lab reported it was positive for rabies. One of my prophylactic series was the result.

Several years later, a backyard saddle horse in Marathon quit eating. I was called and discovered no other symptoms, but the owner had recently run out of good hay and had begun feeding old moldy hay he had scrounged. I assumed the problem to be toxic indigestion after examining the mucosa of the mouth and eyes. I gave a gallon of mineral oil by stomach tube and dextrose with calcium gluconate intravenously. Two days later I was called back. The horse was straining, weak in the hind end, and running a fever. I repeated my previous treatment. I was a little suspicious of rabies, but there had been no cases in the area for two or three years and this horse was in the middle of town in a good V-mesh pen. The next morning he was dead, and the lab reported rabies. I took the series again, but the owner would not. He insisted there was no such thing as rabies. He lucked out.

F. C. (Frank Courtney) Mellard

Mr. Courtney wrote a book, *The Dream of a Youthful Cowboy*, with the help of a son, Rudolph, who had written several books, and Rudolph's wife, Evelyn, an English professor at Sul Ross State University.

He had a ranch south of Marfa, perhaps 20 miles as the crow flies but perhaps 25 or more miles by road. He had divided it between his two sons, Rudolph and Kenneth. He had kept a small portion for his personal use where he ran a small herd of registered, purebred Hereford cattle. If I remember correctly, he was 71 years old when I first came. His primary activity was as a cattle buyer (commission man) for Turkington Brothers of Letts, Iowa. Mostly, if not entirely, he bought high-quality Hereford calves for Iowa and Illinois feeders.

His grandson, Kenneth's son, Courtney Graham Mellard was usually called "little Courtney" as a boy. This was common when referring to the younger of those with the same name. Most of the time it is a misnomer, especially in this case because the grandson grew to be a much bigger man than the old gent.

*   *   *   *   *

When I first came and was trying to build a practice, I often rode with a rancher to save him the expense of a ranch call, although my fee was modest — ten cents a mile on pavement and fifteen cents a mile on dirt roads. This included both automobile expense and my time which wasn't worth much in those early days and travel costs were relatively inexpensive. I was trying to educate them to the services of a veterinarian and hopefully charge enough for my professional service to justify the arrangement. I really didn't like to go with another in their vehicle because I wouldn't have the things I needed, besides being at their mercy as to comings and goings.

Mr. Courtney Mellard frequently insisted I go with him. It was difficult to refuse him. I liked the old gent and respected him, but he was a terror behind the wheel of a pickup. He would be visiting with me, never being at a loss for words, and drift over into the oncoming lane. This was bad, but there being little traffic on Highway 67 towards Presidio at that time, it wasn't as bad as it would be now. Then we would straighten out a ways, begin drifting to the right and off the shoulder, which was even more exciting. There were many small bridges and culverts that had a concrete face that extended up about 16 or 18 inches and that was immediately abutted to the pavement. I think that in many places it was actually narrower than the pavement. It seemed to me that most of the car wrecks on that highway at that time were caused by hitting these concrete faces. He would drift over on the shoulder, and when we got close to one of the obstacles I would pull on the door handle with one hand and point with the other and get a little panicky. His most exciting driving though was his speed. We would leave Marfa at a reasonable speed, and as the conversation became more animated he would speed up. I would press my feet against the floorboard with my hands on the dashboard and point at the speedometer. As soon as I was able to attract his attention, he would slow down very slow and talk bad about those people that drive fast. He would ridicule them harshly, but I never heard him use profanity or vulgarity. I have worked in stockpens with him numerous times when a calf would go the wrong way, butt him or kick him, yet never a curse word. A most remarkable man, as there have been many trials and tribulations that I witnessed. While he was saying his piece about the fast drivers he would be slowing down, finally creeping along, a hazard on the highway, and I would become antsy. I suppose I am, or at least I was, wound a little tight. I didn't like the excessive speed, but the poking along really got on my nerves. However, it wasn't long until he picked up speed again and soon we would be tearing down the highway at breakneck speed. Then he would realize it and slow to a crawl while carrying on another tirade about the speed demons and what a menace they were.

Once off the pavement and on the dirt road to his ranch he sorta let his pickup have its head like he would an old saddle horse that knew its way home. Rocks in the road would have to look out for themselves. Occasionally the pickup would wander off the road and he would jerk the steering wheel much like he would the bridle reins of a horse to get its attention. Then he would usually cram down on the foot feed, that some high-faluting folks call a gas pedal and others that are sticklers for accuracy call an accelerator, kinda like he would spur a horse to wake him up because he strayed off the trail. Every once in awhile he would shift gears whenever he took a notion, regardless of the circumstances. This was more like herding that pickup down the road instead of driving it. Mr. Courtney had spent a lot more time horseback than he had driving a pickup or car.

I was told the grandchildren, Mary Lane and Little Courtney, who often rode with him, were elated when they got their driver's license so they could do the driving instead of Mr. Courtney.

Often when I went with him, we would have to take a side trip to see a rancher or some cattle. This he conveniently forgot to tell me before we started.

I would be told the animal was in the pen that I was going to see. It rarely was. He would open the door of a little feed room, get a bucket half full of cow cake, rattle it and call. The cattle would come eventually. First the bull would be put in his private little shed and fed separately. Then the cows would be allowed to come in the pen and cake scattered carefully for them. The subject would be captured while eating, by putting a saddle rope around her horns. Then she would be snubbed to a post for restraint and I would examine her. The problem would rarely be serious as they were observed so closely. A condition would be nipped in the bud. If medication was needed, of course, I wouldn't have it with me. We would stop by his son, Kenneth's, house. I would have a cup of coffee and Mr. Courtney, a glass of milk. He never smoked or drank coffee or tea, said he didn't need a stimulant. We would eat a cookie or piece of pie and after much discussion of the weather, range conditions, cattle market and everyone's health he would tell Kenneth to get up number so-and-so and he would bring the medicine the next day. Life was a much slower pace then. Mr. Courtney had good, legible horn brands on all his cattle for easy identification, as all were registered purebred Herefords.

The Hereford bull that Mr. Courtney pampered by feeding in a private shed was his pride and joy. He was very fertile, threw good calves, and was very gentle. The pasture was somewhat rocky and hilly and the grass was not too lush, so the bull had to hustle. When he reached the age of sixteen, he was having so much trouble getting around he was shipped to the Turkington Farms in Letts, Iowa, with a load of calves. He bred cows there for at least two years that I know of. The bull never had any eye trouble or other illness, an example of excellent longevity.

*   *   *   *   *

Calves would be contracted by Mr. Courtney for fall delivery. The price, number, sex, and delivery date would be agreed on, and a contract written so that everyone involved would know and remember the terms. Mr. Courtney would usually have a rather large number of calves and from ranchers with the same quality of cattle all delivered the same day. I don't remember him going to the ranch to sort or cull. I think he contracted only with men that he had traded with before, and both knew what to expect.

Calves would come to the railroad stockpens in trucks, then weighed, and counted as soon as possible. This was the pay weight, less an agreed percentage of shrink. There usually was some grumbling as too many trucks arrived too close together, and someone would have to wait. Waiting caused shrinkage.

The calves would be put in separate pens, then the sorting would begin. Most ranchers wanted to leave and deposit their bank drafts but Mr. Courtney often would have them or their men help with the sorting while exclaiming they would never sell to him again. However, he usually paid a little premium, and he could be relied on to fulfill his contract. This was not always the case with some speculators. After hours of sorting, and often he had me in there also getting run over, he would end up with calves that were exceptionally uniform as to sex, size, weight, and color in each group. He knew how many each of the Turkington's buyers wanted.

He would then weigh them as to each load and begin loading railroad cars. Sometimes the cars had not been delivered to the stockpens as promised by the railroad. We would go to the old yellow-with-brown-trim wooden depot and begin harassing the agents, Charlie Bowman and C.L. Bagley. C.L. would start working his telegraph key while Charlie and Courtney began hassling over the number of cars that had been ordered, as well as making out a bill of lading for each load. Then they discussed the weight and number and whether a car and trailer could be used or if two cars were necessary. After one carload was made, extras could be put on another car, called a trailer, at a reduced rate from a car. There was a breaking point when the weight and number required two cars. This is where the process became exciting. I would stand by the big potbellied iron stove and try to warm up, throwing a piece of coal in now and then. I had to wait until the bill of lading was completed before writing health certificates to ascertain numbers and destinations. Occasionally Mr. Courtney would have a problem with the final destination of a group of calves and he would put, "to be diverted en route," which meant I would make the papers to Turkington Brothers, Letts, Iowa.

Soon, C.L. would state the train was on a siding waiting for a passenger or express, refrigerated fruit train to pass. If a train came by highballing[*], C.L. and Charlie would step outside, one on either side of the tracks and watch for hot boxes as the train passed. A little later, C.L. would announce that the train was "in the block," wherever and whatever that was. All I knew was that we could expect it soon and had better get back to the stockpens and get ready to load.

A feeder from Iowa was at the stockpens one day telling me that he had fed these calves for a number of years and wanted to see where they came from and how they were handled. He said he was a farmer raising corn and feeding the calves was a hobby. He and several of his neighbors would each buy a load of calves and would go see each other's from time to time, taking great pride in them. They especially liked the uniformity and quality of the load and did not have to cull any or make any apologies for the cattle Mr. Courtney sent.

It wasn't long until shipping by rail became a thing of the past. The last cattle I loaded on a train were the Clay Mitchell Ranch calves for Maureen Godbold on the Santa Fe Railroad at the Tinaja stockpens about 1970. It was kind of sad for me to see this era pass. There were several reasons for this. One was the poor service the railroads were giving. It took up to seven days for some shipments to arrive in Iowa. The bureaucracy, probably the Interstate Commerce Commission, set a freight rate that the railroads claimed was too low. Therefore, they didn't give livestock priority. Another was the 36-Hour Law. This stipulated that cattle had to be unloaded, fed, watered and rested for 24 hours and could not stay on the train over 36 hours at a time. This may not have been so bad but priority was given to more profitable cargo, such as passengers and refrigerated fruit. The cattle cars would have to sit on a siding and wait.

Another reason was the development of the double deck pots. These trucks could haul twice as many calves and could make the trip in 24 hours or less. Many of the ranchers had scales at the ranch, but more were put in with the coming of the pots. Cattle could be loaded at the ranch and not unloaded until reaching the destination.

They tore down our pretty, colorful, yellow-with-brown-trim depot and built a shabby shack with asphalt shingle sides that soon became trashy. Even that is gone now.

---

[*] Going fast.

Mr. Courtney's granddaughter, Mary Lane, told me on occasion he would drink iced tea. When he did so, everyone would stop and watch him add sugar. She said he would put in an enormous amount and would not stir so that much of the sugar was left in the glass after the tea was finished.

I wonder if the old gent had skimped and scraped so many years putting his outfit together doing without sugar that now that he could afford it, he was going to use it. It was said that many of the old timers didn't make their stake, they starved it out.

Roping a Cow from a Pickup

Kerr Mitchell had a cow with a vaginal prolapse in the pasture that refused to be driven to the pens — she just sulled or balked. He called me, and we attempted to treat her in the pasture. True to form, she would run off each time we got very close. Kerr couldn't rope with his arthritic hand, so he persuaded me to do so while he drove. There are a lot of things that I cannot do, and roping is close to the top of the list, but these were the hard years of the mid-fifties, and I needed any fee I could get so I consented to try.

I tied the rope to the trailer hitch, got in the back of his pickup and we took off dodging yuccas and sacahuiste, but Kerr was being careful to hit every rock and cow trail. I've had some wild rides, but that compared to the best, or worst. We didn't have anyone to haze her and keep her going straight, so each time we would get almost close enough to throw a loop, she would turn. Kerr would turn with her, and I would almost fall out. About the time I regained my balance, we would hit a ditch, and I would fly up. Kerr would get close and he would holler for me to rope her, but I would be tangled up in the rope. I would yell to slow down, and he would just speed up. I finally threw a loop more in desperation than because I had any hope of catching her. Well, to my utter amazement, the cow managed to get her head and all four feet tied up, or should I say, tangled up, in that rope and Kerr stopped just right to keep the rope taut. She was all tied up like a Christmas package. Kerr told everyone that I was the best roper he had ever seen and tried to get me to demonstrate my skill. I acted very humble and declined to show off.

First-Class, High-Quality Sotol

Kerr was known to take a drink now and then. Actually, he drank pretty heavy at times. Sometimes I could tell when he had a snoot full, but not always. Both he and Snotty Barnette could function well under the influence. The fact is, I think they were better cowmen drunk than a lot were sober. Kerr did some cow trading besides his cow-calf ranching, and I am sure that he operated better with a little stimulant. I don't know if he was shrewder or if he caught others off guard, thinking he was too drunk to realize what he was doing and figuring they were getting the best of him.

His father, Tom Mitchell, told him that he would give him $1,000.00 (this was a bunch of money at that time) if he would not drink for a whole year, thinking that if he abstained that long, he would quit. It was said that immediately after collecting the thousand dollars, Kerr got roaring drunk. I use the term *roaring* as a figure of speech, as I never saw him loud, vulgar, or obnoxious at those times.

I arrived at his pens one evening about dark to repair a particularly unpleasant prolapse on a cow. None are very appetizing, but this was huge, stinking and full of screwworms. I sure did hate to tackle it, and Kerr could sense my reluctance. He dug out a gallon jar hidden in an oat barrel. It was a wide mouth jar that originally held phenothiazine drench. He unscrewed the lid, and the fumes made my eyes water. I became tipsy before I took a swig. Kerr insisted this was first-class, high-quality sotol, pointing to the big chunk of charcoal floating in it. He reminded me that the best Kentucky bourbon was aged in wooden casks whose interior had been fired to produce a lining of charcoal.

The wide mouth of the jar made it difficult to take the small discreet sip that I had intended, only to humor him. I ended up with a gulp that took my breath away. When I recovered, the cow didn't look nearly so bad. Kerr's medicine had produced the desired result.

The Santa Fe train that passed through his ranch sometimes made a water stop at Tinaja. In the days when railroad locomotives were steam engines, they had to stop frequently for water. Once, Kerr's beverage supply was low, so he boarded an empty box car going to Presidio. He replenished his supply inside and out and rode the train back. However, it did not stop, so he bailed off while it was moving. The fall skinned him up pretty good, but the worst thing was that it busted his bottle.

George Jones and Angus Bulls

George Jones was a very progressive rancher and had some excellent Hereford cattle. He was like almost all Hereford breeders of the 1940s and had bred for the short, broad head and heavy shoulders with short legs. They weren't described that way, however, they were called blocky. Calf deliveries were a major problem. The conformation was evident in the fetus. Not only was the conformation a problem in delivery, but the birth weights were heavy, which further aggravated the problem.

Angus were said to have small calves at birth. George disliked Angus, but his calving problems were such that he bought a group of Angus bulls to put on his heifers for their first calf. It was a disaster! I spent much of my time at his Quebec pens delivering those black, baldy calves. Many calves would have both front legs and nose showing. His ranch hand would latch onto these and pull. This should have delivered the calf but it didn't. Well, yes, it did but not without disastrous results. A number of the calves didn't survive and many of the heifers had obturator paralysis. The nerves to the hind legs are vulnerable to bruising during the delivery process, especially if it is slow and difficult. At one time, we had twenty-four heifers down. One of the commonly used procedures to treat downers was the cowboy method of digging four holes in the ground for the four legs. This was a good theory but didn't work very well. The method taught in college was a sling, a very elaborate contraption of canvas, leather, metal strip and chains. A tripod of pipes was placed over the cow, and she was raised to a height that just allowed the feet to touch the ground. This was an expensive item, and a frequent cowboy substitution was two tow sacks — one at the heart girth and the other in the flanks. Neither was successful except occasionally with one that could stand after being lifted. We found it best to lower the cow when she would not stand or if she got tired, otherwise the rig would cut her in two. By trial and error, we discovered the best technique was the easiest and most effective. Hobble the hind legs just above the hocks about twelve to sixteen inches apart so they cannot spread eagle and further damage their legs. Allow them to lie on the ground upright, called sternal recumbency. This is a normal position for the cow, the knees are folded and the hind legs bent. Twice a day she should be turned so that the opposite hind leg is under. More turns are desirable if time permits. If the cow will eat and drink and will remain upright without flopping flat on her side, almost all will recover. Actually, it is rare for one not to recover under these circumstances, but if I assure the owner she will recover for certain, she will not. I have not had an opportunity to evaluate all the failures, but a few have been determined to be due to fractures.

George, being the progressive rancher that he was, had purchased bulls from a very prestigious Angus breeder in Arizona. Unfortunately, the Angus people were breeding for the same conformation that Hereford breeders were and this Angus breeder had progressed or regressed to the point his cattle were like George's, and the cross-breeding genetics had compounded the problem. George sold the Angus bulls and never again bred yearling heifers, always giving them another year's growth and maturity. This extra year without raising a calf resulted in a very large cow and much less trouble calving.

A few years later both the Hereford and Angus breeders changed their genetics so that neither breed has much of a problem calving now.

General Boatner

General Boatner was Ben Gearhart's commanding general in the India-Burma-China theater during World War II. He visited Ben at the ranch where Ben had a get-together. I was the only one there who had been a peon, an enlisted man. All the others had been officers, while I had been a Marine corporal. I was being harassed somewhat. Fritz Kahl, who had been a captain in the Army Air Corps, claims that I made the statement that a Marine corporal outranked an Army captain. I don't remember making such a rash statement. I'm sure I was in awe and meek in the presence of all that brass.

However, I do remember General Boatner coming to my rescue, saying that he was the only Marine corporal to have ever been busted to the rank of general in the Army. He had been a corporal in the Marines when he received an appointment to West Point.

Purchase of the Hospital

The Coffield-Gearhart Ranches owned a large ranch in Mexico which they traded for one in Montana. However, it was not an even trade, and it was necessary to raise additional capital. Ben offered to sell me the hospital, lock, stock, and barrel, including the residence with its furniture and fixtures. This was in the first of 1953. I discovered some troubling facts. My professional degree and license had no value as collateral and all lending institutions were reluctant to loan money on the hospital-residence building because they said it had limited marketability, being of value only to a veterinarian. The medicines and instruments as well as the furnishings of both the hospital and residence were not considered to be of any value because they had been used. All these valuations were a completely different story when appraised for tax purposes.

With the help of my father (I thought I would repay him when I sold my calves that fall), I was able to pay the $5,000 for Dr. Gearhart's share of the inventory and the furniture and fixtures of both the hospital and the house. Henry Coffield co-signed a note at the Marfa National Bank for $15,000 which was their limit for my type loan, I was told. There were three $5,000 notes purchased by individuals. Ben's brother, Bill, purchased at least one, perhaps all three. The interest was 6% on the $30,000. The purchase price was a grand total of $35,000 at a time when that was all the money in the world, I thought.

We had been living in a rent house, so in June 1953 when the deal was finally closed, I was able to move my pregnant wife and our daughter, Nancy, into the residence. The first few years had been pretty lean pickings, so we really didn't have much to move except for the many wedding presents that people had been so kind to give us.

Ben's Goat Dogs

Ben was running Angora goats on Brooks, trying to utilize that rough mountain. Eagles and bobcats kept him from getting over-stocked. However, the goats did need to be rounded up to be sheared, vaccinated, and an occasional billy kid castrated. The mountain is so rough, it is very difficult to round up goats — not the easiest to work in the best of circumstances. Some of the gathering had to be done on foot. He bought a couple of high-powered, goat dogs to help. One day I asked how the goat dogs were doing. He said he got rid of them — found out you had to be smarter than the dogs to get work out of them.

Harry's Goats

Harry Langland told me that Fritz Kahl was instrumental in his goat education. Both were foreigners who had emigrated to Texas from Iowa. Fritz was running the Point of Rocks Ranch which is on the west side of Blue Mountain and extends up on that rough son-of-a-gun.

Fritz had gotten a sharp pencil and a long piece of paper and had shown Harry how hair goats (Angora) can get you rich. They utilize country and vegetation that nothing else can, and they will eat anything except meat. They have twins and triplets regularly. You can shear them for the mohair, and buyers just fall all over themselves to buy it. The meat is one of the most delicious. Shearing crews will pay you to come shear your goats just so they can eat the cabrito. Dog men will fight to be allowed to train their dogs for rounding up the goats.

Now Fritz failed to point out a couple of a minor problems. One is that eagles and other predators like cabrito as much as people do, and they will harvest them range delivery. Also, you can weld three of them in a 55-gallon barrel and open it a week later. One will be gone, one will be dead and the other will have screwworms. This was before eradication of this pest.

Harry couldn't wait to buy some of those money makers which he turned loose on "Old Blue." He never saw any of them again.

Lynn "Crit" Crittendon

Lynn Crittendon was a rancher-neighbor of Dr. Ben Gearhart. He was running cattle, but he started raising Specific Pathogen Free (S.P.F.) hogs in a fancy air conditioned house with slated floors that he kept disgustingly clean. Now, everybody knows a hog is supposed to waller in a mud hole. He wouldn't let visitors in his hog house. He even changed clothes to go in. You would-n't think a hog could live under such strict sanitary conditions, but there was very little illness—a veterinarian would starve to death. Once, a big sow did get sick. Lynn and Ben treated her, but she continued to worsen. Finally they called me. We caught her for an examination, and she immediately died. Crit looked at his dead hog, then turned to me and said, "Doc, you're a lot better veterinarian than Ben. He's been trying to kill that sow for two weeks, and you were able to do it in just fifteen minutes."

Postmortem revealed a 3-inch long piece of baling wire in her heart—technically traumatic pericarditis, commonly called hard-ware disease. Not rare in dairy cattle which are fed hay, but not a disease which happens to hogs. Crit's dumb sow couldn't read the book.

We were working cattle in the Valentine country and had a fresh crew. Some had never worked around a Turner squeeze chute before, and Crit was giving them detailed instructions in its use and misuse, telling gory stores of injuries. An experienced man was put on the handle of the neck bar-yoke, and others were cautioned to watch closely how it should be done. Crit stood back and bossed the procedure to see that everybody was doing things correctly. He had rared back on his heels with his arms folded, surveying the situation when a big, heavy, wild cow hit the front end, and the man on the front couldn't close the neck bar. Lynn jumped in to help—bad mistake. He had put his hand in the very place he had been so emphatic to the others not to put theirs. The bar came down and the scissor-like action busted his little finger open like dropping a ripe watermelon on a rock. Jane, his wife, drove him to Alpine to get patched up by a people doctor. Crit did a pretty good job on that finger, but most could do better; even rank amateurs could slice off a finger clean as a whistle.

My Mashed Finger

I was at the Y6 Ranch after the crowd chute had been remod-eled and constructed with pipe. One of the few bad features of pipe pens and the use of pipe to scotch the cows is that the scotch pipe will roll. Almost always, the rolling is to the wrong direction.

Alf and Bodie Means, Lynn Crittendon, Ramon and I were at

the pens working. Actually I don't remember Crit doing any work. Bodie was working the head gate and neck bar of the squeeze chute and putting plastic ear tags in the cows. Alf was working the tail gate of the squeeze and poking the cows to keep them moving forward. Ramon was putting cows in the crowd chute from the crowd or crush pen. I was pregnancy testing and vaccinating, but for the life of me, I can't remember Crit doing anything but talking.

In all fairness to Crit, I oughta tell what he was doing there. He was on his way to Valentine to get his mail and had stopped by to see if Alf needed anything from the city. This was more a courtesy than anything else 'cause there really wasn't much available in this little village. He had on his town clothes (actually they were clean blue jeans), and a person really shouldn't criticize him for not getting in there with those juicy cows that had been eating green grass which was sure enough laxative. The rest of us had to grin and bear it. Although a grimace might be a more correct description of our facial expression.

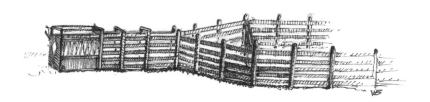

Cattle working pens.
Squeeze chute - crowd chute - crowd pen - holding pen.

Alf and Bodie had their hands full with a cranky cow in the squeeze and Ramon had put a silly old cow in the crowd chute for about the third time, but she kept backing out as the pipe rolled back and forth. I jumped back there to place the pipe so it would hold the cow. By using all the skill and experience that I had acquired, I managed to get the middle finger of my left hand between the upright pipe post and the rolling scotch pipe just as the cow hit it. I guess I must have said unkind things to and about the cow, pipe or the post, perhaps all three. Crit added insult to injury by remarking that if a veterinarian would pay attention only to his job, he might not get hurt. I don't remember my response to his comment, but I know that if looks would kill he would have been badly wounded. I kept on working — I wasn't going to let Crit know how much pain I was in.

The second joint of that finger swelled up pretty bad, and I feel sure it was broken. But, I was busy, going day and night and didn't have time to baby it. Perhaps it is just as well — although the joint is a little big, it works just fine. However, the finger stays cold all the time.

Drenching Sheep

C.M. "Fritz" Kahl sheared his sheep in the fall, and we drenched them shortly thereafter, which was during the baseball World Series. I would open the hood and the pickup windows, have it parked as close as possible with the radio turned up loud so we could hear the game. The engine was left running so the battery would not run down. In 1998, the transistor radios don't use as much juice as the old vacuum tube ones did but we don't seem to get as good of reception in this area.

Sheep were bad about getting stomach worms and would get in trouble if not drenched at least once in the fall. Phenothiazine was the drench of choice for killing the stomach worms, but it was an irritant to most people. Many men could not even be around where it was being used as the fumes would blister their faces. Most of the others would get their hands blistered so that they could not do the actual drenching. The regular type was a thick green suspension that looked like split pea soup. A special Phenothiazine was made to aid in the control of tapeworms and was tinted a reddish color containing lead arsenate. Both types came in glass gallon jars that needed to be shaken to suspend the particles. It would then be poured into a container that was carried into the sheep pen. It was administered with a dose syringe holding two ounces with a six-inch blunt metal nozzle which was inserted into the side of the mouth through the interdental space and gently but firmly eased over the tongue and back to the throat. The mouth and nose were held closed to prevent breathing while the plunger was pushed to deliver the drench. The person holding the sheep had to stabilize the head during the procedure. Three undesirable things could happen: the drench spit out and not swallowed; the procedure not done expediently or was faulty, resulting in the drench being aspirated into the lungs; and a rough insertion causing the nozzle to penetrate the back of the throat and the drench deposited into the tissue. The first resulted in the sheep getting no benefit; the last two resulted in death.

I was called to Girvin one fall to examine a problem. An inexperienced crew had drenched a big bunch (3,000 head, if I remember correctly) of sheep on fields. The back of the throat had been punctured which was revealed on postmortem examination. About 100 head were seen dead and at least twice that number sick.

Beto Bestillas was a good ranch hand. He spoke good English but often mixed it with his native Spanish. He was a strong, excellent worker and very good-natured. A real pleasure to work with. In the hustle and bustle of the work, I would sometimes step on his toes as he held a sheep for me. I would apologize saying, "*Dispensame.*" He would laugh and answer, " '*No* 'cuse me,' *cuando trabajando.*"

Fritz's big old ewes didn't show me much respect and would step on my toes without showing remorse. Now, the toes of shoes and boots are not made to be stepped on. The first 100 times or so was not so bad, but then it began to smart. By the end of the day, the toes were really sore, and being stepped on would bring a grimace and an exclamation. It seemed as if the sheep got bigger and heavier as the day wore on, and the sheep would not just stand quietly but would stomp and twist.

Some men from the oil patch told me about steel-toed shoes. These were really great, except some of the sheep weren't careful and would step up on the foot part that was unprotected by the steel. The drouth of the fifties became worse and the predators more numerous and aggressive, resulting in an end to the sheep ranching in this area. I decided that the shoes would be good protection when working with horses. I always hated to have a horse step on my toe. The toe would hurt right off. It didn't need to be tenderized as with sheep. It always seemed to me that a barefooted horse hurt as bad as one that was shod. A cowboy will often joke with another who has had his foot stepped on saying that it shouldn't hurt because the horse was barefooted.

One day, a great big dun horse carefully and precisely placed his foot on mine, then shifted all his weight onto it and stood there looking pleased with himself. Perhaps some steel-toed shoes are made to withstand 1200 pounds, but mine weren't, and my shoe caved in under his weight. I beat on him, talked harshly to him, but he just stood there with a smile on his face. I finally whacked him upside the head with a metal dental float and got his attention. He looked like I had hurt his feelings, but I really wanted to hurt more than that. He did move his foot off of mine. Sure enough, the dent was a good deep one and was still pressing on my toes, hurting almost as bad as when he was standing on it. I couldn't pull the shoe off. When I finally did, with the help of a big, stout ranch hand, it peeled all the hide off the top of my toes. I never could wear those shoes again. Well, to be honest about it, I didn't try and wasn't even tempted to try.

Cavin Woodward's Pay Day Dandy

Cavin Woodward was the manager of the Lykes Brothers O2 Ranch, south of Alpine on the Brewster-Presidio County line. He was one of my first regular clients and a mighty fine man.

The first road I traveled to his place went down the Casa Piedra road which was paved for the first 18 miles, and turned off using pretty good graded roads with few rocks. Sometime about 1952, a big rain washed this road badly. Part of it was in Presidio County and part in Brewster County, and I guess neither wanted to repair it, 'cause it didn't get done. It became impassable, so then I went farther down the Casa Piedra road maybe another fifteen miles and turned east on a circuitous route. It was a dirt road but still fairly smooth, and I could make pretty good time. Well, doggone if this didn't wash out a year or so later.

Now I had to go by way of Alpine, then south down the unpaved Terlingua road. This wasn't much farther than the way I had been going, but there was a stretch along about Luther Anderson's and the Nevill Ranch that was a booger. It was graded regularly, I guess, but it seems like they stirred up big, sharp rocks every time they did so. Maybe I was just unfortunate to travel it at a bad time.

On one trip back from the ranch about midnight I blew a tire on that bad stretch of road. While I was changing that tire another went flat. Boy, was that exasperating. I had just run out of luck. This road wasn't all that well-traveled to begin with, and this being night, I figured I was here to stay. Pretty soon though a

Mexican came by in a pickup. He had his wife and a bunch of kids in the cab with him. An Anglo may pass you up, but a Mexican never will. I threw the flats in the back end and climbed in after them.

We found an open station right off the bat when we got to Alpine. I unloaded my tires and thanked the man. I had the flat fixed and the blowout replaced. Many stations stayed open all night in those days. Things were tough during the drouth and many had the philosophy that I did, you worked when there was work to be done and were mighty glad of the opportunity. The man running the station had been sleeping on a cot in the doorway, but he came to life right quick when the noisy pickup turned in. He didn't bellyache about being disturbed but was very congenial and acted plumb glad to see us. He was a cheerful cuss and said he was sorry for my problem, but I don't think his heart was in it. I think he mighta been secretly hoping they wouldn't get in too big a hurry to pave that road.

The filling station was at the intersection of Highway 90 and the Terlingua road. The fellow driving the mail hack on his way to Terlingua stopped in to gas up and agreed to haul me back to my pickup. Sure enough, it was still there. You didn't worry then about going off and leaving a vehicle, afraid that it might be stripped. I kinda held my breath as I checked to see if any more tires had gone flat. None had. The driver offered to help, but he had a long ways to go. I said no and thanked him for the ride. I had the tires on in short order and you can bet your boots, I took it easy through the rocks. I got home about an hour or so later. JoAnn was awake and worried.

Cavin Woodward owned a good registered quarter horse stallion named, Pay Day Dandy. After the drouth set in and the pasture pickings got mighty poor, the horse was kept in the pen a good bit of the time. Cavin called early one morning saying the old stud was cut some bad along the backbone.

I put all the goodies I thought I might need in the pickup and a few extras to make it look like I was really coming prepared. The description that the laceration was some bad was an understatement. The cut began at the withers and went back to the hip, running alongside the spinous processes of the vertebra. The cut was down to the bone, the ribs in the thoracic area and the transverse processes of the lumbar vertebra farther back. The muscles were peeled out to the curvature of the ribs and almost to the end of the transverse processes. The whole slab of muscle and hide was hanging down the horse's side. Those who have butchered a deer and cut out the outside backstrap can grasp the extent of the injury. I recommended putting him down. Cavin wouldn't consent.

There was very little bleeding. The wound had been more of a ripping and tearing than a clean cut. The horse was not in shock, nor was he showing any sign of pain, which was remarkable. I was concerned that the nerves and blood vessels had been damaged and the blood supply to the muscles compromised so that it would not heal but would slough. The tissue appeared to be clean of gross debris, but I gently washed it with water to which I had added Quseptic. I then bathed it with Disulfalac. I raised up the mass partially with the help of two ranch hands and began tacking the muscle to the underlying structures with catgut in an attempt to eliminate dead space for serum to collect. I then sutured the skin with retention vertical mattress sutures followed by continuous interlocking sutures for close approximation of the skin margins.

I had the men to ease off on their support and the sutures showed so much tension that I was afraid they would not hold but tear out. A short time before I had used saddle girths to support a belly wound in Clay Espy's horse. We placed one set of girth supports forward around the chest and over the back, but then we were concerned that the back ones would cause him to act up. A tight flank strap is called a bucking strap and causes a rodeo bucking horse to perform. We placed a second set of girth supports around the belly — so far so good, then the real test of putting a third set in the flanks. We gradually tightened them with Mr. Woodward soothing the horse. It worked!

I gave tetanus antitoxin and a whole 10cc vial of penicillin in oil. I left several for twice-a-day injections. The 10cc vial was the size penicillin came at that time. It was so expensive that I used such a low dose, I question whether enough was given. However, in the early use of penicillin, it was so effective that a low dose was often sufficient. I asked that the horse be tied short so that he could not roll.

I came back every few days for several times. The injury healed to my amazement and delight. The area was depressed, atrophied, but he was not ridden because his value was for breeding purposes. Also, he was getting up in years. It was later determined that he was cut by a sharp piece of iron on the frame that held up the roof of his shade.

Later on, the old-timer developed heaves, a breathing problem. We blamed it on the dry, dusty feed and the conditions of the pen. We gave him tender loving care, moistening his feed and dampening his pen. When he got bad we gave him Antiphrine Granules by Haver Glover Labs that helped some. The product was a combination of an antihistamine and a bronchodilator. He sired a couple of more colt crops and was found dead in his pen one afternoon. There was no sign of struggling. Hopefully, he died a quiet death.

Chapter 4

Drouth—Drought

Historically the spelling is drought, and pronounced as such. However, in West Texas it is spelled and pronounced drouth. Dictionaries list this as an alternative spelling.

A controversial discussion is just when does the lack of rain that starts as a dry spell become a drouth? I guess it's a matter of interpretation. Perhaps the size of the area involved may have something to do with it. If a relatively small area is affected it may be called a dry spot. A larger area of relatively short duration is called a dry spell. A drouth is more severe, usually causing widespread hardship. The farmer has crop failure, the rancher has to sell livestock to reduce numbers. This liquidation often causes the price of livestock to fall because of a glut on the market. The combination of drouth and depressed prices causes major financial loss.

Saving has a different meaning in West Texas than the commonly used adage, put something aside for a rainy day. Out here it is "put aside for a dry spell."

The drouth of the fifties sorta sneaked up on us. Rains had been good over most of this part of the country, and there was plenty of grass.

Prices had been going up for sheep and wool, goats and mohair, although I don't remember the figures. Cattle prices also had been increasing. Just before the bust a good age cow would bring $400, even $500 a head. Calves were bringing thirty-five cents a pound at the railroad stockpens scales.

Most expenses were economical compared to livestock prices. Pickups cost less than $1000, gasoline was 18 cents a gallon and 41% cottonseed cake, the range feed at that time, was $30-$40 a ton.

A couple of cowboys who were bachelors told me that on the large ranch where they were working their salaries were $75 a month, living in bunkhouses. When they were at headquarters, there was a cook that fed them at the cook shack. When they were in line camp their groceries were furnished. If several were staying at the place, they took turns cooking. It was said that one man did the cooking until one of the others complained about the food, then he would have to take over. Most didn't want the job, so would eat anything that was put before them. One story went that the cook was fed up with the chore and purposely messed up a batch of biscuits. One of the cowboys popped off on the spur of the moment, without thinking, saying, "These are the hardest, sorriest biscuits I ever tried to eat in my life!" Then realizing what he had said and the consequences, quickly added, "But that's just the way I like 'em."

These men told me the married cowboys were furnished a house with utilities (such as they were) and meat. They were paid $125 a month. The married men were usually older, more experienced, and steady, whereas the bachelors were mostly younger and drifters, men that worked on a ranch for awhile, got itchy feet and moved on.

All the men were furnished saddle horses and saddles although many preferred to ride their own saddle. They were usually allowed to have one or two personal horses that they rode. The ranch would furnish pasturage and also grain when they were being used. Any veterinary expense was their own responsibility.

Some of the more menial work on the ranch was often done by wets. Many of them were excellent cowboys and worked right along with the regular cowboys.

The good prices for livestock and the low expenses were a mixed bag. The combination encouraged many to stay fully stocked, or nearly so, long after they should have lightened up.

Another thing that got many ranchers in trouble was the length of the drouth. Historically, drouths had never lasted over a couple of years. People kept thinking it'll rain anytime, "It always has rained and it always will." But this time it didn't! At least not good grass rains. These are slow-soakers that don't run off but get the ground good and wet — the best ones last several days. But several soft rains close enough together to complement each other will also work. Who'd a thought this would last five years, and in some places at some ranches it was seven?

The straw that really broke the camel's back was the disastrous, sharp drop in prices for livestock. A rancher couldn't afford to sell. An animal wouldn't bring the amount it was mortgaged for. The bottom dropped out of the market when more cattle were shipped than the market could handle. A man leasing country would be completely wiped out. If the land was owned, the mortgage had to be increased, if possible; otherwise, the land had to be sold, or it was foreclosed on by the loan company.

The harsh conditions at the Rough Creek Ranch may have been the beginning of the drouth, but at the time, I just thought it to be the hard old country in a remote rough area.

The first indication I can remember that a drouth might be impending was in the fall of 1951. I was on a call to the Nevill Ranch about 25 miles south of Alpine. Nevill Haynes, the grandson of Captain Nevill, the Texas Ranger who founded the ranch, was the manager. He asked me about the rains in the Marfa-Fort Davis area. I told him they had been plentiful, and all the country was in good shape. I thought this was a true statement. The ranches that I had calves on were in excellent shape, and I was permitted to increase the number that I was allowed to run.

Nevill told me he had very little rain the last two years and was selling all his calves, even his replacement heifers and some of his older mother cows. He complained that the Marfa-Fort Davis area always received more rain than anywhere else.

I didn't think too much about this because the rains are usually local thunderstorms, rarely general rains so there never is an equal amount, even on a single ranch. The big advantage to a large ranch is being able to move stock from a dry area to one that has grass if there is any at all. There have been very few years when all the area is good. On the other hand, there are few when everyone is in a drouth.

Cow prices had been climbing fairly steadily for several years. William "Bill" Allison sold his cow herd at the peak which was in 1952. I obtained permits, tested for brucellosis, and wrote health certificates as the cattle had been sold to a man in Georgia. I argued that he should not sell because prices were still going up. His reply was that prices were too high, having gone up too fast, besides he was getting short on grass as rains had not been too good on his places and some ranches east of the Pecos were already in trouble.

We shipped all the cattle from the Marfa ranch, then all those from the Sheffield ranch and quite a few from the Sonora ranch. He came into the room where I was testing blood for brucellosis one night and informed me that his accountant had told him to quit selling, that any more would be practically given away in income taxes. If I recall correctly, the top income tax bracket at that time was 90%. When the drouth ended and Bill began restocking, I told him that he was the smartest man I knew to have sold out when he did. He replied, no, that if he had really been smart, he would have given the rest of his cows away.

He and my cousin, F.O. "Buster" Edwards, were the only two I knew who sold out at the right time.

Robert Edward Lee Tyler

In the early 1950s, when we thought the drouth was bad, but in reality it was only beginning, a group of us had been having early morning coffee at the Crews Hotel. The Marfa State Bank was in the northeast corner of the building, the hotel entrance was next, then Murphy Bennett's dry cleaning shop, with the post office next to the alley. Mr. Tom Rawls (Don Tomás) was sitting in his pickup waiting for the post office to open. Albert Logan, the postmaster, wouldn't open the door until 7 o'clock. Mr. Tom was anxious to get his mail and get on the road, because it was 60 miles to his Alazan Ranch and all but 18 miles was dirt road. Several of us stopped to talk to the old gent, and as usual, the drouth was the primary topic of conversation. N.B. Chaffin, who was probably the most optimistic rancher I ever knew, spoke up and said, "Well, everyday it doesn't rain means we're one day closer to rain, because it always has and always will." Mr. Tom looked at him very seriously and said, "No, by ———, I remember one time it never did rain." Everyone laughed and scattered. I kept thinking about that statement and asked Mr. Tyler if he knew what was meant. He thought a minute and answered, "Well, he might have had the 1930s in mind that wiped out so many, or 1917-18 that was so dry the good spring at our ranch house dried up and never flowed again, but the worst I ever saw was in 1885-86."

Mr. R.E.L. Tyler was my wife's grandfather and came to the area in 1885. At the time I talked to him he was almost ninety years old but still very mentally alert. He didn't talk much about the old days, but perhaps that might have been my fault for not taking the time to ask questions and listen. I was a young veterinarian full of energy and restless, throwing a pretty wide loop as my practice territory was extensive. However, as the drouth deepened and cattle herds were sold down and many completely sold out, I began to have a lot more time than I could handle. Mr. Tyler got a far away look in his eyes and told me the following.

There had been several years of good rainfall in the area. The grass was stirrup high and lots of running water, springs, and water holes. The area was almost virgin country as the Indians had only recently been controlled and the area opened up and publicized by the coming of the railroad in 1882. Many settlers had been lured by the glowing reports of plentiful grass and water on the free open range.

He said that he was nineteen and his brother, Will, was seventeen when they started from Georgetown, Texas, driving a herd of sheep west. He did not tell me, or if he did I forgot, the exact day they left, but because he would have been twenty years old on September 10, 1884, it was before that date. They drifted along from one watering to the next, letting the sheep and horses graze. They arrived at the Pecos River at Horsehead Crossing in the spring of 1885. The river was at flood stage from either snow melt in the mountains of New Mexico or heavy rains upstream. They had been repeatedly warned to stay clear of cattlemen because of their animosity to sheep. There were several herds of cattle waiting to cross the river when the water receded. The boys were pleasantly surprised at the cattlemen's friendliness who helped them build small rafts and ferry the sheep across the river. While at Comanche Springs (present day Fort Stockton), they were warned that the McCutcheons, who owned or controlled a large ranch in the lower Limpia Creek area, would not allow them to cross their country. They were advised to go by Leoncita Springs and Burgess Springs at Murphysville.

However, they kept to their original plans and when trailing up Limpia Creek, they were met by the McCutcheon men who helped them drive their sheep up the canyon through their ranch. Mr. Tyler was very appreciative of this help and spoke very respectfully of these men. However, I couldn't help but wonder if they were being helpful or just being sure the sheepmen did not stop and squat on their ranch.

Mr. Tyler told me that many had arrived before him and every watering was occupied, although some were beginning to dry up. Part of the squatters had only a few head of sheep or cattle while others claimed to have large numbers. He and his brother were finally able to locate on running water in Merrill Canyon on the south side of Mt. Livermore. I was not told if they just elbowed their way in or leased it from Mr. J.W. Merrill who was one of the few who owned land and had owned Merrill Canyon land since 1881. Mrs. J.W. Merrill told me that her husband had bought his first land with Confederate script issued by the State of Texas to Confederate veterans of the Civil War. He had purchased this script for 10¢ on the dollar, but it was honored by the State at full face value in purchasing land. Rick Tate, great-grandson of A.L. Gage who was the younger brother of E.L. Gage, told me that E.L. Gage had purchased land script from railroad companies at a deep discount to put together his vast land holdings. These companies were given land* by the State of Texas for each mile of track they laid, so that they were land rich but money poor. Therefore, I am not sure that I understood Mrs. Merrill correctly or perhaps both situations occurred.

There was no rain after the arrival of the Tylers, and the creek soon dried up. They were able to get some water to the sheep by the laborious task of digging in the creek bed with a handslip, which is a scoop-like piece of equipment pulled by a horse or mule. Large ones are called fresnos. Water would seep through sand and gravel into the hole. Many of the sheep died of thirst. Then a severe blizzard in the winter of 1885-86 almost completely finished them off.

The remnants of the sheep were sold to E.L. Gage who agreed to buy them if Mr. Tyler would work for him. His brother, Will, went to work for Mr. Haley on his ranch south of Murphysville. The name of the town was later changed to Alpine, but Mr. Tyler always referred to it as Murphysville. The Haley ranch had its principle landmark, Cathedral Mountain, which Mr. Tyler called Haley's Peak.

Except for the blizzard, no moisture fell in 1885 or 1886 until September, 1886. All the water holes dried up as did most of the creeks and springs, for it turned out, most were only wet weather

---

* The number of sections given had varied from place to place and time to time. Sixteen sections were given west of the Pecos during the construction of the railroad across this area. A section is 640 acres.

springs. There were no fences in the area. The railroad fenced their right-of-way in 1888 and shortly thereafter W.F. Mitchell built a drift fence from the bluff at San Esteban tinaja to the railroad east of Marfa. Extensive fencing began in the 1890s when the land began to be homesteaded and bought from the State and the railroad companies. (Fencing data is from *History of Marfa and Presidio County* by Cecilia Thompson.)

When the waterings dried up, the thirsty cattle started drifting. Those that did find water drank too much too quickly and died (water intoxication). Others would bog down in the mud and die while others just milled around places they could smell water until they succumbed. Mr. Tyler stated that a man could walk for miles on the bodies of dead cattle around such places as Antelope Springs.

In the 1950s, Mr. C. E. "Espy" Miller had a ranch west of Valentine on the flat. It extended up in the Sierra Vieja Mountains. The ranch had originally been settled by John Holland because of a good spring of water in a deep narrow canyon which later became known as Holland Canyon. It led to Viejo Pass which provided a passage through the mountains. Mr. Miller said that when he first bought the ranch he was told that a severe drouth, probably the one in 1885-86 had dried up all the surface water in the area. There being no fences at that time, cattle drifted into the canyon from miles around and died, some because they drank too much too quickly, others from weakness, and some starved when the water was fouled by the dead. Legend had it, that it took two years to clear out the carcasses so that the water was accessible. Mr. Holland then built a pipeline out to the flat so that the water could be used and fenced the mouth of the canyon to protect the spring.

The drouth was broken in September, 1886, when it rained several days and nights, and it continued to rain all fall. A big roundup followed to untangle what was left of the herds and bring the cattle back where they belonged. The blizzard had increased the severity of the cattle drift. Mr. Tyler was still working for Mr. Gage. Because he was young and unmarried, he worked the entire roundup from the Rio Grande to the Pecos River although few of Mr. Gage's cattle had drifted east across the mountains. He said the roundup lasted about three months and that it rained on him almost every day. Clear water was running everywhere.

It was a relatively common practice in those days to put your brand on any unbranded animal you could rope. Not an approved practice, but nevertheless common. Often a calf would be branded with the roper's brand regardless of whose brand the cow wore.

Mr. Tyler related that untangling the cattle with cows of one brand followed by a calf with another brand would be very exciting at times. He did not elaborate. Most of the squatters and many of the larger ranchers pulled out because few owned land and did not have the resources to restock. For all practical purposes, it never did rain for many. The next couple of years were good, and livestock were trailed or shipped in by train. Another dry spell set in that lasted a couple of years, but this was not so disastrous because so many people had left the country, and there were not so many livestock. Also, some had dug wells and put up windmills while many dirt tanks (man-made earthen water holes, in central and east Texas, called ponds) had been put in.

These drouths were different from what have been experienced in later times. There was plenty of grass but no water compared to having relatively satisfactory water but no grass.

Struggles Through the Drouth

Bare Ground

Now in the 1950s, the grass disappeared. The small amount of coarse grass that wasn't eaten deteriorated from age, sun and wind. We didn't usually have real genuine West Texas dust storms where the real estate was blowing around. Of course, the dirt blew on the many unpaved streets in town and the vacant lots where loose livestock kept everything eaten down to a nub. Now during the drouth there were considerable bare areas in pastures that contributed to the airborne dirt but most of it developed a hard pan on the surface. This crust prevented penetration by the rain that did fall. A characteristic of a drouth is that rains come as sudden downpours with large raindrops and frequently hail, which compounds the problem by packing the ground. What little rain that fell, ran off, and was of little value to the land. Some dirt tanks stayed full, but the livestock quickly ate the grass near these. San Esteban Lake stayed full and some strategically located, well-maintained Johnson grass fields in overflow areas did well. It was very sad to see the bare ground after the sight of the beautiful gramma grass waving in the breeze of a few years earlier.

Several different attempts were made to slow the run-off. Wire spreaders* were built across draws and overflow flats to catch debris, usually only cow chips, to slow down the water and allow penetration. I'm not sure how successful they were in this purpose, but they were really good about tripping a horse and dumping a rider, working better than prairie dog, badger or gopher holes. Ray Roberts wrapped net wire around yuccas and staked them in washes.

Some would cut notches in a disc plow with a cutting torch. This would be pulled behind a pickup, back and forth, across a flat draw. The procedure was called pitting in an effort to break hard pan surface. It would result in one- to three-inch intermittent cuts in the ground to allow water to soak in. This was a good theory, but the first hard rain filled these up and leveled the ground.

Dirt Spreader Dams

Dirt spreader dams were successful in slowing down the water and spreading it out, and they also helped to control erosion. Earl Hammond was one of the most successful with his complex system of dirt work. Clegg Fowlkes continued to improve his land after buying Earl Hammond's Ranch. Clay Mitchell also had complex systems. The Fletcher Ranch put in extensive work on Long Draw. Joe Mitchell had two systems on his ranch, one on Greenlee Draw near his ranch house and another on Town Draw which drained Marfa. Murphy Bennett had some on the Bandera Ranch, also Ralph Lowe on the Bar C near Kent. Chili Ridley, Sr. had a dandy, good dirt diversion dam across Wild Horse Draw west of Valentine. It threw the water out of the channel and spread it across a tobosa flat. It also irrigated a tobosa flat for Jim White's Chispa Ranch. Unfortunately, some cotton farmers lower down got flooded out when a big rise came down and they harassed Chili until he cut his dike.

---

* Low net wire fences a foot or so high.

Giving 'em the Business

A group of us were visiting at the Jones-Espy Camp at the Bloys Campmeeting. Dr. Burns was the Presbyterian minister in Marfa. It was mentioned that a certain rancher had gotten a pretty good rain. (All rains are good — some are just better than others.) A member of Dr. Burns' congregation said he must be paying the wrong preacher because he hadn't gotten a drop. Dr. Burns answered him, saying, "The Good Book says that it will rain on the just and the unjust. Why don't you get off the fence?"

*   *   *   *   *

We always were hoping and wishing for the hill country and Edwards Plateau to get rain in the winter and spring. We felt that if they got rain in the season they were supposed to, then we would get it in the summer and fall when we were supposed to.

If we had our druthers we would have preferred it to fall in July, August, and September. Of course, if a little came earlier it was always welcome, but it seemed that if there were good rains in May and June, then it would turn off dry the rest of the summer and fall.

The Struggle for Water

Some rough country that wasn't being grazed and had a little grass was watered by running a pipeline and putting in water troughs. It was observed that cattle used the road to these places plus ranch roads through rocky areas as trails, and they would graze out from these areas. Some ranchers would build cattle trails for their use. Some care had to be taken to prevent erosion by careful placement of the trail and building dumps to turn the water out.

Johnny Fitzgerald was ranching the upper part of Merrill Canyon above George Jones' Kelly Ranch on the south side of Mount Livermore. He and J.W. "Skinny" Friend were raising sheep on and around Livermore, and Ben Gearhart was raising goats on nearby Brooks Mountain. All three were feeding eagles, bobcats, and lions. Johnny was hunting lions with his dogs when he wasn't fighting screwworms. When the drouth began to get serious the creek dried up as did the springs and hand dug shallow wells.

Stock just don't do very well without water, not much better than people. He found an old water truck and started hauling water. Now if there is anything more futile than hauling hay during a West Texas drouth, it is hauling water. It is bad enough with a good truck and good roads, but Johnny had access to neither.

C.K. "Kenneth" Smith

It is notoriously difficult to predict the time of calving for heifers due to calve for the first time. Ken had leased the Ford Bell Ranch near Valentine where there was a little grass and drove there every day to feed and check his heifers. The heifers he determined would soon calve, he hauled to me to calve out. I do not recall any of the heifers calving at the ranch unexpectedly or any having to stay in my hospital more than two days. There are cowboys, there are ranchers, and there are cowmen. Ken was a real cowman.

One day, I asked Ken if he thought the cloud formation in the sky called mare's tails was a good sign of rain. He replied, "All signs fail in a drouth, and you don't need any in wet weather. It will rain anyway."

Now, Ken never said much about the drouth we were in, but he definitely was interested in the clouds. He told me that on his way back to town he had been watching a little old cloud about the size of a postage stamp. It wouldn't grow and it wouldn't evaporate, just sat up there high in the sky to tantalize him. A highway patrolman stopped him and made the accusation that he must be drunk the way he was weaving back and forth across the highway.

One day a group of us were admiring a big, fat, barren cow. Ken was looking too, but I'm not saying he was admiring her. His comment was, "I'd be pretty too, if I had never done a day's work." You might not be able to appreciate this statement coming from him unless you knew him. Now, Ken wasn't the ugliest man I ever knew, maybe, but if not, he was a close second. His face wouldn't stop a clock, but it would slow it down considerably. He musta' done an awful lot of hard work! However, he was such a fine man, you really didn't notice his looks.

The cow market in 1955 was bad. A whole lot worse than what was reported in the livestock reports. I don't know why they don't report the averages, just the top prices, and sometimes I think those are exaggerated. A pretty decent cow was only worth about $45.00 a head. Of course, there were some fleshy animals that had been fed heavily brought a little more, but I'm talking about the average commercial range cow that had already gone through three years or more of hard times.

Ken had one of these — actually he had a bunch like that, but I'm talking about a certain one that was very sick. Although medicines and fees were inexpensive at that time, I estimated that it would take about $40.00 to $45.00 to give the cow a chance of survival.

I told Ken that treatment for her was not economically sound. He answered, "Charlie, go ahead. She is worth $85.00 at the PCA (Production Credit Association) as collateral."

Spaying Heifers

Mr. J.E. Baylor had a ranch north of Sierra Blanca. Sometime about the mid-1950s he called me about spaying some heifers.

There were 350 in the group, and Mr. Baylor kept them in the pen off feed and water so they were well-drawn. Mr. Baylor had some heifers spayed in Mexico a few years before, so he knew what was needed. This was during the drouth and depressed prices, and he needed to lighten up some more on this ranch and didn't have traps to hold them. He wanted them finished as soon as possible so that he could turn them out in a big pasture to recuperate. Later, they would be shipped when they were completely healed.

I don't remember the reason he wanted them spayed; it could have been to increase the price. Often the price spread between steers and heifers was three cents a pound, and usually spaying would reduce this to only one cent and other times a spayed heifer would bring the same as a steer. Another reason he may have wanted them spayed was so he could pasture them in a national forest. Usually several ranchers would have permits to run a certain number of cattle in the forest for a specified time at a set fee per head. A problem to this was that bulls were turned out to breed cows. If you didn't want your heifers bred, they needed to be spayed.

Mr. Baylor had modified his crowd chute and had plenty of help. Woodrow Mills loaned me his generator to run electric clippers and he went with me to run it and clip the hair at the incision site in the left flank. There were a couple of men to wash and dry the area and swab it with alcohol and a couple of big strong men to grab each heifer's tail and almost lift the hind legs off the ground as I made the skin incision. I would then poke my fingers through the belly wall, stretch the muscles apart and insert my entire hand and wrist. I would grasp an ovary and excise it with long, curved, blunt-pointed scissors, then repeat with the opposite ovary. I would extract my hand and discard the ovaries and go to the next heifer as Stuart "Button" Jones sutured the skin with a quick figure 8, using cotton string from a big roll that was in common use in grocery stores at that time.

The modified chute held three heifers that I operated on and three heifers being prepped so that no time was lost waiting. After I finished the first, I would operate on the second, then, the third, and suture the third while Button sutured the second. These three would then be turned out and the next three moved into position. I had a large-mouth gallon jar to which I periodically added sulfanilamide powder from a 25-pound container. I would dip my hand in the powder and carry a portion into the heifer's side and abdomen as I operated.

We pretty much used up the whole day but all 350 were spayed, fed and watered, and turned out. Mr. Baylor rounded them up in a couple of weeks, removed the cotton sutures, and shipped them. He reported all had recovered promptly and never missed a lick. Our hands were very sore for a few days but Woodrow's were much the worst. The ranch was very sandy, and this being the spring windy season, the cattle's hair was full of sand which dulled clipper blades so that they had to be sharpened on a whet rock very frequently.

*   *   *   *   *

Mr. Baylor had some heifers spayed on his ranch in Mexico and exported them to the United States. There were 500 head in the stockyards in El Paso when he was approached by a man who had heard about them and that they were for sale. Mr. Baylor said he told the man that they were spayed, had just crossed from Mexico, and quoted an asking price. The price and conditions were agreed on, and they were paid for. That night while sitting in the restaurant at the Del Norte Hotel, he overheard the man asking another where he could find bulls for 500 heifers. Mr. Baylor's suspicions were aroused. He went to the table and asked if the bulls were intended for the heifers they had just traded on. The answer was in the affirmative, so Mr. Baylor asked if he heard him tell that they were spayed. The man admitted that he had, so Mr. Baylor explained what the term *spay* meant and the heifers could not be bred. The man was distressed, and Mr. Baylor bought them back.

Postmortems

Truman Foster was the manager of the Balmorhea Ranches, a division of Clayton Anderson, a big cotton firm. Their primary operation in this area was cotton farming, but they owned considerable ranch land adjacent to their irrigated cotton fields. I was told they also had cotton gins, cottonseed oil mills, and were big in the brokerage business.

The ranch ran Hereford cattle successfully. The ranch land surrounded the Balmorhea lake which impounded some rainfall runoff and water from springs.

During the drouth of the fifties the rain was particularly sparse in that watershed, and the lake water level dropped drastically. The newly exposed shoreline produced a bumper crop of cocklebur plants. The small plants are very toxic to cattle, and these were eaten because the pastures were dry with little grass. I was called because of a serious death loss in the cattle. Postmortem examinations and observing the nearby plants that showed to have been eaten, revealed the diagnosis. Death is so sudden there is no hope of treatment; therefore, the cattle were moved from that pasture.

*   *   *   *   *

During the drouth of the fifties, Truman had to turn cattle onto one of the irrigated alfalfa fields that usually was allowed to mature to be cut and baled for hay because the range land was so dry and short. Many started breathing hard, and when the attempt was made to treat them, they usually died from the effort. Those that survived the stress of being caught and treated soon died anyway. A year or so before, Truman had pneumonia in some of his cows that we treated with Sulmet boluses orally and penicillin in oil intramuscularly. This was the ultimate in medication at that time and worked very well in the pneumonia cattle. However, it wasn't working on these cows, so Truman called me in a panic. There were several dead near the road that I posted. This revealed the lung problem of pulmonary emphysema, properly pulmonary adenomatosis, but is commonly called *cow asthma.* I accused Truman of letting his cows smoke cigarettes. He didn't think that was funny. I didn't know what had caused the asthma, because bloat and scours had been the only problems that I had seen with lush alfalfa. When in doubt, change pastures. They were eased onto an old cotton field with some dead weeds and old grass. The trouble soon stopped, and I found in the literature later that sometimes, moving cattle from dry pasture to lush will cause this. What a dilemma — leave them in the dry, hard pasture and let them starve or move them onto good feed and they die anyway.

Hollywood Comes to Marfa

The filming of the movie, *Giant,* in the area came at a good time. We were suffering from a drouth and severe economic depression in 1955, and the money the company was spending provided a much needed boost to the economy.

The well-known actors, Elizabeth Taylor, Rock Hudson, James Dean, and Chill Wills, attracted sightseers and the curious. I didn't personally follow the activity very closely. I wasn't all that impressed with movie actors. During World War II when I was in the Marine paratroops at Camp Gillespie, near San Diego they filmed a movie about us. It was never released because we didn't jump in the islands. The main actor was a big man who grabbed my parachute and threw it around and sat on it, not showing it the respect that I thought it deserved. He walked off and left it laying on the ground at an inconvenient place for me to retrieve it, never acknowledging my presence. I was plumb put out at him. A major asked if I wanted to repack it before jumping. Well, there wasn't time to do so and hardly enough time to readjust the harness. I really wanted to make the jump. I always enjoyed the thrill, but perhaps I had another reason. I wouldn't admit it to anyone, but I secretly thought that maybe the filming crew would center on me as I left the plane, floated down and landed, making me the hero. I did have a serious talk with the Lord as I jumped regarding the opening of the parachute. As it turned out, I ended up at the opposite side of the field, completely out of the scene. However, I guess it was just as well because a gust of wind caught the chute, and I made a very undignified landing.

During the filming of *Giant*, I worked with some of the horse handlers whose names have faded from my memory. The most popular actor among the local men was Chill Wills who frequented the beer joints at night and was a real down-to-earth fellow.

The structure built to represent the ranch house for the filming was on a tobosa grass flat in front of the Worth Evans' Ryan Ranch house. I don't think the tobosa had been green for at least three years. The director wanted green grass so the Marfa Fire Department sprayed it with water for days. The effort was a failure, and eventually it was sprayed with green paint. It looked realistic. I don't know what the product was, but it didn't damage the grass and it washed off when it finally rained.

Mr. Frank Inn was an animal trainer who came to Marfa with the movie crew. He brought several dogs with him. They had no active part but were in the background on a number of scenes. He brought them back and forth from the set in a station wagon automobile that had a tailgate that opened on the back end. After shooting one, day Mr. Inn called his dogs to jump in the back of his vehicle. A big hound missed and hit his abdomen on the tailgate. The bladder was full and ruptured from the impact. Uremic poisoning developed, making a very sick dog. Dr. Stover, a physician, took an x-ray for me, as I had not yet purchased one. This confirmed the diagnosis and surgery was performed.

Mr. Inn would stop by the hospital each afternoon during the slow, stormy recovery. JoAnn asked him to train our pet toy fox terrier, Zeke. He had already been around Zeke enough for his evaluation, and he was too diplomatic to tell us the reason for declining. He may have thought he was too hard-headed or possibly too dumb. Some time later he told me that his primary income was obedience training and that he enjoyed an enviable reputation because he was careful to screen prospects. He felt he could evaluate a dog quickly. One day he saw a small nondescript cur in my cages that had been left for euthanasia. The dog was healthy, but the owners were moving. They could not take it and had been unable to give it away. There was no animal shelter in the area at that time. Frank fooled with the little dog and quickly became interested. We obtained permission from the owners for him to take the dog which responded remarkably fast, learning to jump and sit in a chair, sit upright with folded front legs, crawl on its belly, and roll. Mr. Inn named the dog, Marfa, and it soon became an active member of the troop, returning to Hollywood with the other dogs.

The filming company for Giant had brought several horses. One in particular was said to be a very valuable, trained horse. This was the big, black horse from the East that was brought to the Texas ranch by the movie characters played by Rock Hudson and Elizabeth Taylor. One day after shooting a scene, the horses were fed and watered. Shortly thereafter, this horse developed colic. I was called about dark when he became violent, pawing, lying down, and rolling. I worked with him all night. He would become easy, and the situation would look encouraging. A small amount of gas would be passed and a little urine, but each time he would relapse. About sunup he finally had a good bowel movement, and passed a quantity of urine, and began to nibble on feed. I had thought the case was hopeless a couple of hours before but had been reluctant to recommend euthanasia because all the men were cussing and crying over the value. He was insured for a substantial sum, and they were worried over the insurance company investigation as to the cause. They also assured me that he was so well trained, he was irreplaceable.

While the men were bemoaning these matters, I was concerned for the horse. I've seen many animals and quite a few men in pain of various degrees, but I think a horse with colic is the most pitiful thing I have ever witnessed, especially the severe form that resists my efforts to relieve him. The sweating, trembling, labored breathing with flared nostrils, kicking at his belly, front legs buckling, going down and rolling in spite of our efforts to keep him on his feet, his groans with expiratory grunts — are all heartrending. I never felt so helpless and inadequate as when a horse continued to suffer after I had done everything I could.

When this horse finally was easy and out of pain, I could feel no sense of triumph, only that of relief and thankfulness. I was completely exhausted emotionally.

Another Side of Veterinary Medicine

Otis Kimball ranched north of Alpine and sold his cows in 1954 or perhaps it was 1955 to a man in West Virginia. That state required both a brucellosis and a tuberculosis test. This testing was not a problem because our area was clean, so the possibility of a reactor was almost nil. I could take blood samples, test the blood that night, and do the paperwork so that the cattle could be shipped the next morning, if only brucellosis testing was needed. Tuberculosis testing took longer because it required an injection of test material (tuberculin) intradermally (in the skin) in the caudal fold of the tail. This site would then need to be examined 72 hours later for a reaction.

Otis did not have any grass in his holding traps and very little in his big pastures, which was the reason for selling. No hay was grown locally, so the expense of hauling added to the price of the hay made it very costly to feed.

Arrangements were made with the buyer so that he would keep the cattle in quarantine and be tested on arrival at the destination, if the West Virginia state officials would permit this. I telephoned the State Veterinarian for permission. This was a big deal in those days. I rarely phoned long distance. Instead, I would write a letter sent with a three-cent stamp. But, in this case, time was of the essence, and I felt like I could make my case better in conversation than in a letter. I cried on his shoulder, explaining our predicament and describing in detail the cleanliness of our area and how disease-free our cattle were. His reply was their area was pretty dirty and if ours was so clean, the cattle would have no natural resistance to their diseases and would soon all get sick. I thought I had really put my foot in my mouth and quickly back-pedaled, apologizing for bothering him and stating we would test as required.

More Drouth Stories

The first commercial hotshot (electric shockprod) for use on cattle was made of a fiber material covered with a heavy coat of shellac. It was not very sturdy, but it did have the advantage of not causing the user to suffer a shock if it developed a short. The next hotshot was all metal with a rubber cover on the handle for insulation. Although this was much sturdier, the rubber cover on the handle would soon crack and shorts would develop due to wear and tear.

About 1956, when the lack of grass and depressed prices were at their worst, Kerr Mitchell was forced to sell his cattle. There never had been a dry spell to last this long, and a lot of ranchers had hung on too long. We were loading some cattle on a truck at his ranch, and they frequently had to be encouraged to go up the loading chute ramp. Kerr was using an old, worn-out, metal hot-shot whose rubber handle was in pretty bad condition. In the hustle and bustle of the work, he would frequently get shocked. He would squall like a scalded dog and jump up in the air. Ordinarily, most of us would have thrown the thing away, but these were hard times. Kerr didn't quit, never missed a lick. We would laugh at him, but he couldn't see the humor of the situation.

Kerr tried irrigating some of his country at the Tinaja section house on the Santa Fe Railroad that ran through his ranch, growing hay for his drouth stricken cattle. This wasn't profitable, and he sold this part of his ranch to Mac Benge. Soon after selling his cattle, it began raining and his country got very good. He began looking for cattle to restock. There were no local cattle for sale and none close by. The closest quality Hereford cattle he could find were in northern New Mexico and cost an arm and a leg. The widespread drouth had caused extensive dispersal of herds. This is one of the trials of ranching: when you are forced to sell, cattle are cheap because others are having to do it also, and when you want to buy, they are expensive because others are restocking too.

Kerr and several others tried sending their cattle to Oklahoma and other areas to grass. This did not work out for most. There is a saying about ranching in this area, "You don't feed hay, you don't haul water, and when cattle leave your ranch, they should belong to someone else." I personally didn't adhere to this, to my regret. I sent cattle to grass in Montana, and I hauled water to the dry Brushy Canyon place of my father's in south Brewster County. Do what I say, not what I do! Another saying that was discovered to have merit was, "You don't move cattle east or south."

*   *   *   *   *

I tested a trainload of prime age cows in 1955 for the disease, brucellosis, at the railroad stockpens in Valentine. They were being shipped to a buyer in Alabama. I was told they averaged $45 a head. They were all good quality, young, Hereford cows but were very thin, being the last remnants of several herds.

There were some exceptionally good cows belonging to Cole and Alf Means that had been on feed at Lobo either at the Clarence Bell place or Buddy Griffin's. Both men had irrigated fields of sorghum they had cut and put into trench silos. The Means' cows had been fed this, supplemented with milo and cottonseed meal. They had hoped to hang onto the group as a foundation to rebuild their herd when it started raining again, but they had given up. I understood that many of the thinner, weaker cows in this shipment only brought $40 a head, whereas the Means' cows sold much better. I was concerned that many of the thin cows might be too weak to make the trip, but they were loaded with plenty of room to allow them to lie down. I never heard how they made the trip.

*   *   *   *   *

Claude Lee had the Antelope Springs Ranch. He finally gave up in the fall of 1955, sold the last of his cattle and horses, shut down his windmills, and would have closed his gates except that a county road ran right through the middle of his property and was not fenced.

He had a government rain gauge and kept the official rainfall record. He sent in the record and moved the gauge to his house in town, explaining that he was going out of business. The officials wrote him, thanking him for his cooperation and said they understood the reason — only one place in the U.S. had recorded less rain, Death Valley, California.

*   *   *   *   *

Some of the cattle on a few ranches appeared to be doing fairly well where no animal should. It was explained by saying the cattle had learned to crack the rocks and get the kernels out.

*   *   *   *   *

I was told that one year during the worst of the drouth, someone in Van Horn asked Calvin Jones who ranched northeast of there in the Delaware Mountains if he thought his cows were bred up. He replied, "I hope not." When questioned, he explained that an open, dry cow can live on pretty lean pickins, but a cow nursing a calf has a tough row to hoe, and both may die.

*   *   *   *   *

They told of a tourist visiting in the Big Bend Park who stopped in Study Butte to gas up. He surveyed the harsh, barren landscape and asked if this country was good for anything. The gas attendant said, "Oh yeah, this is cow country." The fellow asked how cattle could make a living where there was no grass and blessed little of anything besides rocks. He was told the cattle turned the rocks over and licked the moss off the underside. The tourist wandered out and turned over a bunch of rocks, came back and said he didn't see any moss. The attendant said the cattle had already cleaned up the rocks down here where it was flat and easy to get to — the man needed to climb up on that mountain and check the rocks there. The high, rough, steep mountain to the north didn't look inviting on a hot, summer day. The man just shook his head, got in his car and drove off.

*   *   *   *   *

Pat Mulloy and his wife lived in Fort Davis, and Pat drove back and forth to the Jeff Ranch. He was one of the few who received some rain during the drouth of the fifties. The Barrel Springs Ranch belonging to Frieda Gillett was another. Pat would tell when he got a rain, but as the area became drier and the situation worsened with other ranchers hurting so badly, they began to avoid him. People would rejoice in another's good fortune up to a point, but let's face it, the adage that "misery loves company" has more truth than many of us care to admit. Pat finally stopped telling of his rains. When questioned he would give a little head motion that was non-committal. Pat later acquired the reputation of not admitting to a rain. Actually he never denied getting one — he just was reluctant to say anything. When I heard someone ridicule Pat for his silence, I would try to explain the reason he was silent. Pat had managed to maintain his cow herd and was one of the few good clients that I had during those hard days.

Dilemma

Stuart "Button" Jones had the Lake Ranch south of Marfa. Stuart was running sheep and doing fairly well until the drouth became serious for him about 1953. When the grass began to play out, it revealed a heavy stand of lechuguilla which the sheep began eating and dying. Stuart hired crews of wet Mexicans to grub the lechuguilla. This was an act of futility, but when a person is in trouble, he will grasp at straws. He would attempt to drive sheep away from the lechuguilla patches horseback. The only thing this was successful in accomplishing was to cripple horses with the thorns.

Stuart and I were going to the ranch in his pickup with my little black bag and had stopped to open a gate. We saw a porcupine. It was the first I had seen away from the Davis Mountains. Stuart got his 30-30 rifle from the rack behind his seat and started to shoot it when we realized it was eating lechuguilla. We knew that deer pawed it up and javelinas rooted it up to eat the white crown or heart, but this was our first experience with porcupines eating it. This one dug at the base with his long claws, then ate the heart. We watched a long time and did not disturb him. I suppose this goes to show there is something good with almost anything.

The reason Stuart was going to kill the porcupine was because a calf will smell one and gets its nose full of quills, then its mother will not let it nurse. A horse will paw one and get quills in the foot, sometimes going into joints or tendons, causing them to be crippled. Dogs often get quills in their muzzle and mouth. Also, porcupine will eat the bark from a tree, killing it. They especially like fruit trees.

We went on to the headquarters, and I was able to locate the lechuguilla thorn and extract it from the pastern of a horse. One of the wets watching showed me his chest where a piece of lechuguilla had stuck in. It takes some degree of skill to grub the plant, and even then an occasional awkward blow will cause the center piece to fly up. This one had stabbed him in the chest and the point had broken off in him. He had already worn it a few days, and it was becoming more painful. The other Mexicans had attempted to pick it out with the point of a pocket knife but had been unsuccessful. He didn't want to be taken to town to a doctor for fear of being caught by the chotas and deported. This was one of the many times I was faced with this dilemma.

Pressure to Practice Human Medicine

A veterinarian is sometimes faced with a dilemma, perhaps more so in this sparsely settled area where physicians are few and far between, especially at an isolated ranch with a sick or injured wet Mexican, who if taken to town to a doctor would be deported. Penicillin sensitivity or allergy was particularly a problem, as it can be very deadly. I was often pressured to give someone a penicillin injection when it first became economical for me to carry it routinely on calls. When the pressure became too great, I would produce a large gauge calcium chloride needle. This needle is approximately the diameter of a kitchen match and some 6 or 8 inches in length. It had a small curl at the end which frequently occurs when the needle becomes dull by bumping a piece of metal. This little hook is referred to as a fish hook. I would then take a large 60cc syringe and attach the needle, take the bottle of penicillin, and ask the subject to drop his pants and bend over. No one ever called my bluff.

Birth Defects

The drouth of the fifties produced some interesting phenomena. I don't know how much was caused by the drouth and how much from genetic problems connected to the snorter dwarf syndrome. One interesting case was a two-headed calf. I had a terrible time delivering it. Had I known what it was, I may have been able to do a caesarean, although by the time it was determined, it was too late. I had that head frozen and stored in the locker plant with the intentions of having it mounted when I could afford it. However, I saw so many the next few years that I became disenchanted with them and threw the frozen one away, hoping to never see another.

I blamed much of the problem on the drouth because the nutritional value of old dry grass is lost, causing mineral and vitamin deficiencies, and the lack of forage often caused the eating of toxic plants. We have an abundance in this area, so it is often a challenge to diagnose the cause of death, illness, abortion, birth defects, or poor doers.*

Some other birth defects were lambs with a second small mouth in their cheek, no tail, extra legs, or a horn in the middle of the forehead. Calves were found with receding or protruding lower jaw, short forelegs, very small eyeballs, or skin with hair on the cornea of the eye. The most difficult to deliver, either by the

---

* No known problem — they just don't grow out or gain properly.

normal birth canal or by C-section, was shistosomas reflexus. The fetus is inside out. The legs and skin are inside, with the heart, lungs, and abdominal contents outside. This anomaly is repulsive in appearance. The joints of the legs, neck and spine are frozen and they will not bend; therefore, it is difficult to deliver. Hydrocephalus, a large head with excessive fluid in the ventricles of the brain, usually necessitates embryotomy.

Stargazers

Early in the drouth, we began to see many calves that were weak at birth. They would lie flat, making no effort to stand or nurse even when assisted. They were non-responsive to treatment and died within two or three days. Their eyes would be wide open with a blank, unseeing stare. C.K. Smith called them stargazers. I assumed the problem to be vitamin A deficiency because there was none in what little grass there was and none in the 41% cottonseed cake being fed.

After some trial and error, it was determined that a two cc (ml) dose of the injectable vitamin A given intramuscularly to the pregnant cow a few days before parturition was effective in prevention. This product was a concentrated form of cod liver oil containing 100,000 units of vitamin A per cc in a 10cc vial at a cost of $10.00 per vial. It was a great day when vitamin A was synthesized.

Unusual Problems with Plants

Mesquite

When I first came to the area, a common sight in the south part of the county near the Rio Grande River was Mexicans with burros gathering ripe mesquite beans in tow sacks. These would be stored in an adobe building for subsequent feeding to milk goats and burros mainly, but also to milk cows and horses, if the family was prosperous enough to have them.

Cattle grazed some on the leaves, but I don't know how much they actually ate or how much nutritive value there was. Some years when there was a good bloom crop, the cattle would really get a boost from them.

The beans were a valuable source of feed for livestock, primarily cattle. They caused some major problems with impactions in horses some years. Many ranchers said it was caused by the ripe beans falling on the ground, then being rained on and fermenting. Personally, I think the problem was caused by them being too high a percentage of the diet or because they were not completely ripe.

When beans are ripe they are sweet, having a high sugar content. I expected laminitis, founder, but did not see it caused by beans. The impactions rarely caused colic, usually only constipation with the resulting lethargy and lack of appetite caused by the absorption of toxins from the stagnant gut. My treatment was mineral oil by stomach tube and small, somewhat frequent injections of the laxative, cascara sagrada. I was always afraid of carbachol, that it might cause gut contractions to be too violent. After treatment, the horse was slowly walked.

I would perform a rectal examination if there was no bowel movement in 24 to 36 hours and attempted to massage the mass with fear and trembling, always afraid of rupturing a gut. Sometimes the abdominal wall would be soft, and when I could feel the mass, I would knead it from the outside, hoping to help in breaking down the mass and mixing the oil with it. I allowed access to water but not feed until the horse had a good bowel movement. When economics permitted, I gave intravenous lactated Ringer's solution liberally. I occasionally gave an enema if I thought the mass was far enough back in the gut that the water would reach it without having to give much.

Cattle in the Pecos River valley had a nervous toxic syndrome called *jaw and tongue,* named for the chewing gum type of symptoms produced by the over consumption of mesquite beans. I never saw this problem west of the Davis Mountains. I think it was because the Pecos valley had a thicker, heavier stand of mesquite trees with many more available beans. The mesquites in Presidio and Brewster Counties were scrawny and sparser. Probably there were some other pickings, such as catclaw leaves and beans, blackbrush leaves, salt cedar, a few weeds and a little bunch grass. It's rather surprising what cattle can find to eat in the desert if given plenty of room.

*   *   *   *   *

A poor, sorry-looking, little steer calf maybe six weeks or two months old was hauled to my place about the middle of the 1950s.

The eyes were sunken and the skin was hard, obviously dehydrated and emaciated. The rancher's small children had been riding horseback with him in the pasture when this calf was discovered lying near a water trough. He pulled his rifle out of the saddle scabbard and started to shoot the little fellow to put it out of its misery, but the children began squalling and begging to save it. A short time before, their pet dog had suffered strychnine poisoning, and I managed to save it. Those kids thought I could work miracles.

I examined the calf with the use of a stomach tube, discovering a blockage in the esophagus about midway in the neck. The area was swollen and hard. I suspected a mesquite limb was hung there, it being a common problem. I could not possibly reach it with forceps. The only way was an esophagotomy. This term is used for the surgical procedure whereby an incision is made through the neck into the esophagus. Sometime during my college days in surgery, I had gotten the impression that this was not possible in animals. The wound would not heal, so food material would leak into the surrounding tissue, resulting in infection and death.

I asked for them to leave it, that I would do what I could. I didn't want them to see me perform euthanasia. Those tear-stained little faces looked up at me, each was gently stroking the side of the calf and asked to stay while it was treated. The father agreed. He didn't help me a bit.

I decided to do the esophagotomy. The calf was a goner anyway, so there was nothing to lose. I figured the kids would take out as soon as I began the incision.

Because it was semicomatose, no general anesthetic was needed, only local infiltration of procaine. The site was clipped and scrubbed, then painted with Tincture of Phe-mer-nite. I began the incision hesitantly, but the children made no move. I proceeded to make a generous cut, perhaps ten inches long, then began to separate the skin from the underlying tissue by blunt dissection. The father suddenly remembered there was something he needed to do in his pickup. I continued to separate tissues down to the esophagus. There must have been six or eight thorns protruding from the surface of it, with some leakage from the holes made by them. I opened the esophagus at the upper part of the lump and pulled out a length of mesquite limb tangled with grass. The little tykes grabbed the stinking mess with a triumphant shout of glee. They ran to show it to their father.

I inserted a stomach tube down the throat into the esophagus past the incision and into the stomach. It was all clear. I carefully sutured the esophagus and surrounding tissue with catgut after smearing sulfa powder and penicillin throughout the area. I put a needle with a tube attached into the exposed jugular vein and began a slow intravenous drip while I closed the remaining tissue and skin. I pumped in milk replacer before I removed the stomach tube. The children helped move him onto a heating pad and cover him with a blanket.

The calf made an uneventful recovery. I later operated on a number of calves with similar problems and an occasional cow with choke that I could not relieve with a tube. I wish that I had known that I could perform this operation a few years before when I had so much trouble with bones and deer horns, but most of these were before the cost of penicillin was economical, so the success rate may not have been very good.

Dagger and Soap Yucca

There are two common plants of the genus Yucca. The larger of the two is more common in the lower elevations and called spanish daggers or usually simply daggers. The Mexicans called them *palmas*, which is also the name for the large palm trees of the lower Rio Grande Valley.

The higher elevations, such as the Marfa Basin, have a few dagger plants, but the more common is the plant we generally called yucca. It is sometimes called the soap yucca because the early Mexicans and Anglos used the heart or center to make a homemade soap. The Mexicans call it *palmilla*, that is, a little palm.

Both plants have very nutritious blooms. One of the favorite treatments for retained placentas was feeding these blooms. Any sick animal was often fed these because they were very palatable and easy to eat, besides being nutritious. I never had an analysis, but I think they must have also been high in vitamin A. Some years the bloom crop was very good, and the smaller palmilla would really be of value. The larger, palma dagger blooms were high and difficult for cattle to reach. Ted Harper would ride horseback and pull down dagger blooms for his cattle with a pole equipped with a hook on the end.

The heart is not edible in either plant, but both cattle and horses would sometimes eat the dead dried leaves, or blades, as they are often called. They have no nutritive value but are of benefit by providing fiber bulk to the diet and in alleviating hunger.

I only saw cattle eat the green blades on the yucca one time, that being during this severe drouth.

I diagnosed toxicity in several yearlings and two-year-old cattle on the Nopal Ranch that had symptoms of either lechuguilla or sacahuiste bloom (*Nolina texana*) poisoning (they have similar symptoms), yet neither plant was present. However, there were a large number of yucca that showed evidence of having been grazed. This was the only time I suspected this plant of being toxic, but it was the only time I saw the green blades so heavily grazed. A large number of plants were killed by being stripped of leaves.

Oak Poisoning

Charlie Thomas was ranching in the Glass Mountains north of Marathon. He had been a client when he ranched south of Marfa on the Murray Cripple Mill Ranch. He had run out of grass and moved to a Glass Mountain ranch during the drouth of the fifties, which was kinda like jumping out of the frying pan into the fire. He had heard of hill country ranchers feeding their goats by cutting limbs from oak trees for them to eat the leaves. Oak trees were plentiful on this ranch, so he put Mexicans to cutting off limbs for his cattle. Two cows had died, and several others had developed black, tarry diarrhea. This was the only oak poisoning I saw in the mountains, but it was the only time I knew of that an effort was made to feed it.

* * * * *

I don't remember any significant poisoning by the plants I usually considered the worse offenders, that is, the three kinds of loco, senecio, and psilostrophe. It was too dry for these plants to be numerous during the drouth.

Sotol

Sotol is a large, grass-like plant with long tapering leaves that have prickly edges. It closely resembles sacahuiste. The stalk arises from the center of the plant and is grazed while it is small until it becomes coarse. This stalk reaches several feet in height. The blooms are small compared to dagger and yucca blooms. The entire stalk and blooms are tall and slender, giving rise to the name *desert candle*. I never knew the bloom to be gathered for livestock feed. The heart or head of the sotol is an excellent feed. The leaves were cut off with a machete or axe and the heart cut from the roots with a grubbing hoe, or it was pried up with a crowbar. These may be broken open on the spot for livestock or may be loaded and hauled to a place of feeding. If left to ferment, it is especially palatable, and it was said animals would come quite a distance when the odor was detected.

Indians and early Mexican settlers roasted the hearts for food. It was eaten as it came from the roasting pit, or it was ground into a flour which was later made into a cake or tortilla. The juice was fermented to make a very potent alcoholic beverage. A sophisticated method of marketing this drink was to place it in a wide-mouth jar to which was added a piece of charcoal supposedly to absorb impurities. It was usually sold in old recycled whiskey bottles.

The leaves were not eaten because of the saw-like serrated edges. Occasionally I would see a horse with a fetid, purulent, nasal discharge. If only one nostril was affected, I would be suspicious of foreign material, especially if sotol was being fed. Sometimes a piece of leaf from the head would hang up in the throat, and violent coughing would force it into the back of the nose. Sometimes, only a bad breath and chronic cough would be the result of a leaf hung on the soft palate. The passage of a stomach tube through the nostril would usually dislodge it. If not, and a scratch on the tube or a feeling of rasping would show it was not dislodged, I would suture a piece of flannel cloth on the end of the tube and rotate it as it was inserted. Often the rough, saw-like edges would cause it hang on the cloth, and it could then be extracted. A few times this turned out to be a piece of catclaw limb.

The problem was less common in cattle than in horses, but stomach tube treatments in cattle often resolved a chronic nasal discharge or chronic cough, even though I rarely saw a foreign object.

Dr. Ben Gearhart rigged a knife-like apparatus to the front wheel of his vehicle and drove through a thick stand of sotol to break it up. This had limited success. Some weird things were tried during the drouth of the fifties.

Supplemental Feeding

I was told the origin of the term *cow cake* was from the original method of extracting oil from cottonseed kernels by a hydraulic press after they had been separated from the hulls. This method resulted in large, thick cakes that had to be broken in pieces or ground into meal in order to be fed.

When supplemental feeding became common, the cottonseed meal was tightly pressed into range cubes that were still called cow cake. These were firm and fed on the ground. They were cylindrical, about ¾ inch in diameter and in various lengths usually 1 to 1½ inches. Regardless of shape, they were commonly called range cubes. This was a 41% protein product.

The man doing the feeding would count the number of cattle that came to his call. He would then calculate the amount to be put out, usually one to three pounds per head, depending upon the range conditions and the owner's pocketbook. If he was feeding alone, he would take the 100-pound sack, open it, carry it on his hip, and call, while walking in a big circle, pouring the feed. This would spread out the feed so that cows had a chance to eat without being fought off by an aggressive one. If two were feeding, one would drive while the other poured out the feed from the back of a pickup which was referred to as the feed wagon. When I came to the area, I only knew of one place where the feeding was still being done from a wagon pulled by a team of horses and that was at Clay Espy's Poor Farm Ranch. The man feeding was Lara.

Some would use a feeder to dispense the range cubes. This was a box that was open at the top where the cake was poured in. It fell on a tilted screen that led to a small funnel or trough that protruded over the side of the pickup truck bed. A rope allowed the driver to open a door, allowing the feed to pour out.

The first cubes were fairly soft and crumbled somewhat with

handling. The screen was to allow small pieces to fall into a tray and be saved, because if it fell on the ground it would be lost, the cows unable to pick it up. These screenings were called *siftings*. This would be fed in troughs to milk cows and any cattle kept in a pen for any reason.

A process was later developed to completely remove all the oil by use of a chemical solvent. This was called *New Process* and resulted in a very dry fine powder that could not be pressed into a cube. Molasses was added so that it would hold together.

One of the first feed mills to make a range cube this way produced an almond shaped cube. The first cube that was objectionable because of the soft texture was replaced by a cube so hard cattle had a great deal of difficulty eating it. It was pitiful to watch a hungry cow wallow a piece in her mouth trying to chew it.

Some help finally came from the government with a grain-assisted program of corn and milo. Most of this was fed by grinding and mixing with cottonseed meal to make a range cube. Some added alfalfa leaf meal, minerals, and vitamins, besides the molasses. Later, urea was added as formulations became more sophisticated. Most of this was a 20% protein product, but varied from 10% to 38% according to the recipe.

During the drouth some attempts were made in feeding cottonseed meal and salt loose in troughs. This salt and meal was a good theory. It was a method to feed the meal with the salt to limit the consumption. Several days' supply could be put in troughs, then individuals would eat some, then drink water, and go back to pasture. This was economical to mix and feed. A major problem with this occurred in sheep. Ewes would develop beautiful udders, but there was no milk in them. The baby lambs would starve to death. I don't remember salt and meal being fed to cows with calves. The problem I saw with it in cattle was that a wind storm would blow the fine meal out of the trough, leaving the coarser, heavier salt with just enough meal to flavor it. Yearlings that had laid out during the wind storm and had become very hungry, would eat this, resulting in salt poisoning which was often fatal.

The yellow pigment of cottonseed meal has caused me some frustration over the years. It was erroneously thought by many to be carotene, the precursor of vitamin A. It will stain the fat and fibrous connective tissue, an icterus or jaundice color. At times I have been tempted to think of lechuguilla or sacahuiste poisoning and other times red blood cell destruction or muscle damage. This was more likely to occur when fed for long periods in a drouth.

Empty cake sacks (tow, burlap, gunny) were sold back to a feed dealer or to a bag company to be cleaned, mended, and resold to the feed mills. The paper sacks used later had little resale value.

A joke was circulated during the drouth of the fifties about a big rancher who was as dry as everyone else who showed up driving a brand new Cadillac. People were shocked that he could afford such a luxury. When questioned, he answered, "I sold my cake sacks!"

*   *   *   *   *

Prickly pear that the Mexicans called *nopal* was fed sparingly in this area. Most of our pear was coarse and fibrous and had big thorns that were difficult to burn. Much of it was a low scrubby plant. Some of the area had a little better pear and was burned using a pear burner. This was a backpack container of kerosene with a pump-up, air pressure dispenser. It was similar to, if not identical to, herbicide and insecticide backpack sprayers.

Feeding pear was limited and never practical as in the south Texas area near Laredo where my friend and classmate, Dr. Ben Hopson, fed it and referred to it as South Texas Alfalfa. When labor and fuel were relatively inexpensive, it was fed routinely. The men burning the pear wore metal leggins for protection against rattlesnakes. One of the chief disadvantages to the practice was that many cattle would then eat pear that had not been burned. This resulted in pear mouth. The tongue and lips would get so full of thorns they couldn't eat. During the fifties we had pear mouth problems with cattle, sheep, and goats, even though they had never been fed the plant. The hungry animals would eat, or try to eat, pear that had not been burnt. Screwworms would get in the sore lips, further complicating matters. I was often called to diagnose and recommend a treatment for pear mouth, blue-tongue, virus soremouth, and screwworms, all of which were common in sheep.

Hay

Alfalfa hay was rarely fed. The cost, because of transportation, was considered prohibitive except for a few saddle horses, milk cows, and sick individuals as well as heifers in the maternity pen.

Hay traps had been common, but the only ones I knew to be still actively harvested were on the X Ranch near Kent, on Clay Mitchell's ranch south of Marfa, and on the J.W. Merrill ranch west of Fort Davis. These were overflow, gramma grass draws that were fenced to keep cattle out and the grass allowed to grow. It would be mowed by a side sickle mower and baled on the X Ranch and by Clay Mitchell. The Merrill ranch raked and hauled it to the barn loose stack. Tobosa grass was said to have been used in the past, but Dr. Ben Gearhart tried it during the fifties unsuccessfully. Most ranchers had abandoned the native grass hay traps and had planted Johnson grass in them when I came to the area.

Bar ditches were mowed by the highway department using side sickle mowers. Many ranchers adjacent to the places that grew lush grass would harvest this. Dick Swartz on the Merrill ranch was one of the more diligent in utilizing this grass. Later, the highway department changed to rotary mowers that shredded the grass and made it impossible to harvest.

There was a fairly good stand of Johnson grass in some bar ditches in good years, and Mexicans would cut it by hand with a machete, load it on a burro, and haul it to town. I was always amazed at the amount they could load on a burro. Some would cut it with a scythe and haul it to town in a two-wheel cart pulled by a burro. However, the *ricos*, the rich ones, would haul it in a pickup. Many burros, milk cows, calves, and a few horses would be staked in bar ditches to graze. Often they were tied to a fence post with a long rope. My hospital-residence was at first fenced and had cattle guards in two places to keep out stray animals but allow vehicles to have access.

Johnson grass fields were commonplace. Kerr Mitchell had a cement diversion dam across Alamito Creek in his Rancheria pasture and irrigated about ten acres of Johnson grass when the creek ran. Most that grew Johnson grass would allow it to become mature and rank to increase volume. This would decrease palatability and increase waste as it became coarse, but an ole hungry cow would clean it up. Kerr would cut his at an ideal stage of growth, and it made excellent hay. I fed it to my sick horses and cattle in the hospital with good results.

Ray Roberts at the Pruett Ranch northeast of Marfa on the Catto-Gage Ranches had a large Johnson grass field in the Greenlee Draw below his house. He raised large amounts of hay that was used on this ranch and other Catto-Gage Ranches in the Alpine and Marathon areas.

Clay Mitchell had several fields irrigated by a rather elaborate series of dirt, diversion dikes. This took some degree of skill to implement so that the water would be spread evenly, not cause erosion, and not be washed out by a cloudburst. Clay had several draws that flowed into the ranch. Long Draw originated on the Love and Petan Ranches and flowed by the Fletcher house and through that ranch and completely through Clay's ranch. The Sauz Draw and the Big Trestle draws also drained large areas. Maureen Godbold, Clay's daughter, claimed Clay had more interest in the dirt work and tinkering with the haying equipment than he did in his cattle. However, he was a very successful rancher and had good Hereford cattle.

Ben Avant had a Johnson grass field west of Marfa on the Big Trestle Draw. Ben was what I considered an old man. It was quite a sight to see him following his plow horse as he worked that field. I guess he was one of the last men that I saw working a plow horse, perhaps the last. It had been common in the Brazos River bottoms near College Station. It seemed as if most of the horses that we treated in veterinary school were plow horses.

Ben Avant always wore his hat uncreased, the brim flat, and had it square on his head, never cocked to one side. Most men creased the crown, curled the brim and wore it at an angle. I guess Berry Hart at Kent had the brim of his hat folded up against the crown to the most extreme of anyone I can remember. Several wore it cocked to one side, some almost to an extreme.

One of Ben Gearhart's greatest claims to fame came from his tobosa grass haying. We had been told that old timers would mow and put up tobosa grass hay. By doing so for several years, the clumps, lumps, and holes would level out and the old coarse grass would not be allowed to become stemmy, leaving only good fresh growth. Ben's equipment didn't last that long. He tore up all the side sickle mowers, rakes and balers that he could beg, borrow, buy, or steal. I can personally vouch for the fact that this was the worst hay I have ever seen in my life. It was full of dirt, cow chips, and the toughest, coarsest grass stems imaginable. He brought some to me to feed sick animals here in the hospital. He was as proud of those bales of hay as my daughter, Nancy, when she presented me with mud pies as a child. Ben claimed if you soaked the hay overnight in a water trough, it would soften up, and cattle would eat it. I tried overnight, over a weekend, and over a week. I never was able to get anything to eat it. However, the bales did make good braces for propping up a downer cow.

Woodrow Mills was one of the most resourceful ranchers coping with the drouth of the 1950s. He sprayed tobosa grass with molasses. He purchased molasses and stored it in tanks at the ranch. He would put some in a cattle sprayer, then add water and agitate it well to get it thoroughly mixed. He would drive to one side of a pasture, call the cattle to him and spread cake on the ground. While they were eating, he would then drive hurriedly to the other side and spray the grass where there was a good thick stand of tobosa. He had to finish promptly because the cattle would come to the sound as soon as they finished the cake. He would have to stop when the cattle came, as they would get in the spray and get covered with molasses—what a mess that was! There was quite an art to the correct mixture and its application. If it was too thick, it wouldn't go through the spray nozzle, and if it were too weak or applied too lightly, the cattle wouldn't eat the tobosa. If everything was done just right, the cattle would get reasonably full, and the area would be almost black because only the old stumps would remain. Woody said that when it finally did rain, these eaten off areas were prime grazing places, as all the old coarse stems were gone and the cattle had nice fresh tender grass.

Almost all the nutritive value was in the molasses because the tobosa was old, but cattle, which are ruminants, need the roughage, and they would not otherwise eat the dry, tough grass. He also burned prickly pear to feed, but the molasses spraying was his claim to fame.

My Efforts to Cope

Nineteen of my regular clients sold all their livestock, discharged their employees, and locked their gates. Neighbors would check on things and attempt to keep out poachers. This was a significant number because I didn't have a large number of clients at that time.

There was a severe reduction in the number of livestock among those who were able to continue to operate. The first cattle to be sold were the older cows. These were the ones in which almost all the cancer eye cases occurred. This surgery was a high percentage of my practice in those days. The number of heifers bred for replacements was much fewer. These constituted most of my obstetrics. These factors severely curtailed my practice. Small animal practice was negligible.

I was very frustrated during these early years because I could not persuade the ranchers to pregnancy test. Most claimed they could determine if a cow was pregnant by looking and that by using eyeball diagnosis they had 95% calf crops. Perhaps some did have the exceptional calving percentages in that era of limited supplemental feeding, but I found there were a lot more 95% calf crops in coffee shops and beer joints than there were on the ranches.

The drouth-depressed prices of the 1950s had a big influence on my life. Many friends and a number of good clients went bankrupt. Several ranches changed hands. Some of the businesses in Marfa were forced to close their doors. My own personal finances were a disaster. There was a drastic change in the socio-economics of the area.

I sharpened hypodermic needles, scalpel blades, scissors, and clipper blades. I purchased chemicals in bulk, such as calcium gluconate, dextrose, sodium iodide, procaine HCl, chloral hydrate, magnesium sulfate, sulfonamides, atropine sulfate, gentian violet, acrifavine, potassium permanganate, and petrolatum. Distilled water was bought in five-gallon containers and mineral oil in 55-gallon drums. I saved, cleaned, and sterilized bottles, jars, vials, stoppers, and lids. I salvaged pump-type spray bottles from old Windex containers to administer thin liquids. Oil-type squirt cans were used with thicker liquids, and soda straws were used to blow and apply powders.

I mixed medicines, prepared and sterilized injectable fluids. Most pharmaceuticals used at that time were not so sophisticated. Oral medications were often put in gelatin capsules of various sizes and administered with a balling gun. Some were mixed with molasses or honey and placed on the tongue. Liquids by mouth were often given to large animals with a drench syringe, while larger quantities were mixed with water or mineral oil and given by stomach tube.

Cotton and silk sewing thread, as well as fishing line, were frequently used as suture material. These efforts were not highly rewarding, but some expense was saved. It taught me to be careful, but probably more important, it kept me busy so I would not brood on the inactivity and the resulting financial difficulties.

I tried maintaining a satellite clinic in each of Van Horn, Balmorhea, Fort Stockton, and Sanderson. I went to each of these places once a week but quickly saw that it was unprofitable. I then tried one day a month, but this was not very profitable either. However, I met many people and made friends who later became good clients. I only did this during my off-season, as I was usually better off staying in my office during the calving and shipping seasons, even though there was precious little to do.

As the drouth became worse and livestock prices lower, finances became tight, and often when we passed an ice cream place we became silent. I think Nancy's first words were at a time like this when she commented, "No money, no money."

I felt then and sometimes I still feel a little self-pity because these hard times deprived me of the practice and income during a time of my life that I thought should have been the most productive. Yet, perhaps this was really a blessing in disguise, as I was able to spend much time with my family in those early, precious, formative years of our marriage and our daughters' lives. Also, it may have taught all of us a lesson in thrift and gave me a good work ethic, although some would say I became a workaholic. Actually I just did what needed to be done when it was needed.

Later, it was difficult to find the time to be with them when my practice consumed almost twenty-four hours a day. Sometimes my days and nights would run together and my wife, JoAnn, would drive me while I slept, when I was overcome with fatigue.

We received some help from my parents. They would bring us canned goods that they bought on sale in case lots in San Angelo. Some of it was off brands, not very good quality and not very palatable, but we couldn't be too choosy.

JoAnn's father, Jim Tyler, kept our vehicles running at no

charge long after they were worn out. Dr. Stover, our physician, and Dr. Roy Slaton, the dentist, charged so little, it was almost gratis. Dr. John Pate in Alpine operated on both girls, tonsillectomies, at no charge. JoAnn and I set a personal budget of $125 a month for living expenses. Nothing was purchased on credit. Drugs and supplies were purchased only when I had the money.

Thoroughbred race horses were a problem for me in clinic duty at college. They were high strung, and most of their trainers and owners were also. Of course, there are exceptions as I learned later, but my first impressions and prejudices were hard to overcome. These horses seemed to be more susceptible to diseases, injury, and infection.

Hogs were another animal that I disliked. Their squeal was one of the most irritating sounds I ever heard, and their manure had the most repulsive odor. Most that I had known were fed garbage which may or may not have contributed to the odor. Another reason I disliked this animal may have been because they are most difficult to hold on to. They don't have any good handles. The greased pig contests that had been popular in my youth seemed to be a waste of time to grease those rascals. How anyone can tie those little short, stout legs with a *bosal de morrano* (hog knot), as a double half hitch is called, amazed me. It was paradoxical that these two animals were instrumental in my surviving the drouth, and thereby changing my attitude towards them.

The conditions caused many large animal veterinarians to abandon their country practice in the southwest. Actually there weren't very many to begin with. Because of the scarcity of large animal vets (and I would like to think, my reputation) it was not uncommon for horses, sometimes truckloads, to be brought to me from long distances, occasionally from New Mexico and Arizona. There were especially those wanting a standing castration and those needing a cryptorchid operation.

I finally reached a point during this time when I could no longer hold on. I could not support my wife and two little girls and also make payments on my notes. I had borrowed from the Marfa National Bank to purchase the veterinary hospital-residence and also from the Marfa Production Credit Association to buy calves that had lost money.

I had contacted friends at Texas A&M, Oklahoma A&M and Missouri State University. All three institutions had been encouraging as to a position on the veterinary school staff. A classmate, Elliot, had asked me to come to Houston in a small animal practice. I did not want to leave the area or quit practicing on large animals.

A job (not a position!) became available as a ranch veterinarian-livestock manager on a cattle and hog operation at Leon Farms near Fort Stockton. JoAnn wasn't enthusiastic about moving there, to put it mildly, and I wasn't anxious to become more closely involved with hogs than I was already, but when things are really hard you do what you have to do.

I contacted the ranchers that had co-signed my notes and asked their permission to close my practice and move there. Some said not to be in too big a hurry, but I told them I had probably put it off too long already.

Six local ranchers who were still holding on called me to the Paisano Hotel one night to the W.B. Mitchell's sons' office. This was Hayes and Joe Mitchell's place. George Jones, C.K. "Ken" Smith, his brother, T.E. "Tio" Smith and Kerr Mitchell were also there. They asked me to stock vaccines and other livestock remedies. They said they would buy these things from me and encourage others to do so. Then at the end of each month, I was to tell them how much additional funds I needed, and they would make up a kitty.

The nearest veterinarians were in El Paso, Odessa, San Angelo, and Del Rio. I didn't want to leave these men without a veterinarian, but I didn't have the funds to stock these items. Neither did I want to go in competition with the O.M. Franklin Company store here in town. This was not only a retail store but also the distributing point for a Franklin territory that extended from Sierra Blanca to Odessa, to San Angelo to San Antonio, down to Corpus Christi and Brownsville. Dr. A.J. Hoffman was the veterinarian in charge and had been with the company since its beginning in 1917 and had been in Marfa all that time. I went to him and told my story. He said there was no problem, that he would stock me on a consignment basis, and if I had an opportunity to sell more than I had in stock to send them to him and he would give me credit for the sale. I objected, saying that he could not do this, that it would get him in trouble with the company. He emphatically replied that he could do as he pleased because he owned the company! I learned later that he did own considerable stock in the company and had the freedom to operate as he saw fit.

The ranchers were true to their word, and my income from sales was sufficient so that I never had to ask for supplemental income.

Ralph Lowe and the Bar C Ranch Horses

Charlie Donaldson was a cowboy in the sandhills north of Odessa, Texas. Ralph Lowe, an oilman in Midland, bought a ranch in Colorado, and Charlie went up there to run the operation. In 1952, the ranch was sold and the Bar C Ranch near Kent, Texas was purchased. Charlie moved with the change in ownership.

When the ranch was stocked, good Hereford cows were bought at a time when a person should be selling instead of buying, but we didn't know that at the time. Don't they say that hindsight is 20-20? Times had been good, lots of rain, lots of grass, and cow prices had been going up and were at historic highs. We didn't know that the bubble was about to bust. The rains stopped. The grass disappeared. The price of feed went up, and the need for it increased while the price of cows went down.

Shortly after Charlie Donaldson came to the Kent ranch, Ralph Lowe bought some valuable thoroughbred race horses to be bred and raised on the ranch. Tex Sutton was brought in from Kentucky to care for the horses.

I took a dim view of all this because in my limited experience, these horses had been high strung, hyper-excitable, difficult to handle, and subject to injury and infection. However, the Lowe horses, the Reynolds Brothers' horses at the X Ranch near Kent, and those of Morgan Chaney at the San Francisco Ranch south of Marathon became a substantial part of my practice.

A foal was born with a severe bilateral inguinal hernia. I told Tex the only way I felt comfortable in repairing this was to include castration. We called Mr. Lowe who reluctantly gave his permission because the colt had excellent bloodlines and was potentially a valuable breeding animal. The surgery went well. The colt grew out and developed into a winning racehorse on the west coast. Mr. Lowe kept us posted on the horse's victories. I'm not sure if this was to show the success of the surgery or to chide us for having castrated him. Tex was sympathetic with our decision and rationalized that he probably would have been a hardheaded, hard-to-handle colt that would have necessitated castration anyway.

A few years later, Charlie and I were pregnancy testing cows when Tex came to us saying that a mare was having trouble foaling. We went to see her, and the colt's nose and both forefeet were out. Tex said he had tried to pull on the feet but nothing came. He was really excited because the colt was still alive and he was telling us all about how the mare and stud were out of so-and-so by such-and-such which didn't impress us. I wrapped the front feet with a gunny sack, applied obstetrical chains and attached the cattle calf puller. I thought Tex would have a stroke. "You can't do that to horses!" I told him I was going to do it or go back to Charlie's cows and kept right on pulling. When the legs were exposed, I moved the sacks and chains higher. The colt slipped right on out. The legs weren't hurt and he was up nursing soon with Tex still shaking his head and muttering, "You just can't do that to horses."

A very valuable mare died. Tex and I called Mr. Lowe to notify him. He said there wasn't any need for a postmortem as he accepted my diagnosis of a twisted gut. He didn't carry insurance on the horses because he felt the premiums on the number he had would not be cost effective. He thought he would be better off to self-insure. Mr. Lowe told us that it was too bad, but he had just completed a high producing oil well which would ease the pain of the loss.

On another occasion of a death loss, his reply to our report was that he had just shut down a duster, a dry hole, that cost him two hundred-fifty thousand dollars, so the loss of this horse was insignificant. I have always believed that ranchers and dry land farmers were the most resilient and philosophical people to adversity, but oilmen have got to be on a par.

The X Ranch Horses

The Reynolds brothers, John, Watt, and Will, owned the X Ranch at Kent, Texas. They arrived at their Gardner Place division from Fort Worth one day when Johnny Stewart, their horseman, and I were examining a thoroughbred filly foal. She had a high fever, loud, difficult breathing, profuse salivation, and nasal discharge. She was so weak that examination of the four-month-old filly was possible without sedation, which would have been dangerous in her condition.

I finally thought I could see something deep in her throat, and with considerable effort I was able to force my hand and arm deep enough to grasp a mesquite limb about fourteen inches long that she had tried to swallow. When it came out and we released her, she went down, as I had cut off her wind with my hand and arm so deep. A few pumps on her chest caused her to start breathing and she revived, but there was considerable bleeding. I knew by this there was quite a bit of tissue damage from the mesquite thorns, and the high fever showed that the torn area was infected.

Penicillin was injected in the muscle and sulfas given intravenously. I had seen recoveries in calves with this but did not think she could. I told the owners there was a poor chance of survival and no hope that she would be able to race because of the throat damage, even if she lived. The best we could hope for was use as a brood mare.

The Reynolds brothers watched quietly and thoughtfully, expressing their appreciation for my efforts. I left medication for Johnny to continue treating her because this was almost 100 miles from my office. Johnny told me she made a complete recovery and won a number of races, defying my prediction. I was told they named her "Mrs. W.D." for their mother. I wondered if their mother had suffered some type of throat problem or respiratory arrest at some time.

The thoroughbred stallion that was used to breed the mares at the Gardner was kept at the headquarters in a nice stall with adjacent exercise pen so that he could go in and out at will. The mares would be brought to him to be bred. He was the meanest looking and acting horse that I ever saw. When we drove up to his pen, he would greet us by squealing, rearing, and pawing the air, then charging towards me with teeth bared and eyes blazing. I was really scared of that horse, but Johnny Stewart would walk in the pen, snap on a halter shank and ignore the threats.

I was thankful that the owners only wanted stomach tube deworming and vaccinations once a year. At that time, two injections of sleeping sickness and tetanus vaccines were supposed to be given as boosters, but I only gave him one. I was concerned

that I might not be immunizing him properly, but later the rec-
ommendation was changed to a single booster once a year.

Morgan and Frances Chaney's Horses

Morgan Chaney and his wife, Frances, were two very remarkable people. They came from New London, Connecticut. They
had known Tom Mix well. Tom Mix was a real cowboy who had
become a Hollywood movie actor. He was not an actor or singer
turned cowboy for the movies. Perhaps you may ascertain from
this that he was my boyhood hero. He was! He was killed in a
fire attempting to rescue others. This may have had much to do
with my respect and friendship that I had for the Chaneys. Any
friend of Tom Mix was a friend of mine. However, this was not
all together the case, as I enjoyed their companionship.

Frances was an excellent cook and always fed me really well.
They were both good conversationalists and were so appreciative
of my services. I'm glad that I knew and visited with them at a
time when my practice was very slow, informal and relaxed.
Thus, I had the time to enjoy them as friends as well as clients.

Much of the ranch was on top of a high limestone mesa.
Morgan raised thoroughbred race horses. It seemed to me to be
the worst place possible to do so. There was grass, mostly Chino,
but lots of daggers, palmilla yuccas, catclaw, and ocotillo. But the
thing that really bothered me was the large amount of lechuguilla
which has crippled more horses than anything except barbed wire
and rocks. Rocks were also plentiful, mostly the slick rock common to limestone hills. When a colt was two years old, it was sent
up north to go into race training. Morgan explained that the main
expense of running horses was in the training and that many
broke down on the track after major expense was invested in
them. His philosophy was that a horse raised in this country was
tough, hearty, and had good feet and legs. Any that made it to
two years old would not break down in training or on the track.
He claimed his theory worked.

I had seen wild cows necked to burros and a few colts that kept
fighting a halter also necked to burros, but Morgan halter-broke
all his young horses this way. He used a bigger donkey than our
little Mexican burros and used an elaborate harness and halter rig
to buckle the two animals together while they were being held in

a specially constructed chute. They would be turned out into a big pen until the colt settled down and behaved. Then they would be turned out in a pasture together for a while. He said he never had a colt to slip out or choke down with that rig. A colt would squeal and kick at the donkey and occasionally the donkey would bite the colt. The donkeys did a good job. All the colts were easy to handle and lead.

Morgan was one of the few men who had good gentle horses to castrate. Also, we castrated his horses first class. The preparation included use of a casting harness, intravenous anesthetic containing chloral hydrate, magnesium sulfate and pentobarbital, a thorough surgical scrub, and tincture of iodine prep. I had my instruments in a disinfectant solution, and I scrubbed my hands, which was customary. Although at the Chaney ranch, I could do a much better job since I didn't have to throw and tie the horse, and I had more time. I used sterile sulfas in the incision and followed with tetanus antitoxin and penicillin as it became available. I was always thankful to get a good report.

Other Thoroughbred Horses

I had to modify my opinion of thoroughbred horses when Rube Evans moved here with his thoroughbred polo horses. They called them ponies, but I think this was more a common expression than descriptive. Rube used these horses for ranch work with any and all cowboys riding them. I never had any trouble handling them and they had no more problems than most ranch horses.

Rube took his polo playing pretty serious. He claimed that when he graduated from New Mexico Military Institute he was given a second lieutenant commission in the U.S. Army and a Ph.D. in polo playing.

* * * * *

Bart Evans was a student at Sul Ross and was a polo player with several thoroughbred polo ponies that he worked with when classes permitted. He was much like Rube Evans and treated his horses like horses. However, he would not allow me to use a twitch on their upper lip when I passed a stomach tube to deworm them. Instead, he would locate a rough rock about the size of a ping-pong ball, put it in the horse's ear and grasp it, applying pressure as needed to keep the horse quiet. This was a new version of twisting of the ear.

Hogs

Almost all the hogs in the early days of my practice were those kept on the ranch, one or two sows to raise pigs for home consumption. I didn't like them. They were kept in a small pen, most of which was a mud puddle wallow. There was no way they could be handled without getting filthy. The high-pitched squeal would nearly blow the top of my head off, and the odor of their manure was just awful. They were fed the house garbage plus a little corn that was soaked and soured. The Spanish goat is said to eat anything except meat. Well, the hog takes this one step further, eating anything that doesn't eat them first.

During the last years of my practice, hogs were no longer kept on ranches nor were chickens and milk cows, except for an occasional dogie cow, to raise orphan calves. It was even a rarity for people to fatten a calf for meat. The chickens and milk cows were no longer kept because it was cheaper and certainly a lot more convenient to buy milk, butter, eggs, and fryers at the store with transportation so easy. Barnyard hogs and fattening calves were still being kept until the local locker plants all closed.

There was a fellow down Limpia Canyon from Fort Davis who had a pretty good hog operation. They suddenly started dying, and he called me. I examined a few and posted a couple that all had typical textbook symptoms and lesions of hog cholera. Hog cholera caused considerable economic loss until it was eradicated. It was a fearsome, highly deadly viral disease that affected hogs only. He had been careful to feed only shipped-in commercial hog feed and purchased his boars from carefully selected breeders.

He had gone on a vacation and his help thought they were economizing and fed scraps from butcher shops and garbage from restaurants. Actually these were only cafes in this little town — none of the establishments could be dignified by calling them a restaurant. They were very pleased with themselves and bragged to the boss saying how they had saved him on his feed bill. The owner stopped the practice immediately, but it was too late. Some of the scraps or garbage had been contaminated, and hogs started dying.

This was one of the few times I telephoned for vaccine or medicine in those early days. Trans Texas Airlines had a regular route stop at the old Marfa Army Air Base. I received the vaccine promptly, which consisted of two injections, one of a live virus to stimulate immunity and a second of antiserum to prevent serious illness and death. The death loss stopped very soon. I had worn old clothes that I burned together with the empty vaccine bottles. I boiled all the equipment that had been used. The live virus and serum method of vaccination produced almost immediate immunity, whereas the killed vaccine took longer. However, this live virus could contaminate clean premises.

Fortunately, it did not spread, and this was the only hog cholera that I saw. I encouraged all to vaccinate with Crystal Violet, a brand of killed vaccine. I used this vaccine on a large, Chandler family, hog operation.

The Chandler family was very successful farming cotton in the area between Balmorhea and Pecos, known as the Pecos Valley. Cotton farming was very profitable in the Pecos Valley during the fifties. Cotton thrives on hot dry weather if it is irrigated. Irrigation water had recently been tapped with wells, and virgin grassland started to be farmed. It was very productive at first, much of it producing five bales to the acre.

The price of cattle had gone down drastically during the drouth, but hog prices held up fairly well, so the family put in a 500 sow operation. They called me to see if I would take care of their operation. I needed the income and told them I would be glad to. The man they got to take care of the hogs was a *bracero*, a Mexican national, who had been processed and was legal. This man was very knowledgeable regarding hogs. He could do almost anything except read and write or speak English. He was very congenial and hardworking. He taught me a great deal. I don't know if he was one of their farm hands and they just lucked out or if they recruited him in Mexico.

The first group of baby pigs to be weaned was placed in new pens on fresh ground. There were good feed and water troughs with no muddy wallow. I thought this ideal until the dry condition of the white powdery soil caused a dust problem, resulting in a high incidence of dust pneumonia.

The first major outbreak occurred rather suddenly with several deaths and a large number sick. Previously we had treated most illnesses with sulfamethazine solution added to the feed or mixed with the water. But we discovered this was not practical in the baby pigs, as they were neither eating nor drinking. We tried giving it as a drench by mouth with poor results. I had not used penicillin in hogs yet, but its price had been reduced somewhat. Also, a new antibiotic, streptomycin, had recently become available, but I had not read of its use in hogs. I had just received a shipment and because of a misunderstanding, more came than the small amount I had intended. I did not know the dosage, safety or efficacy in hogs, but in those days new drugs were being developed and made available with little testing and less information. Many of us felt our way along, especially those of us in isolated areas. At that time there were little or no legal ramifications to a drug's use or misuse.

I began treating the pigs, chalking them with one color for penicillin and another for the streptomycin, using different size doses. I was trying to determine the best drug for the least cost.

The work was rather hectic because of the large number of pigs being presented to me by several handlers. I accidentally added streptomycin to a 60cc syringe that was half full of penicillin. I was afraid this was a disaster, but the drugs were too expensive to discard. I was concerned that this combination might be toxic, so I administered a minimum dose and put an obvious mark on them so they would be easy to identify. It was late when I finished, but I took the time to check this group especially carefully. All were still alive with no evidence of a reaction.

This hog operation was seventy miles from my office, but I was there at daylight, anxious to see the results. The group that received the combination was already better: several eating and drinking and no death loss. There was little if any improvement in the other two groups, and a few had died. I retreated the entire bunch with the combination. All responded extremely well, and the cost was less than had been anticipated.

I began using the combination on cattle routinely, with excellent results. I was very tentative in my use in horses, dogs and cats but soon gained confidence in its safety and efficacy. A major drug company, Pfizer, soon marketed this combination under the trade name, Combiotic. This product did not have the exact same proportions and was more expensive than mine, so I continued to use and dispense my formulation. Gradually the company reduced their price, and my practice became too busy for me to mix mine. Streptomycin was soon marketed as dihydrostrepto-mycin. The Federal Drug Administration removed this drug from the approved list in the mid-eighties.

The hog operation was very profitable for both the owners and me for several years until atrophic rhinitis occurred and became increasingly severe, so the operation was terminated.

The Joe Bishop Cow

Joe Bishop sent word to me to come see a sick cow at his Jap Camp place. This was down the Casa Piedra road just past the end of the pavement about a mile. The cow was in a little chicken coop type of pen, flimsy. The cow was badly tucked up (gut empty) and hollow-eyed. Her tongue was out about a foot and swollen. "What do ya think, Doc?" I answered, "Looks bad, doesn't she?" "Now, Doc, what'll it cost to fix her up?" I replied, "Mr. Joe, I don't know what's wrong with her. We'll have to snub her to a post and examine her, then treat accordingly." He kept asking questions, and I finally told him it would cost $5.00 to examine her, another $5.00 if I gave an intravenous bottle of sodium iodide if she had *woody tongue*, and another $2.50 if I passed a stomach tube to give her some water and a little gruel. She had about a 50-50 chance of survival as weak as she was. Also, he already had $4.00 for my trip of 20 miles from town. He said she wasn't worth it, so I offered to take her for the vet bill, thinking this would call his bluff. He agreed and offered to loan me his trailer to take her back to the hospital. In fairness to Joe, I should mention that this was during the worst days of the drouth, and the cow probably wasn't worth more than $45 if she was at a market. That was a problem at this time because the only practi-cal way to get a cow the 200 to 250 miles to a market was by send-ing a truck load at a time.

It was a pitiful little homemade affair with sides about 4 feet high. I hooked onto it and backed up to the gate of the pen, opened it and the trailer gate, then spooked the cow, who stum-bled in. I closed the trailer gate, said my goodbyes, and took off for town poking along slowly, hoping the trailer would make it.

Shortly after I went onto the main Presidio highway, a carload of drunks passed me, yelling and honking. The cow jumped out of the trailer and ran or rather wobbled down the lane. I drove up beside her and penned her to the fence. I put a rope on her horns, snubbed her to a post, then backed the trailer up against her tightly until she jumped in again. I tied her head down so she couldn't jump out again and made it to the hospital. I determined that she did have woody tongue, and she responded to treatment just like they're supposed to.

I hauled her to Dick Swartz's ranch where I had a pasturing agreement. I examined her and was surprised that she was about four months pregnant and should calve in the spring. It always amazed me how much a cow could go through without aborting. Also, sodium iodide will usually make a cow abort except when you want it to, then it never does.

That summer she still hadn't produced a calf. I examined her, and she was open. That fall, when I examined my other cows, she was pregnant again. Next spring she looked a little tucked up. I examined, and she wasn't pregnant. That fall, she was pregnant, and against conventional wisdom, I decided to give her another chance. The next spring, Dick called me saying that he had shot my cow and explained. While riding his pasture he had seen the cow hooking a dead calf. He rode over and observed that she had recently calved and decided that the calf was stillborn, and the cow was trying to make it get up by hooking with her long horns. A few days later he was in his pickup truck and saw her hooking another cow's calf that was not dead, not gently but viciously. He got out his 30-30 rifle and shot the bitch. I agreed he had done the right thing.

I had just about convinced Dick of the value of pregnancy testing, and I was afraid this little episode might throw a wrench in the works, undoing all my progress. However, Dick had let me check a little bunch of cows that hadn't had a calf that year and they had either calved or failed to calve according to my test results. This, together with the results of his entire herd the next year, made a believer out of him. He hadn't been bashful about telling everyone the benefits of the tests.

Off-Duty

Meeting the Southern Pacific passenger train in the evenings was a big event. The steam locomotive with the large drive wheels, the rush of the steam release. I didn't understand why this was done, but it certainly was spectacular. The steam whistle and the bell were never quite equaled by the horn of the later diesel engines. Observing passengers getting off and others boarding, using the small step placed for their use. The conductor calling, "All aboard." Speculating where and why the travelers were going or had been. Negro Chaney with the baggage and mail cart. The chug as the train began to move and increasing clicky-clack as the wheels passed over the joints of the rails. This was exciting.

Some very special occasions during the hard years of the drouth were celebrated by going to the Palace Theater or the Drive-In theater (which was next to the cemetery) with popcorn and a root beer soda pop. Another treat was a hamburger at Sixto's, but the greatest was a Mexican supper at Carolina's. Sometimes an ice cream cone eaten while riding up and down the main street.

We spent many hours together on hikes — actually we were only strolling along, prowling. JoAnn would fix a picnic lunch that Nancy, Janet and I would help her eat. JoAnn walked with us until one day on Carpenter Mountain she found four rattlesnakes beside the trail that the girls and I had just passed. That was the last time she went walking with us. She sat in the pickup, reading and worrying about us.

Indian artifacts have intrigued me as long as I can remember. The ability of people to survive in this arid area amazed me, but most of the evidence of their presence showed they were nomadic and probably only came during the rainy season. I was able to find a fairly nice collection.

Miller Robison owned the San Esteban Ranch that had a big lake that stayed full even in the worst of the drouth because what little rain fell came in gully washers and ran off the barren land. He sold fishing memberships but gave me one in exchange for treating his animals.

Manny Howard gave us access to a little dam with a nice pool of water a few miles down Alamito Creek. We would catch perch and fry them on the spot. Nancy and Janet would swim and wade in the water.

Visiting

Early in my practice, Dr. Gearhart suggested that I join the ranchers for early morning coffee at the Crews Hotel. His purpose was two-fold, first, to become acquainted and second, to educate them on services I could perform. These proved to be a definite advantage and served the intended purpose, but my entertainment was not the least of the benefits. Some very colorful stories and interesting management, political, and philosophical theories were expounded. I'm sure much of what these old timers discussed influenced my practice and my life.

I continued to join them after I married and until the financial situation of the drouth resulted in my no longer feeling comfortable in spending the small amount for coffee, especially on the days when I felt it was my turn to pick up the tab. I may have been a little self-conscious and paid more than my share. Soon, the Crews Hotel closed, a casualty of the drouth.

Henry Coffield and Clyde McFarland were regulars. N.B. "Nat" Chaffin, Joe Bunton when he was here from his ranch in Mexico, Ingram Mills, George Jones, Frank Jones, Worth Evans were frequent.

Visiting was always a great pastime, especially in the early days but almost always in conjunction with my professional calls. We did belong to a bridge club that was more a social gathering than a serious card game.

After the hospital and residence were purchased in 1953 and we moved there, I often invited clients into our kitchen which was so handy for coffee or ice tea and a snack during consultations, which were gratis, as I considered them educational and practice builders. They were informal visits, and many that were friends were invited to a meal with us. Later the pressures of the practice prevented this.

Mr. Espy Miller, who ranched west of Valentine, was visiting in the kitchen when my younger daughter, Janet, joined us. She was a little tyke and had not yet started school. She climbed up in a chair opposite him, rested her elbows on the table with her chin in her hands, and studied him a long time. She finally said, "You have a lot of hair in your ears." He politely acknowledged the fact. JoAnn and I were embarrassed, and I immediately began talking to hide it. Soon she commented, "You sure have bushy eyebrows." Espy said, "They are, aren't they?" He didn't seem disturbed, but JoAnn and I both were, and Janet was hustled off to a back room before she could make any more comments.

Along in the 1950s, we had a Methodist preacher who was raised country and liked to go on calls with me. Rev. Tomlinson made a pretty good hand, too. We returned one afternoon, not yet having eaten, so JoAnn prepared us a meal. She did that a lot, making meals at awkward hours when I came in late, often dragging someone in with me.

Janet hadn't started school yet and she got up from her nap and joined us, climbing up in her favorite chair. She looked at Rev. Tomlinson a long time very seriously, finally telling him very emphatically that he shouldn't yell in church, that it was God's house. He did have a tendency to get rather loud when making a point. He asked, "Do I really sound that loud?" She replied, "You sure do, I can't sleep." The preacher didn't seem perturbed, but told her, "Now, if I get too loud, you hold up your hand, and I'll be quieter." Janet agreed that she would and was satisfied. JoAnn and I were mortified. We felt that Rev. Tomlinson assumed we had been raking him over the coals after church each Sunday, criticizing his sermon. After that we sat with Janet between us, ready to grab her hand if she started to raise it. She never did, but the sermons were a little more subdued after that.

Hunting Rabbits

There were enormous numbers of jack rabbits in the fifties. Some speculated that the numbers were caused by a natural cycle, but others thought it was because of vigorous control of predators, especially coyotes and eagles. There were many sheep and goats in the area at that time. Also, many thought they preyed on baby calves and newborn foals. Other predators were also hunted, such as lions, bobcats, and fox.

The drouth of the fifties caused the grass to vanish and the other plants to diminish. This absence of cover allowed the rabbits to be revealed as there were fewer places to hide. Extension agents advised that rabbits ate a large amount of grass for their size, and it was said twenty-five rabbits would eat as much as one cow. The large numbers of rabbits made a major impact because of the small amount of grass. Rabbits also have a destructive method of eating, in that they bite off the grass near the ground and eat the tender nutritious portion and discard the upper bulk. C.K. Smith furnished ammo and a pickup to his grandson, Sammy Humphreys, and some of his friends to hunt rabbits. They claimed to have killed 800 one weekend. I don't doubt this as there were very large numbers.

The drouth had reduced my practice drastically, and I had a lot of idle time. I often took my family jack rabbit hunting as most ranchers would allow me, even encourage me. JoAnn, Nancy, and Janet became very good shots. I possessed a semi-automatic 22-rifle but bought a single shot one. I wanted them to become adept at loading and ejecting. Also the slow, methodical procedures improved marksmanship, but the principle reason was to be frugal with ammunition. There is a tendency to fire many rounds when it's so easy just to pull the trigger.

Reading

I soon realized that graduation and obtaining my license to practice was only the beginning of my education. I have often said that I wish that I was as smart as the day I graduated. I suppose that published articles on poison plants was what I concentrated on most at first, although my limited practice (not by choice, just not yet developed) allowed me to read extensively regarding each case. I subscribed to all veterinary journals that were printed at that time and a few human medical journals, looking for broad subjects, particularly pharmaceuticals and especially antibiotics that were being developed so rapidly. This may seem like extensive reading, but the so-called information explosion was only beginning. I still had a great deal of free time which really increased as the drouth reduced my practice that had only recently began to expand. Television was in its infancy and not available in Marfa. Radio reception was never really good in these mountains until late in the evenings, and even then such shows as *Amos and Andy, The Inner Sanctum, Fibber Magee and Molly, Bob Hope*, and *Red Skelton* did not use much of the evening.

Big Band music could be enjoyed while reading. I read a great deal for enjoyment, by writers such as Mark Twain, O'Henry, Rudyard Kipling, Zane Gray, Rudolph Mellard, Winston Churchill's books on World War II and many other historical books such as *The Great River*.

Chapter 5

Shortly After the Drouth

In the late 1950s, when it finally began raining, Mike Shurley was riding with his father, Bill, in a pickup at the ranch. He was a pretty big kid and often rode with his dad. As they rode along, he began asking Bill what something was that he was seeing in the pasture. Bill would answer sacahuiste, cardentia*, dagger, yucca, and so forth. Each time Mike would answer, "No, that!" Bill finally stopped the pickup and had Mike show him the object in question. Mike got out of the pickup, walked over and pointed directly at some green grass. Poor little kid. He was six, maybe eight years old, and had never seen green grass out in the pasture.

*   *   *   *   *

C.K. "Kenneth" Smith was always a strong supporter of the Highland Hereford Bull Sale and always had bulls consigned to the sale. After he sold out, he kept only two registered cows, Miss Puritan and Miss Starr. These he pastured with the county agent and good friend, Jim Bob Steen. He also would buy good bull prospects from other registered breeders as calves, grow them out and fit them, then consign them to the sale. The sale auctioneer once commented that Ken was a remarkable breeder having only two cows, yet five bulls to consign. Ken replied, "That's nothing. I heard old timers tell that in the early days, there were men that came to this country with nothing but two old oxen pulling a wagon—yet, they had 100 calves that fall."

Electronic Ejaculator

Sometime in the late 1950s, an electronic ejaculator was developed at the Southwest Research Center in San Antonio by Dr. Marden. I was told the original purpose was to collect semen from monkeys. A severe freeze in Colorado had frozen the scro-

---

* Also called cardenche, cholla or cane cactus.

187

tum of many bulls, and there was a question as to whether this resulted in infertility. Colorado State University at Fort Collins invited Dr. Marden to come and attempt to modify his instrument for use on bulls. He was successful, and many bulls were tested, revealing a rather high percentage of infertile bulls, although I understand that the frozen scrotums did not seem to be the cause.

The results of this testing became known to Joe Lane, and, being the progressive rancher that he was, he urged me to offer this service. The instrument cost $500 which was quite a sum at that time for me since I was poor as a church mouse, still suffering from the effects of the drouth. There was other equipment that was also needed, but another problem was the distance to Fort Collins, Colorado which was the only place to receive instruction. I told Joe there was no way I could do it. He persisted, and when the Colorado State team held a short course at the veterinary college at Texas A&M, I went. I believe there were 8 or 10 of us in attendance, several of whom were instructors at the college or associated with the Agricultural Extension Service.

I was thoroughly convinced of the value and practicality, even though it necessitated an electric generator, incubator box, and microscope, besides the ejaculator and other minor items. The college, Woodrow Sharpe from Castroville, and I ordered ejaculators. Therefore, to the best of my knowledge, I had one of the first three in Texas, at Joe's prodding. It was not only a profitable venture for me, but an invaluable service to the area ranchers. We all had Joe to thank.

A Not-So-Typical Work, Thankfully

The Circle Dot Ranch in Terrell County northeast of Sanderson was one of the ranches that had restocked after we thought the drouth had broken, then experienced dry times. The ranch was negotiating with a man in South Dakota for the sale of a substantial number of cows to lighten their stocking rate. They requested that I determine my fees for complying with the health regulations for the shipment so that a selling price could be determined.

This was another instance where an extravagant telephone call replaced the letter with the three-cent stamp because everyone was in a panic to hurry things up. So I called the State Veterinarian in South Dakota for their requirements. He stated that brucellosis and tuberculosis testing, in addition to the customary standard health certificate would be necessary. I calculated my charges for the tests per head plus two calls to the ranch because I would need to return in 72 hours to inspect the injection site for the tuberculosis test.

A selling price was quickly agreed on, and I was notified of the date the cows would be available. I took the blood for the brucellosis test and made the tuberculin injection. The night before I was due to return to read the TB tests, I received a call from a client wanting me to test a large number of cows the next day for pregnancy. I had a very tight schedule and did not think I could work these into it. But it would be a nice income, and I hated to lose out as I was still deeply in debt from the drouth years. The Circle Dot was about 150 miles from Marfa, and the potential pregnancy testing was in the opposite direction.

Fritz Kahl agreed to fly me. There was no landing strip at the ranch, but the nearby county road would serve the purpose. The rancher met the plane, and we went with him to the working pens. Reading the test required that the cows be run through the chute and that I feel of each individual at the base of the tail. This was time consuming, but we got along pretty well and were on schedule when we returned to the plane. Lo and Behold! The blooming county road maintenance crew had been there and torn up the road. They had left a little passage way next to the fence for vehicles, but there was no way we could take off. We had to cool our heels until they returned. I think the rancher went and hustled them back. I don't remember how long we waited, but it was too long and I missed the cow work that I had hoped to do. Every time after that when traveling the dirt roads in Terrell County and I hit a chuckhole, I would think evil thoughts towards the county road maintenance crew.

To add insult to injury, I soon afterwards received a letter from South Dakota raking me over the coals for not having complied with their requirements that all Texas cattle be sprayed with CoRal insecticide before entering South Dakota. I was mad as a wet hen because I had talked to them only a short time before and nothing was said regarding CoRal. Their letter stated the cows would be kept in quarantine, and they would no longer honor my health certificates. I wrote a hot letter but called the Texas State Veterinarian before sending it. He sympathized with me stating the new regulation had only been instituted the day before my health certificate date. He explained that a large shipment of freshly dehorned and castrated steers had been shipped there from San Antonio. They were full of screwworm eggs that hatched, causing worm cases which spread rapidly. Screwworms were unknown in that cold climate, but the introduction in the summertime had caused a widespread epidemic. The people in the area didn't know how to prevent and watch for cases, much less how to treat them. Actually, there were no screwworm medicines available in that area. He said relations between the two states were strained, and it would probably be best to let things cool off. If I absolutely needed to ship cattle to South Dakota within the next six months to call him.

Brucellosis Testing for Eradication

A nationwide program for the eradication of brucellosis was started in the late 1950s. We were told this area was first to begin testing in the state of Texas. This necessitated drawing a blood sample (from the jugular vein at that time) into a numbered glass tube and applying a numbered metal eartag to the ear. And, we would usually put a chalk mark number on the side or back for easy, temporary identification. Many ranchers refused to have government men do this and insisted on my services. I was compensated on a per head basis.

Truman Foster would put his cows in cotton fields after the cotton had been picked. Before mechanical pickers, the picking was by hand and many bollies* and leaves remained in the fields besides weeds and annual grasses. This provided excellent grazing for relatively short periods. There were no working pens in these fields, and cattle would be driven horseback from field to field.

Because there were no permanent pens in these cotton fields, temporary, makeshift facilities were constructed. Well, maybe not constructed, thrown together may more clearly describe the technique. There were few squeeze chutes in the fifties, and portable ones were very rare. Most of the time we used a headgate made by Keezy Kimball of Alpine. It consisted of 2×8 lumber with ropes and pulleys and had a hay rake tine for a spring. This was tied to

---

* Immature cotton bolls.

the front of the crowd chute with ropes. This headgate was to catch each cow's head.

One day the ropes holding the headgate broke after the head was caught, and the cow charged off wearing the headgate like a necklace. We did not have a horse. Escapees would be driven on foot back to the pens for a second attempt. This cow did not cooperate, just trying to get into our shirt or hip pocket, depending upon whether we tried to stand our ground or were running from her. We finally hemmed her against the fence with the use of several pickups. We tested her and retrieved the headgate.

The next work, H. McDermott was horseback beside the chute, ready to rope any that escaped. A big, stout, crossbred brahma-type cow with long horns hit the front of the chute going ninety to nothing and Truman, who was working the headgate, missed her, but H. was ready and roped her. He had a big loop to go over the long horns and caught the cow pretty deep, giving the cow lots of leverage. The rope was tied hard and fast to the saddle horn so that when the cow hit the end of the rope, something was bound to give. It was the saddle girth. The saddle was jerked off the horse, and it flew through the air with H. still riding it. It hit the ground, bounced a little, and the cow never slowed down. H. hung on while being pulled across the big lot with us yelling encouragement to "Ride her, cowboy!"

The Wooden Headgate

This headgate was a time saver, but I had more than my share of problems with it. I didn't have the time or opportunity to visit with others who used it. Perhaps they had equal problems.

A cow that initially escaped from the chute was an aggravation but usually no injury resulted. I would stand to one side, out of the way, until the head was caught in the scissor-like headgate. Then a man would stabilize it with nose tongs and the neck bent to one side. I would then squat down in front, insert the bleeding needle into the jugular vein, and allow blood to flow into the glass test tube.

The fast and furious pace, together with fatigue late in the day, caused some wrecks. Sometimes the nose tongs would slip out, a kink in its rope would straighten or break. This would allow the head to swing around, causing a horn to jab me or the cow's head to slam into mine. The cow's head was harder! On occasion, the rope holding the neck bars closed would slip or break, releasing the cow that would then run over me.

I guess the worst injury was once when the rope holding the headgate to the front of the chute broke suddenly, and the cow with the headgate still on her came through on top of me. It probably wouldn't have been so bad if both sides had come loose, but instead, one side held fast while the cow jumped around trying to get away. She stomped me pretty good. I was lean at the time, and I suppose I should have had a ruptured spleen. I was sore all over. How can you limp when all parts are hurting? I still had a pen full of cows to test that had been a problem to gather. Therefore, I felt I had to finish. The first few were painfully slow until I began to work the soreness out. I was able to finish and drove back home. I was really glad there were no patients waiting. I thought I had recovered until I climbed out of the pickup. I was so stiff I could hardly walk. I walked around a little, then unloaded the blood samples and equipment. I centrifuged the blood and ran the tests. The plate agglutination tests were still being performed, and I was pleased that all three dilutions were negative. I called the rancher to report the results, and we breathed a sigh of relief.

I went in the house and announced that I was taking a bath. JoAnn's comment was that it wouldn't be a waste of time, that I really needed it. I filled the tub with water as hot as I could stand it and soaked until the water got cold, then I let it out and refilled with hot water. I fell asleep in the tub and JoAnn awakened me. I took four aspirin, ate supper, and went to bed. Morning came too soon. I started to take another hot soaking bath but realized I just had time to load the pickup, take my previous day's samples by the trailer with the portable state-federal lab and be on my way to another herd of cattle.

Very little brucellosis was found in the area, but the hassle of retesting periodically was a possibility that kept us on edge until the blood was tested. Of course, I could not be completely at ease until the state-federal laboratory confirmed my tests.

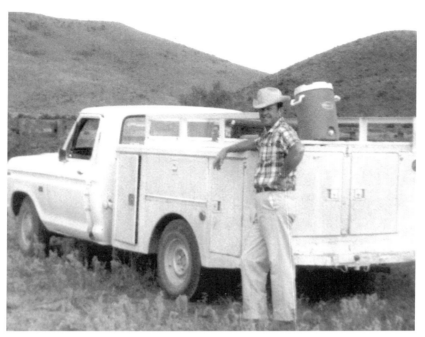

Practice pickup.

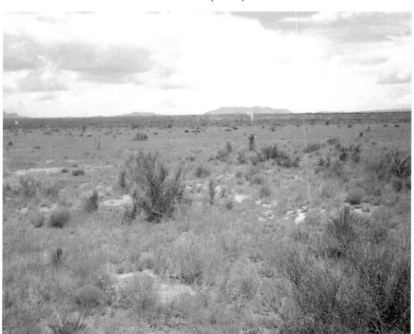

Marfa Plateau.

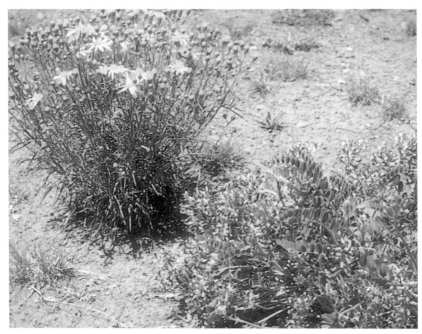

Senecio (left) and loco (right).

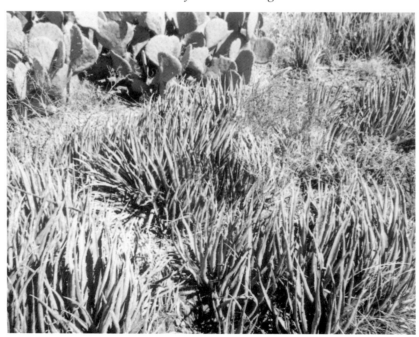

Lechuguilla with prickly pear in background.

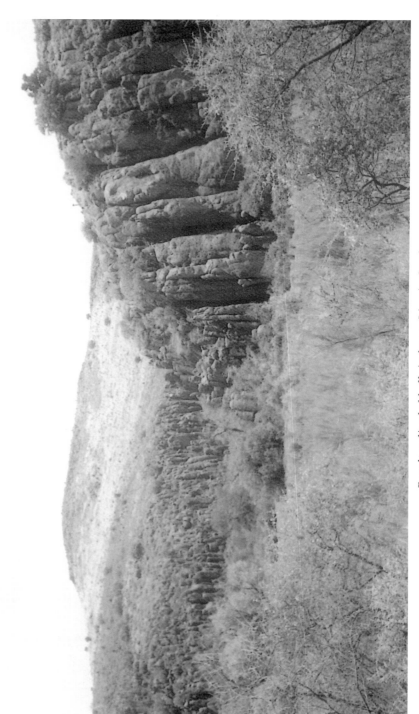

Basalt palisade bluffs in lower Limpia Creek.

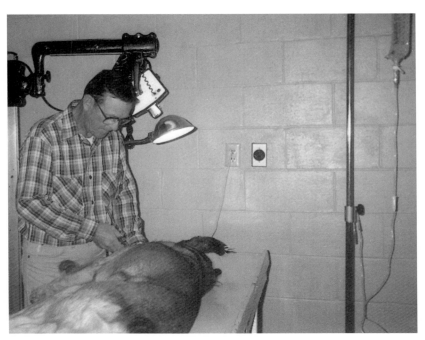

Starting an intravenous.

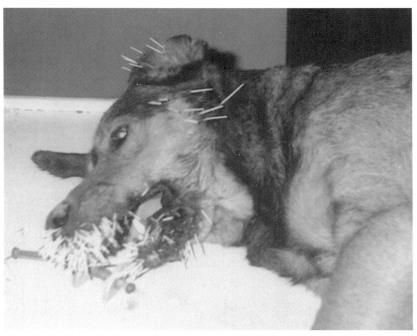

Porcupine quills.

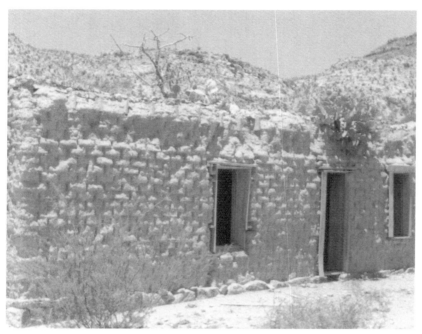

Victim of the drouth.

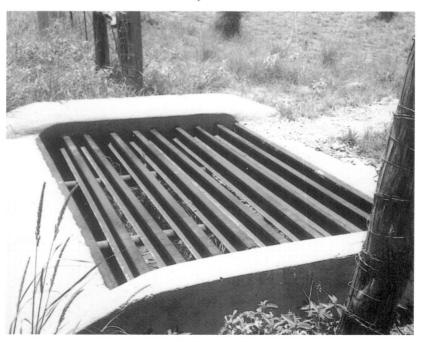

Cattle guard.

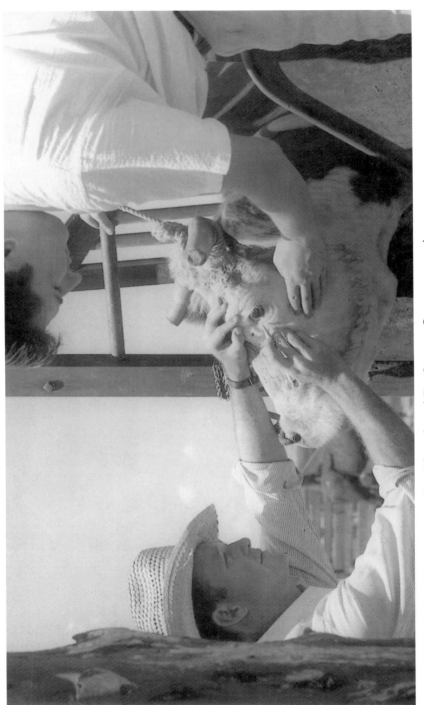

Dr. Edwards and Dr. Queen - Cancer eye seminar.

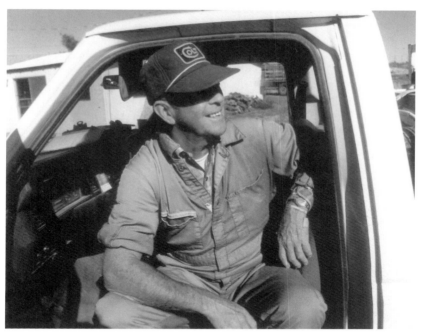

Watching a cowboy running from a fighting cow.

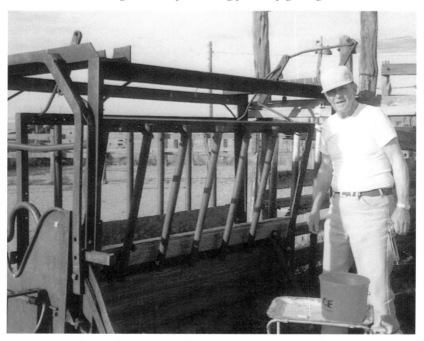

Ready for first cow beside Turner squeeze chute.

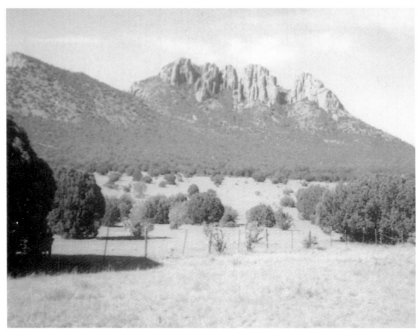

Sawtooth Mountain near Rockpile.

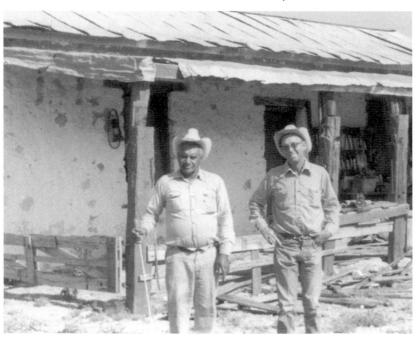

A couple of cowhands at the Post Headquarters:
Blas Payne (left) and Bubber Mathers.

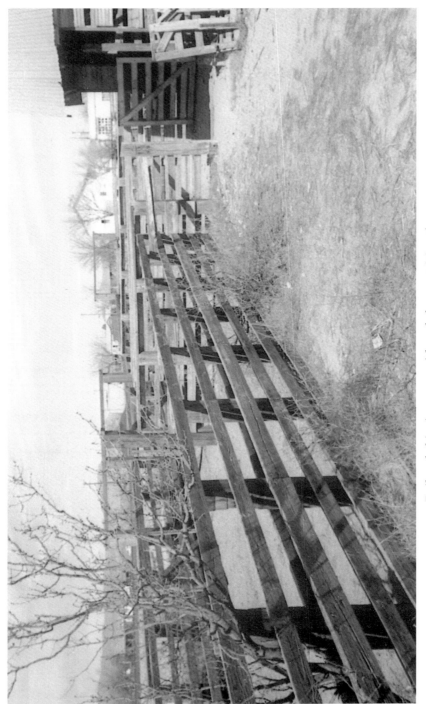

Railroad shipping pens with scale house at Marathon.

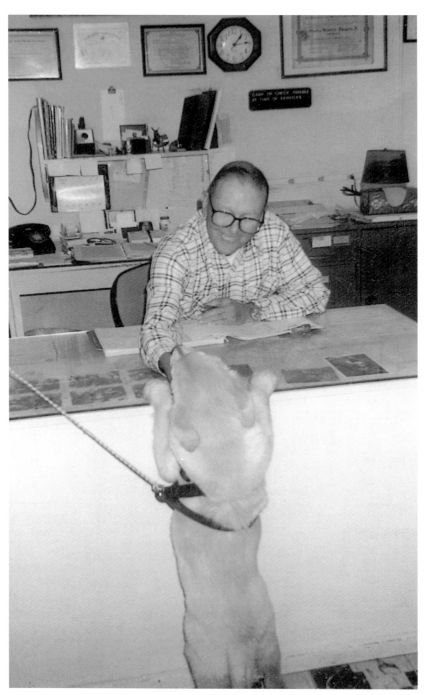

Consultation.

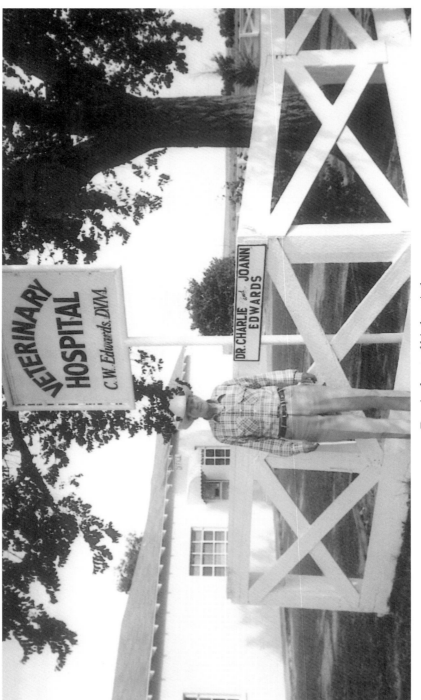

Doc in front of his hospital.

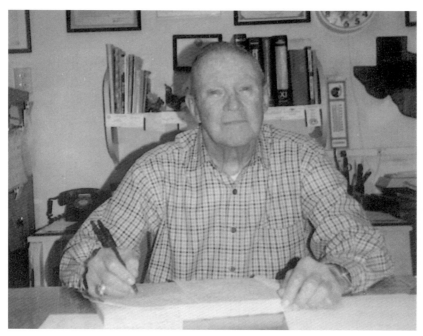

Doc at reception desk doing bookwork.

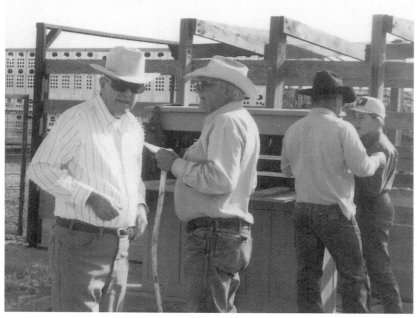

Shipping calves at the Brite Ranch on a "pot" truck.
(left to right) Doc, Jim White, Mac White, Raphael White.

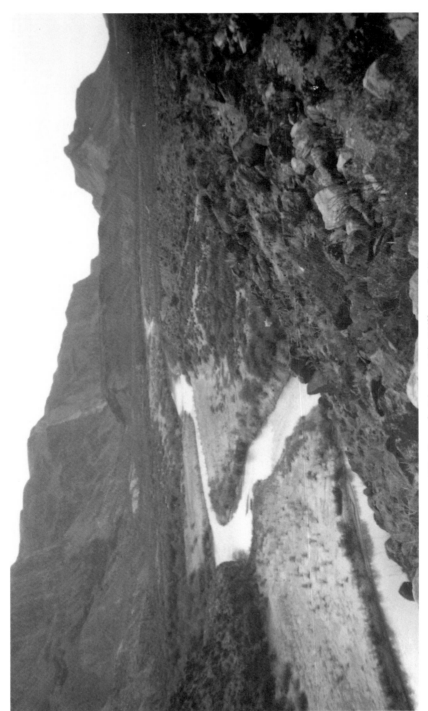

Rio Grande River at Big Hill near Lajitas.

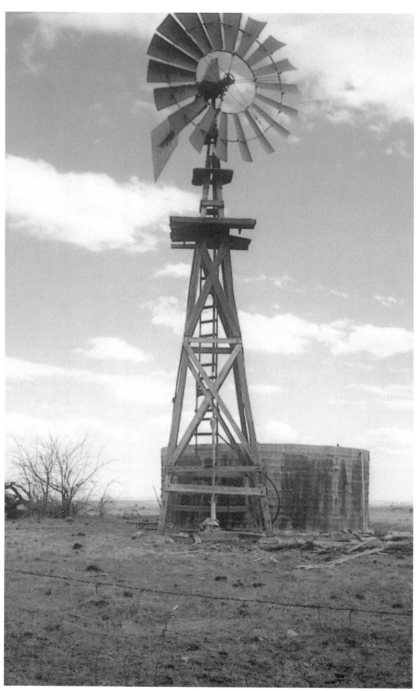

Windmill and storage tank.

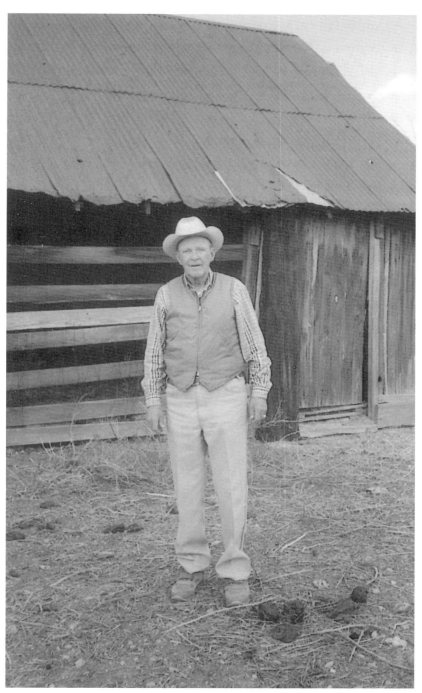

Rare luxury, a calving shed.

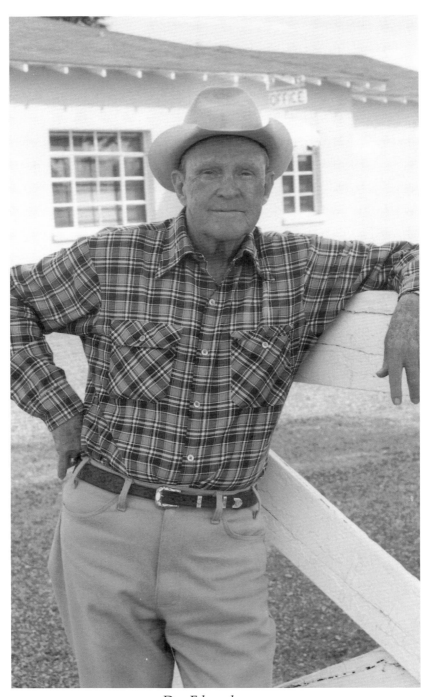

Doc Edwards now.

Chapter 6

Up to My Armpits

Much of the time I was up to my armpits either figuratively or literally. The large number of animals and the distances caused such long days and short nights that at times I felt like I was going twenty-four hours a day, seven days a week.

Actually, I was up to my armpits delivering a calf, treating a retained afterbirth, or down a cow's throat extracting a foreign object — in addition to the time spent palpating for pregnancy.

Palpation is the diagnosis of a condition or state by touching or feeling with the hands. In a cow country this term is frequently applied to the procedure when a veterinarian inserts the hand and usually the arm, sometimes up to the shoulder, into the rectum in order to feel the uterus for evidence of pregnancy. We first called it pregnancy testing or checking.

My first introduction to the procedure was at John Tarleton Agricultural College at Stephenville by Dr. Verne A. Scott, the elder, in 1942. He was a professor at the college, teaching Animal Husbandry and Dairy Husbandry. He was also the college veterinarian. He was the inspector at the local locker plant which was a small slaughter house, that butchered, packaged, froze and stored meat. His private practice was limited to spare time which usually meant night calls. I worked with him in my spare time. It probably hurt my grades, but I did not think of their importance except to pass and get on with other things, concentrating only on that which interested me and which I thought would be valuable. Dr. Scott impressed on me the value of pregnancy diagnosis and allowed me to have hands-on experience. I also was *privileged* to hold the calcium gluconate bottle on a cold winter night or wallow around in a pig pen delivering babies since his hands were much too large, and mine were just the right size. He didn't pay me, but I was introduced to the practical aspects of veterinary medicine and gained valuable experience as he explained procedures. Mrs.

Scott often fed me, and sometimes I would get a midnight snack.

In the Big Bend-Davis Mountain area the calf crop percentages were exceptionally good, although I discovered they weren't quite as good in most cases as many of the claims that were made. However, I could elicit no interest and didn't really push it until the drouth of the fifties caused many to begin selling cattle to reduce their numbers. I still couldn't get much interest as they doubted my accuracy and suspected that it would cause abortion, if not by my hand, just the stress of putting a cow through the chute. There were a few ranchers in the rough country and especially along the river who felt, like my father did, that a cow should not have a calf every year, because if she does, it will be a little scrawny thing and no account. However, if she rests a year, she will produce a good calf.

When the drouth ended and ranchers began restocking, a definite interest was shown in pregnancy determination. I'm not sure of all the factors, but locally, Dick Swartz in Fort Davis, where I had been pregnancy palpating for several years, was very vocal in telling of my success with his cows.

Cole and Alf Means in Valentine, Bill Donnell in Marathon, and J.M. "Manny" Fowlkes in the Van Horn area were all influential men who were some of the first to use and advocate my service. They, together with Dr. Ben Gearhart, had much to do with the acceptance of the practice.

While I Was Working

A group of deer hunters were watching me check cows. They had their noses wrinkled up. One, a dentist, commented that it was sure nasty work. I answered that it wasn't nearly as bad as sticking one's hand in a person's mouth. He thought a moment and agreed.

I tried to convince those that believed it to be very repulsive, that it was only grass and water. It wasn't dirty until it got on the ground.

I was testing cows with one hand and smoking with the other. My father watched a few minutes, finally saying, "I hope I never want a cigarette that bad!"

I was pregnancy testing heifers in a Turner squeeze chute at the

McMinn pens for Jim White. Now Jim had watched me do this for some time and knew that I had done it many years at different ranches all over the area. He said kinda serious-like, "Charlie, if you die before I do, I'm going to have a picture chiseled on your tombstone showing you up to your armpit in the rear end of a cow that was trapped in an old worn out Turner squeeze chute. There won't be any need for a name, everyone will know who it is!"

Once in a while somebody would run a bull or steer in while I was working fast and furious. Everybody would have a big laugh when I became frustrated because I couldn't find the plumbing. Occasionally, rocks were put in the rectum. These pranks didn't usually bother me because a break with a little humor makes the work pleasant. Of course, when it was done repeatedly it ceased to be funny, and I would declare that the next would cost the ranch an extra $10. This would put a stop to it. I found a tin can and a bottle on occasion. These didn't upset me, but once a prickly pear leaf stuck a thorn in my finger, and I wouldn't test her. How they got it in there was beyond me.

Freemartins would cause me some concern. They are uncommon, so I'm not expecting them. They have the external genitalia of a female but no ovaries, uterus or cervix.

When I first began practice, the available glove-sleeve combination, called a large animal obstetrical glove, was thick, heavy rubber. I tried to use it for calf deliveries, especially when it was very cold, but I was unable to get a good grip on parts of the calf. I would try to use it when pregnancy palpating, but I could not distinguish the features and determine pregnancy except when the fetus was very large, so I soon abandoned any attempt to use it and worked with bare hands and arms.

When I was checking with bare arms, a delay would really be miserable with the cold and wind on my wet arm. If the delay was very long, the manure on my arm would dry. Most delays were short, when a cow balked or two tried to get in at the same time. Other times the delay could be long, caused by a cow trying to crawl over the side or turning around so the crowd chute had to be emptied and reloaded. The longest delay was caused by a cow flipping over backwards and laying on her back in the bottom of the narrow chute.

Although the discomfort—no, downright pain—of the cold and drying was bad, the numbness of my fingers was worse. I would think there was no feeling at all in my fingers until I stuck my hand in the lubricating liquid hitting the jagged pieces of ice. Yet when I entered a cow, I could not distinguish the structures and would have to let my hand warm up to regain my sense of touch.

Some would ask the problem, and others would say there had to be one as I was taking so long. I would try to get a very questioning expression on my face, but there was usually someone who saw through my charade and tell the others that I was just dawdling to warm up while the rest of them were freezing.

The worst thing about testing with bare arms was the irritation. I shaved my arms to reduce the friction which helped some, but the arms would get red and chapped even to the point of some blood seepage. I would use one arm until it became too painful, then change to the other, back and forth.

Although I suffered while working, the pain at night when I was trying to sleep was really bad. I tried soaking them at night and bathing them with various products to soothe them, but I never found anything really effective. Camphophenique worked about as well as anything.

A plastic, shoulder length glove became available that was made for artificial insemination use. This was a one-size-fits-all glove. I only knew one man whose hand and arm were large enough for it — Big Sam Mathers, a cowboy who lived in Marathon.

Some companies began making smaller gloves so that I could work its finger over mine to make a reasonably good fit. I was sent a sample that was ideal, but I lost the name of the manufacturer and distributor before I had a chance to order.

The Pitman-Moore Labs marketed an obstetrical lubricant named Lubrivet. This was excellent for both obstetrical procedures and pregnancy testing, much better than only soapy water.

I was often asked how many cows that I could pregnancy check in a day. Most of the time this was only idle curiosity but sometimes a very serious question by telephone. Some rancher would have a large number of cows that he wanted tested as quickly as possible. He had heard of my ability and was making a legitimate inquiry.

The answer I would give was between 35 and 1035 depending

upon the facilities, the available help, the breed of cattle and the stage of pregnancy. It was also important to know what he called a day. Was he talking about an eight-hour day or a twenty-four hour day and, if it included night, whether it was moonlight or dark nights. Cattle worked well by moonlight but poorly by most truck headlights because it usually blinded them.

35 Head All Day

Soon after pregnancy testing began to be accepted by the ranchers in the late fifties, I was called one evening by a man who had 38 cows in the pen that he sure wanted to know if they were pregnant. I had an appointment north of Van Horn for the next morning. I thought I would whip by and test these cows right quick because they were near the highway fairly close to Van Horn. I called my appointment who said to go ahead because he could wait a little while, and besides he was a friend of the man needing his cows worked.

I arrived about good daylight to find a couple of cowboys waiting. The cows were crossbred Brahma-Hereford that had a reputation for being a little bit excitable. They had gotten restless during the night when a norther had blown in. Cows and horses are a lot like people when it comes to a cold wind — they get upset. Well, they didn't want to go in that crowd pen that led to the crowd chute, and we probably weren't as patient with them as we should have been because they hit the side of the pen and splintered the old rotten boards, escaping into the relatively small shipping trap.

We gathered up the pieces of boards and borrowed a few nails here and there. We scrounged some baling wire and patched up the hole pretty good. The cows were gathered and put back in the pen. We let them settle down and put a little cottonseed cake in the crowd pen that led to the crowd chute which was made of boards, but held only one cow at a time. There was no squeeze chute as they were few and far between at this time. We had stuck four fence posts in the front end to block it. We eased a cow in and put another post behind to scotch her. I climbed the side and hopped down behind her. I put a big chalk mark on her rump to show if she was pregnant. We repeated this on the six or eight other cows that were in the crowd pen. We started to fill it again, but I guess the remaining cows saw what I had done to the first bunch and didn't want any part of it. They broke out our patch, making the hole larger and splintering the boards badly. We borrowed a few boards here and there to patch the hole and penned the cows again. This time, the old salty cow that had busted out in the lead each time before did it again, and the rest followed her. There wasn't enough left to fix the gap, so we went to town and bought some boards and nails which we used to patch that hole real well.

The ole wild cow wasn't in the bunch this time when they were gathered, and we were able to work two crowd pen loads. Lo and behold, if the cows didn't tear up a whole new place. I was about ready to call it quits, but the men said the boss had told them to have those cows pregnancy tested, and that's what they were going to do, come hell or high water. They went back to town for more lumber and brought back some hamburgers. We ate and patched the pens. We were able to check some more cows before they tore the whole side of the pens down and escaped.

We had now tested 29 of the original 38 head. We patched the pens again. The cowboys had brought a good load of lumber the last time, but now the cows wouldn't go in the pen. We only had outlaws that were spoiled. We talked it over and decided because it was getting late in the day, to just head and heel the cows, stretch them out on the ground and I would palpate them lying on my belly. I really wasn't eager to do it because I had done it a few times. It is really awkward — my arm doesn't bend in the right direction for this position. We finally got 35 head tested. Two cows were watched as they jumped the fence into the big pasture and ran off. The first ole snaky cow was never seen again, so we assumed that she had also.

It was getting late so I didn't go on to my other call. It was not a very profitable day for me having tested 35 cows at fifty cents a head and driven 120 miles, 60 each way, which was included in the per head charge at that time.

My First 1000-Cow Day (Late 1950s)

Cavin Woodward was the ranch manager of the Lykes Brothers' O2 Ranch, south of Alpine. He had good rains at the end of the drouth of the 1950s and grew a good stand of grass. He had sold almost all the cattle off the ranch during that prolonged dry spell and needed to restock. He bought a bunch of good quality Hereford calves and turned the bulls on them. However, the next summer it didn't rain, and the grass disappeared. When the grass was green and tall it obscured the fact that much of the turf had been lost.

Cavin chose as many of the better heifers as he thought the ranch would winter and contracted the rest for late November delivery. The buyer showed up on the delivery date and after looking them over, offered a nice premium for the pregnant ones. The ranch owners were called, and they told Cavin to do what he thought best. I was called that night and told the heifers were in the pen, with the buyer and his trucks waiting. Cavin was not only a friend but had been a good client all during the drouth, having me treat the good quarter horses that he raised.

I was in a tight spot, having a morning appointment to test cows for Bill Sohl and an afternoon appointment to test at the Altuda pens for the Catto-Gage Ranch. I called Bill who said being late wouldn't hurt because the cattle hadn't been penned. I then called Travis Roberts of the Catto-Gage Ranch who said Cavin was a friend; besides, they had missed too many cows when they rounded up and needed to make another sweep.

I called Cavin back telling him I would be there at first light and he said he would be ready. It was still dark as pitch when I arrived and set up my outfit. The ranch hands started easing a few into the chute with the help of pickup headlights. This is kinda slow going because some cattle are blinded, and others spook at the shadows. However, we had worked a pretty fair number and had made a good dent in them by sunup. As soon as the chalk marks could be seen, Cavin started sorting them horseback. He was riding a good cutting horse. I finished up a little before noon and stopped by the cook shack for a cup of coffee, a piece of fried meat, and a big chunk of camp bread.

I got to Bill Sohl's place, south of Alpine, just as the men were finishing their meal. Fortunately, they had eaten early and we went right to work. These cows worked good. Charolais aren't as easy to pregnancy test as Herefords, but these had gone through the chute often and knew the way.

I arrived at the Altuda pens a little later than I had hoped for but not as late as I was fearful of. The men were well-rested and congenial. Travis Roberts always had a good crew of men. Some were his regular ranch hands, and others were day workers. I think a couple may have been friends helping out. Swapping out was done a lot in those days. The ones I remember being there that day were Biddy Martin, Guy Lee and Big Sam Mathers. All were grown men and knew their jobs, a pleasure to work with. They had moved a Turner squeeze chute from the Arnold place. It was not a portable chute in the sense that it had wheels. The men had cocked up one end and backed a pickup under it, and the chute was scooted into the bed of the truck. Along about sundown, men would take turns eating a snack from their sack lunch while the rest of us kept at it. This was before I started carrying emergency rations, so Guy Lee shared some of his fried deer meat and cold biscuits, besides pouring me a cup of coffee in the lid of his thermos. Now, I've eaten some good meals in my life, being fortunate to have lived and practiced in the cow country of West Texas and eaten meals prepared by many ranchwomen and camp cooks, but this fixed by Maisie, Guy's wife, was as good as it comes. I especially liked venison, and this was cooked just right. I ate with one hand while I pregnancy tested with the other, hardly missing a lick. I never once made the mistake of getting my hands mixed up.

These cows weren't used to being worked through a chute. I guess that was the reason it was a little slow, but when the sun went down, things went a lot faster. There was a full moon, and it was already high in the sky. It was a relatively warm evening for November, with no wind blowing. This was my first good size cow work by moonlight, and I learned that it was almost ideal if there was a good crew that wasn't give out.

I had pregnancy palpated almost 1100 head. There were a few under 500 head at the O2 Ranch, a few under 300 at Bill Sohls, and a few over 300 at Altuda, the exact numbers escape me. When I say we worked over a thousand head in one day, I'm not talking about an eight-hour shift. In ranch country, a day is from can 'til can't. I had stretched it a little farther, but still it was well within the 24-hour day.

There were several factors involved in my being able to test that number, even though I had to move twice. Good men and a fair set of facilities, maybe not ideal, but adequate. The cows were well bred up[*] and in an advanced stage. The heifers weren't too

---

[*] High percentage of pregnancy.

bad for being yearlings, but even those weren't real late, the bulls having been picked up the first of August. All in all, a very satisfying day. The fact they weren't interested in the stage of pregnancy made the work go faster.

Ted Gray

The first time I met Ted Gray was at the 06 Ranch house on the north side of Alpine. I knocked and he called, "Come in." He was sprawled in a large leather chair with his boots propped up on a foot stool looking a little lordly. He had his hat and spurs on. I introduced myself, standing with hat in hand because I was raised to remove my hat in the house. I don't know why he had his on. Perhaps it was because he had spent so much of his life in a cow camp where the hat was the first thing on in the morning and the last thing off at night. Maybe he was a little restless waiting for me, although, it was exactly the appointed time. It was my policy to make every effort to be on time and especially so when meeting someone for the first time. An early arrival could be a little awkward in certain circumstances and being late could be worse for that all important first impression. However, my rule for promptness was much like my inflexible rule not to allow anything to prevent my going to church Sunday mornings. By having this strict rule, I was able to attend about half the time. Being a veterinarian, the ox got in the ditch quite often.

Ted and I looked at each other a few seconds not saying anything, just sizing up one another. His wife, Addie, had been to my hospital a few times with a pet. She was a very gracious lady and had impressed me very favorably. Ted had an excellent reputation, and I had heard many good things about him. But I guess I was studying him as much as he was me. I was proud of my ability to evaluate someone on sight. Sometimes I would be disappointed when they spoke, but not this time. He unwrapped himself, stood and walked across the room with his hand out and greeted me warmly.

He said the cattle should be in the pens or close by. He had his horse in a trailer hitched to his pickup, and he pulled out with me following. We went a few miles north on Highway 118, turned off just across the Musquiz Creek bridge, and went east a ways on a dirt ranch road. The herd was in sight as we arrived at the corrals. Ted unloaded his horse, tightened the saddle cinch, mounted and went to meet the herd to help pen them. I stayed out of the way so as not to spook them. Almost all the ranchers and cowboys were good horsemen, but Ted Gray and Joe Lane were two of the most graceful riders, in my estimation. I never failed to admire their ability. I guess being mounted on a good horse helped, but I believe they would have looked good on Mark Twain's genuine Mexican plug. The herd was penned in short order. It was plain that the men knew what they were doing. The cattle were strung out and allowed to drift through the gate slowly and smoothly. No yelling, just an occasional slap of a rope on leather leggins—very professional, a thing of beauty. The fact that the cows were gentle helped. Not an outlaw in the bunch. I suppose not everyone can appreciate this action, but I have witnessed so many wrecks at a time like this, that I thoroughly admired it. The gate was kept open for me, and I drove in beside the squeeze chute and set up shop. I was ready to begin pregnancy testing when the first cow was brought in.

Things were going nicely when Otis Kimball drove up and joined us. The usual social amenities were exchanged. However, Otis would not shake my hand that I had been checking cows with. In fact, almost no one would. Although sometimes a person would call my bluff and offer to do so, then I would have to back off. Now, Otis had been in it up to his boot tops, many times, but he declined my extended hand with just a little negative twist of his head and a faint grin. He watched the operation a while and commented that I didn't test his cows as quickly and smoothly as I was doing Ted's.

Ted introduced me to his friends at a restaurant in Alpine one evening; saying I was the best veterinarian in West Texas. However, it was the extra special ability of Ted Gray and his caliber of cowmen that made me look good. I felt very humble with that comment coming from him.

Ted, along with other directors of the First National Bank in Alpine, came to help and give moral support when we broke ground for our new Marfa National Bank building in May, 1983. We were going into this undertaking with fear and trembling because of the cost, and we needed a boost to our morale.

Chapter 7

Some Memorable Workdays

Faith Cattle Co.

I was driving from ranch to ranch because of the large number of cows to be tested in October and November. There were some occasions when the cows would be kept in the pen until I got there, while the cowboys and ranch hands ate, rested and sometimes even slept, as I might arrive during the night. Night time work was much smoother and quicker than most would realize, especially if there was a moon. I am referring to pregnancy testing, as I need little light, only to find the cow and the men to work the cows into the chute. My work is by feel, and besides, it is always dark in the inside of a cow.

The Faith Cattle Company owned by Wesley West was part of the old West-Pyle Cattle Company after it was dissolved. The Crawford shipping pens were one of the best sets of working pens in the area. There was a bunkhouse and large shed that usually housed vehicles and equipment, but during cow works it was emptied and the chuck wagon and cook occupied it. The pens had good alleys for moving cattle from pen to pen and into a couple of smaller crowd pens leading to the crowd chute. Cows never had an opportunity to turn back and get spoiled.

Many cowboys in the Fort Stockton-Sanderson area were working in the oil patch because the pay was good, but their first love was cowboying. They liked riding good horses, a good bunkhouse, good chuck, and the fellowship of a bunch of good men. They knew and liked the foreman, Jim Dulaney, who was a good cowboy and a good man. Mr. West was often at these works and was pleasant and friendly and didn't throw his weight around. There often were two or three men for every position in the pens. One set of men would work while another group drank coffee, ate, played cards, horsed around, and even napped. No man ever got tired as there would be someone pestering him to take his place. Lots of joking and kidding but never any maliciousness. I never asked and was never told if this big group of men was drawing a salary, but I strongly suspect this was their vacation from their roughneck work.

One particular night, I arrived just after dark on a bright moonlit night. The temperature was perfect, light jacket weather with a slight breeze. The men were all rested and ready to go. There were right at 850 cows in the pen, and I had another ranch to work the next day. I had eaten sardines and crackers and had drunk coffee from my thermos around noon between ranches, but only had water since. While I worked, men brought me biscuits, fried meat and coffee with lots of good bull. We went through those cows in a little under eight hours, and I left there about sun up to the next ranch. I was young and able to go long hours on coffee and cigarettes. I may be paying the price now at age 77, but I have no regrets. Few men have been as fortunate as I to live and work in such beautiful country, do what I love, work with such good people, and still make a comfortable living for a wonderful, caring family.

Another time at the Faith Cattle Company, at the headquarter pens we pregnancy tested 600 cows in four hours. I use the term "we" although I was the only one actually testing. The men putting the cattle through the chutes were the ones doing the hardest work, as I had learned to work in a more or less relaxed manner usually doing only the pregnancy palpation when help was plentiful, so I didn't have to vaccinate or help with the squeeze chute.

Maureen Godbold

Maureen Godbold had her father's place, the Clay Mitchell Ranch. She was a good ranch manager but was not satisfied with her ability to pick replacement heifers and had been having trouble getting her yearling heifers pregnant. Jim Bob Steen, the county agent, and I went to the ranch to look at her heifer calves and make some recommendations. The result was that Jim Bob picked out all her replacements and we recommended an increased feeding program, beginning immediately after weaning, with a small daily amount. Then, increasing it shortly before the bulls were put with them. Also, she had been using yearling bulls as was customary. We suggested that she also put a few two-year-old bulls, that were experienced, with them.

I routinely performed a semen evaluation on her bulls shortly before breeding. We chose only the ones that tested the best to go with these heifers and recommended they be rotated every ten days to two weeks during the breeding season.

I pregnancy palpated that fall finding a 100% pregnancy in the eighty heifers, all but two of them were to calve in the first 60 days. Maureen was well pleased, but the problem was she wanted 100% every year and that just doesn't happen in mature cows, much less in heifers.

Jim Bob's choice of heifers resulted in fewer calving problems also.

Graveyard Pens

Susan Combs and Gene West were operating the Post Ranch as the Maravillas Cattle Company. Susan was a descendant of the old gent who put together several ranches in the Marathon area back in the early days.

We were at the graveyard pens. This set of working pens was situated next to the Marathon cemetery. A cemetery used to be called a graveyard and these pens were of that vintage.

Bud Coffey, the foreman from the Headquarters Ranch, Blas Payne and Tootie Garlick, along with some day workers (cowboys who worked on a temporary basis), were pushing cows through the chutes while I was pregnancy testing and vaccinating them. These were pretty sorry pens. There were 250 head of Hereford cows, and every one tested out pregnant! I have found excellent pregnancy rates many times, but this was the only time I found 100% in a significant number. I attribute this success to Gene West because of his knowledge and skill as a manager to have produced such spectacular results.

Needless to say, we didn't set any speed records in those pens, but we got the job done, and everyone was in a good humor, in spite of the fact that we had been two hours late getting started because of a fog.

There are fogs, and then there are fogs. This was a humdinger! The trap was only 160 acres, but cowboys kept losing cows they were driving and getting lost themselves as visibility was only a few yards. Their sense of direction was lost, only the bellowing of the cattle and the hollering of the cowboys kinda kept the bunch together.

We joked about the fog and speculated on when the pens were built and who built them. I said I thought perhaps the Irishmen and Chinamen building the railroad in 1882 had built them with discarded lumber as a joke in their spare time while they were resting.

Bud Coffey said he felt sure Noah built them with lumber from the Ark so he could pair up his animals because they had become separated from each other in their rush to get off that boat and onto dry land. Actually, they didn't know what dry was until they got introduced to the Big Bend of Texas. I guess Bud didn't really have to top my explanation, but they say the first liar doesn't have a chance.

Actually, the pens weren't in too bad of condition as compared to some I have worked in, but it gave us something to talk about. The pens were only used a couple of days in the year, so there wasn't much need for them to be very fancy. They were serviceable and that's what counted.

Charlie Donaldson

Charlie Donaldson had always been able to have a high percentage of his cows bred. His desire to have a 100% pregnancy rate in at least one pasture had almost become an obsession with him. One could almost see him wince when I called a cow open. He acted as if it were an affront to his ability as a cow man.

We were testing 400 head at the pens on top and had tested quite a few, and all had been pregnant when we stopped for lunch. Betty, Charlie's wife, had brought lunch to us as she usually did, and as always, it was welcome and delicious.

I engorged myself, really shamefully, but it was so good I couldn't stop eating. The fact that Charlie had worked the hound out of me had really stimulated my appetite! I took a lot of ribbing on the amount I ate, but what was bad was that I started finding some open cows when we started testing after lunch. Charlie was upset because he wanted that 100% pregnancy so bad. He said he never would feed me again until we had finished the work.

Jim Phillips

James "Jim" Phillips was manager of the 101 Ranch of the Bowman Family, Mt. Ord Ranch of Mrs. McLean, and the Petan Ranch of McLean Bowman, grandson of Mrs. McLean. He also pastured steers on at least one ranch, the Kerr Mitchell ranch and had yearlings in feedlots. This would have been spread pretty thin for a man of ordinary capabilities, but Jim seemed to handle it with ease. He was a pleasure to work with because of his personality, but also because of his knowledge and skill as a cowman. He always made me look good as a veterinarian, especially when I was pregnancy testing cows by palpation. All of the cow works went well, and several times I pregnancy tested over a 1000 cows in a day for Jim.

There was one very memorable day at the Flat Corrals on the Petan Ranch. The cowboys had gone out early and were at the backside of the pasture by the time they could see and had the herd strung out, bringing them into the pens well before sunup. As the first cattle entered the corrals, they were immediately started through the cutting chute. Jim stood above the two cutting gates and sorted them three ways: steers, heifers, and cows. The cows were funneled to me through alleys, crowd pens, crowd chute and then into the squeeze chute. I had set up my lubricant for my arm, the chalk to mark the cows, vaccine, and syringes. Jim had set up a lawn chair and a couple of thermoses of coffee for me as was his custom. There were two men in front, one was working the headgate and checking eyes on the right side, while the other man was checking eyes on the left and putting a chalk circle around any eye that needed surgery later. One man was working the squeeze and chalking according to the state of pregnancy. A fourth man was working the tailgate and vaccinating. One of the main reasons Jim could accomplish so much so efficiently was because he always had a good bunch of men working for him. Harry Wells was one of the best.

Jim had weighed the calves and loaded them on trucks by noon. The cook at the chuck wagon* had chow ready. We ate and went back to work, as it was too cold to lounge around and shoot

---

* Although it was still called a chuck wagon, actually it was a pickup truck with a chuck box mounted on the back.

the bull. I glanced over my shoulder occasionally to observe Jim standing on top of the cutting chute sorting the cows I had worked, separating the shippers from the keepers and those that were to be put in a trap to have their eyes treated at a later date. Sometime along in the middle of the afternoon or so, Jim sent a Mexican to see how many cows were left to be palpated. He returned and reported there were *bastante*. This Spanish word lit-

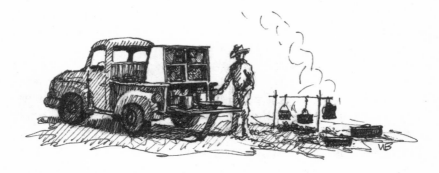

Modern chuck wagon.

erally means "enough," but also is used to indicate a large number or amount. When I first began to practice, a wet was helping me during a surgical procedure. I had a fair sized incision open and I asked the Mexican to put some sulfanilamide powder in it before I closed it. He was pouring a rather generous amount and I wanted him to stop by saying that was enough. I said *bastante*, which he interpreted as meaning much more and he emptied the whole dern thing in there, much to my distress. Needless to say, I never made that mistake again. We assumed there were many more. Since we had originally planned on a two-day work anyway and he had been working his men pretty hard, Jim said they could use a little rest. We stopped for the day after we emptied the crowd chute, crowd pen, and holding pen. I arrived early the next morning and he reported we had worked 1064 head and only had 255 more. I was disappointed that we had stopped, because we could easily have finished, and it would have been great for my ego. I could have bragged that I tested 1319 head in one day.

Cole and Alf Means

The Means family came to the area sometime about 1884 when Mr. John Z. Means drove a herd of cattle from San Saba accompanied by a wagon driven by his wife and pulled by oxen. Alf, one of the grandsons, still has the old ox yoke.

Mr. Means had several boys. Each ended up with a ranch of their own, with Mr. Cole having the Y6 Ranch. Alf joined his father here after his discharge from the Army following World War II. He lived in the old original adobe ranch house with his wife, Ruth. Two boys and a girl were born to this union, Alfred G. "Bodie" Jr., Craig and Debbie. Mr. Cole lived in a nice new house on top of the hill. Alf and Ruth later moved here, and Bodie and his bride, Mickey, moved into the old house.

Mr. Cole and Alf had much to do with the success of my practice. Their friendship and encouragement were very important. Furthermore, they were some of the first to allow me to pregnancy test their cows. Their endorsement had a great deal to do with its acceptance in the area, because they were well known and highly respected. They were two of the finest men I ever knew and truly a pleasure to work for and work with. Bodie and Craig have grown to be equally fine men. A truly remarkable family.

A meal at the Y6 Ranch was always very special. There were many ranchwomen that fed me over the years, but I think that I ate at Ruth Means' table more than at any other place. Perhaps she pampered me more by fixing things that I especially liked. She always prepared delicious food, and I was made to feel like a very special, honored guest.

Many meals were eaten in the old headquarters house at the foot of the hill and many more at the new house on top of the hill. These were delightful meals, and I enjoyed the comfort and fellowship of the table. The meal was always begun with a blessing, which added to the occasion. Perhaps they had one at every meal. They did every time I was present, whether at the ranch house or at some working pens in the pasture. I'm ashamed to admit we only returned thanks at my house when company was present or the family was visiting.

We always removed our boots before going in the house. This was notable because it showed respect for the house, but also because their condition from working cattle really wasn't suitable to wear in the house. Also in a little selfish aspect, my old tired feet needed the rest.

I never saw any sibling squabbling or quarreling. The way both boys treated their sister, Debbie, was truly remarkable, always acting as if she were a guest of honor. She in turn always acted the perfect lady.

Ruth would bring us hot meals when we tested cattle at the working pens at Four Corners and at Double Wells. The trip to Double Wells was farther, but the roads were better and there was only one gate. The road to Four Corners in the early days was over a rough, rocky hill. Later, a more circuitous road was used, which was much smoother, yet it did have two gates. They weren't wire gaps but regular gates, and they didn't drag badly. Earlier years, we worked in the fall, then later, when Bodie and Craig were big enough to help, the work was put off until the Christmas holidays so they could enjoy it when they were home from school. Actually, I think they really did enjoy working as much as Alf and I did. I almost always enjoyed working cattle, especially with a congenial crew that knew how to work. Those boys knew how to work. Alf was probably a good teacher, but I think a lot of it was bred into them, as they came from a long line of cowmen.

It always amazed me how Ruth prepared a meal, loaded it in a pickup, and drove to the pens. It would still be hot, even on a cold day. She would then spread it out and serve it on the tailgate. Ruth would bring me a thermos of hot coffee, because she knew I liked it so much, even though she brought ice tea for the rest as that was their preference. One time a blizzard was blowing and Ruth had to fight them off my coffee.

Later the testing period was changed to late summer and early fall. Then Ruth would prepare the food and place it in an ice chest for us.

One year the Y6 Ranch had an exceptionally dry, hard year, and the grass was short. Cole and Alf arranged to pasture their cattle out, there being three different ranches that would accept some. I was approached to divide them so that the calving interval on each ranch would be bunched, and they could bring the pairs home in a group and release the pasture. They reported that all calved "as advertised," and they were well-pleased. This happened when I was first trying to get pregnancy testing accepted.

They talked to many, far and wide, of my work and of the safety to the cows.

*   *   *   *   *

J.M. "Manny" Fowlkes bought about 200 head of crossbred cows from Cole and Alf Means who told him I had pregnancy tested the cows and they were all open. Manny came into my office the next year and told me not a single one of those cows had a calf. He said that they had told him they were open, but he could look at them and tell they all had a calf in them big as a dog. He said he thought to himself, "Charlie may know how to treat a sick animal, but he doesn't know doodley-squat about telling whether a cow is pregnant or not."

Manny was well-known and well-liked, and he loved to tell about those open cows and break out laughing. I had a number of ranchers call me from a distance asking if I was the vet Manny was talking about. If so, they wanted me to test their cows. He was one of my best advocates. In defense of his eyeball diagnosis, he was familiar with and accustomed to Hereford cattle whose rear end and belly are relatively tight and smooth when open, but in advanced pregnancy both structures would be larger and looser. Brahma cows and their crosses, as these cattle were, have a tendency to have a big belly and a large, loose rear end, even when open.

Testing Without a Squeeze Chute or Headgate

The early days of pregnancy palpating were under some rather crude conditions. Squeeze chutes and even head gates were pretty scarce. I was working at Dick and Alice Swartz's Merrill Ranch in a long, wooden crowd chute. We would put cedar posts across at the front end, about 4 or 5 to block it, move a cow up to it and then put another post behind her. A space was left for me and a couple more posts, placed to hold up the next cow. I would climb up on the fence while the front cow was let out and the next cow moved up. This gave me plenty of good exercise, so I didn't need a fancy gym set at home. I would sit on the narrow top board which was uncomfortable, but it really wouldn't have been so bad if they had been good new ones instead of the old ones with splinters.

We weren't setting any speed records but were getting along pretty good. These were big ole gentle Hereford cows, so we were working them quietly. I was deep inside the front cow up to the hilt, when the cow behind spooked. She broke the posts and came on top of me. She was riding the front cow with me between. She wouldn't just stand there but kept trying to climb on over. She couldn't make it though, because my hip pockets wouldn't hold her feet. José Escobedo, a big, strong, Mexican ranch hand, came over the fence and grabbed her tail, and pulled the cow off me. My arm in the front cow was still holding me up, but when she was turned loose, and my arm came out, I collapsed on the ground. I soon caught my breath, wobbled around a little, and gingerly climbed up on the fence. Needless to say, the operation slowed down considerably as I eased up and down the fence and was particularly gentle with the cows. It was fortunate that there were only a few more head left, because each was torture. I was kinda disappointed in the x-rays not showing broken ribs. I was cautioned just to take it easy for a few days. No need to worry about that; I sure took it easy!

The Mix-up

There were still quite a few of the ranchers that would not pregnancy test after it had been accepted by many. One of the older ranchers bought a herd of cows as replacements when he grew some grass. The man selling wasn't too anxious to have the cows tested and badmouthed the practice. He stated these cows were exposed* and claimed he always had a good calf crop.

When the new owner got these cows home and looked them over after they had a chance to fill up,† he began to have his doubts. He gave them a little more time and still didn't like their looks, so he got a couple of friends to look at them. These men agreed that a lot of them were questionable as to their pregnancy status and encouraged that they be pregnancy checked.

I always put a chalk mark on cows to designate which were open and which were pregnant as most would go into a large pen together after leaving the test chute. He didn't want those chalk marks all over his cattle. Actually, they were kind of generous,

---

* Had bulls with them.
† Cattle being worked and shipped often will shrink by losing their belly because they hadn't been eating properly.

especially in those early days.

His set up was such that the cattle could be separated easily as they left the chute. The open, non-pregnant cows were put in a little pen and the pregnant ones in a larger pen next to the group not yet tested. There were about 600 head all together, and we had worked about half of them when suddenly a ranch hand let out a squall. The gate between the tested and untested cattle had been knocked open, and the two groups had co-mingled. The rancher was thoroughly disgusted and threw the outside gate open to turn everything loose and quit. I couldn't handle this and finally convinced him to let me retest those at no charge. He reluctantly let his men pen the cows again and didn't object to my putting chalk marks on them this time. It was after dark when we finished, and I was beginning to regret my offer to retest at no charge. He didn't offer to pay me a little extra. I think, no, I know he was unhappy because I had found too many open. For several years, I insisted, no chalk mark, no test. Also, I carried pieces of rope to secure every gate of any consequence.

Procaine Penicillin in Aqueous Suspension

This penicillin was developed probably in the early sixties. It was an aqueous suspension with good syringe ability, quite an improvement over the penicillin in oil that we had been using. The product was marketed in 10cc vials with each cc containing 300,000 units. It was supposed to maintain a therapeutic blood level for 24 hours, but I always preferred to give it twice a day when possible. Refrigeration was required.

A person called from Van Horn, 75 miles from Marfa, and described a sick cow. I could not possibly go, as too many patients were waiting. At that time there were few veterinarians, so another could not be called. The man didn't have a way to haul her. I hoped penicillin might help. I wrapped a few bottles of penicillin and a screwtop can filled with water that I had frozen. This would keep the penicillin cold, and I sent it on the bus with instructions to keep it in the refrigerator and to give 10cc twice a day in the muscle until all was given. About two weeks later he called and said the cow had made a quick recovery and had seemed to be well when the little bottles of white stuff was used up. He said that he had only given about half of the liquid in the can, but the cow sure was getting hard to treat now! Poor man, he was giving only water.

The demand for penicillin decreased rapidly in late spring, and the cost dropped also, but in the fall, both the demand and the cost increased quickly. I thought of an easy way to double my money. I bought extra refrigerators and purchased 1000 of the 10cc vials at what had been the historical low price. I was very smug. Penicillin is produced by a fermentation process of the yeast, *penicillium*. Schenley, the whisky distillers, put in three large fermentation vats, producing penicillin in large quantities and flooded the market. The resulting price war caused me to take a whipping.

Morumide

George Jones came in my office once, complaining that his ranch hand said the milk cow had badly chapped teats. I recommended and dispensed a jar of Morumide ointment, a Massengill company product, containing cod liver oil and sulfanilamide. George opened the jar, smelled it and tested it by rubbing a little on his hands. Few cowmen would use anything on their livestock that they hadn't checked out on themselves. He then asked if it was any good. I went into a long spiel on its many uses and virtues. He grunted and left with it.

A few days later, he came back saying that it hadn't helped the cow a bit. I was shocked and finally asked if it had been applied liberally twice a day with gentle massage like I had recommended. He said no, that when he had got back to the ranch, a colt that was being broken and trailing a rope had gotten tangled up in it and rope burned all four pasterns badly, and they had used the Morumide on him. He was in the pen next to the cow, and if the product was as good as I said it was, it should have cured the cow which was just across the fence. He gave his deep, little belly laugh.

Dick Swartz and the Grasshoppers

Dick had a grasshopper plague. I had heard of locust plagues, but this is the only one I experienced. They appeared suddenly one morning. We never knew where they came from. Could they have migrated into the area or suddenly emerged from eggs? A few times I have seen grasshoppers cover the pavement for a short distance but did not seem to be a problem in the pasture. These covered the highway for over two miles and extended well into the pasture on both sides. The pens where we had planned to work were in the middle of this mass. We opened the gate and turned the cows out that had been penned the afternoon before. There was quite a noise. We speculated whether it was caused by chewing, hopping, or flying. Dick telephoned a crop duster in Pecos who stated he could load an insecticide to treat the area from the air and come, but it would be the next morning. The enormous numbers would devour the grass soon. That afternoon a cloud came up, and a moderately severe hailstorm came. It killed almost all the grasshoppers but did not badly damage the green, pliable grass. The accompanying rain washed the grasshoppers into deep drifts against fences and small bushes, and into dirt tanks. Dick called off the aerial spraying and began to be concerned about the piles of dead, decaying grasshoppers causing a stinking mess, contaminating the area. A day or two later large numbers of buzzards appeared and in a few days had consumed all the dead grasshoppers. The massive number of grasshoppers was really frightening. The enormous number of buzzards was unreal, and where they all came from suddenly was as much a mystery as the appearance of the grasshoppers.

Heat at Carrizo Springs Ranch

1958 had been a good year for grass rains on Mesquite, Cibolo and Cienagita Ranches in Presidio County owned by Hamilton "Ham," Russ, and Tucker White. The ranches had been vacated or nearly so during the drouth. They contracted to buy two-year-old Santa Gertrudis heifers from Red Nunley. The contract called for a certain number subject to my pregnancy examination on January 10, 1959 at the Nunley-Briscoe Ranch between Carrizo Springs and Laredo.

Russ flew Tucker and me to Del Rio where we spent the night with Jim White, Sr. and Mamacita, as Mrs. White was known. Russ was a good pilot and flew very conservatively, not taking any risks. The weather was good, and the flight was smooth. We flew over Mexico on a direct route from Marfa to Del Rio.

Several years later Russ flew the route and was intercepted by

US Fighter planes that directed and escorted him to Laughlin Air Force Field. This was during the Cold War with Russia, shortly after the Cuban crisis. He had been picked up by radar coming out of Mexico. They raked him over the coals. Needless to say, he never took this route again.

Ham drove us to the ranch early the next morning, arriving there about daylight.

Red Nunley had got the option to have his veterinarian verify any pregnancy diagnosis that he questioned. Ben Hopson, D.V.M. from Laredo, was his representative. Ben and I had been classmates and good friends in veterinary school. When this was discovered there was some good-natured joking that neither the buyer nor the seller had a chance with two friends checking each other.

The ranch had excellent facilities, the best I had ever seen at that time. There were good high fences of heavy lumber with well-constructed gates. The crowd chute was partitioned into a series of one cow units by sliding gates that blocked off each cow. There was a good squeeze chute at the front end, a little past a cutting gate. Non-pregnant heifers would be sorted off by this gate, not having to go through the squeeze chute, where the pregnant ones were being branded by the White family.

This setup was a major disadvantage to me. My technique had been to test through the side of a squeeze chute with the cow's head caught and sides squeezed. This way I could test with a minimum of effort. Here, the arrangement necessitated the cow being tested in the partition before the cutting gate. A bar was put behind the cow to give me room to stand behind her. This meant I had to climb up the side of the chute to allow the next cow to come in. The side of the chute was high so that I had no problem getting out of reach of the heifer's horns, but the climbing up and down with boots slick with juicy cow manure was a real challenge after about a hundred head or so. They were being fed prickly pear which caused loose stools.

By this time of the year, the Marfa area had cold weather for 6 to 8 weeks, and I had become acclimated to it. Here at this ranch, it felt like the middle of summer. In fact, the official temperature was 89 degrees in nearby Laredo that day. To make matters worse, there was a large branding fire upwind from me. I had never seen such a large fire before, but this was brush country and wood was plentiful. Around Marfa wood was scarce, and accordingly, very small fires were built. These small fires resulted in difficulty in heating very many branding irons at one time, as some would get pushed out and not get hot. A person that had many things going so that some were neglected was said to have too many irons in the fire. This outfit had no such problem, plenty of hot irons.

The trade had been for a certain number of heifers. There were a total of 500 head in the herd. We had been working quite a while when it became apparent that we weren't getting enough cattle to test pregnant. Another hang up was that the prettiest, slickest, deep cherry red cattle were the pregnant ones while the more slender, long-legged, burnt haircoat were open. Red was having a fit, calling on Ben to double-check a number of the ones I called open. Ben agreed with all my diagnoses. Red called a halt to the test and was about to call off the trade. He was seriously believing there was funny business going on. Ben took him to one side and assured him that the cattle in the best condition are more likely to become pregnant. He finally agreed that this was true but insisted the trade was for a certain number and because trucks were there for that number, if he couldn't sell that many, he wasn't going to sell any.

Red and the White brothers got in a huddle and it was agreed that the original number would be accepted with the heifers that were not pregnant at a reduced price. I had welcomed the break as I was exhausted, climbing up and down in that heat. I had gotten my second wind by the time they settled their differences, and I was able to finish the entire herd. There have not been many times in my life that I was as tired and a cold beer tasted as good as that night after testing those 500 head in the heat.

On the Spot

Mr. W. A. Foley was a fine old gent who I really enjoyed. We didn't get much work done, but we sure got in some good visiting. He owned a ranch about 10 miles west of Valentine and another on the east edge of town where he lived. He had a daughter named Lou who was married to Chilton Ridley, nicknamed "Chili." Their son, Alton, was called "Chili Bean."

Mr. Foley sold his cattle and leased the ranches to John Moore and John's son-in-law, Lynn Crittendon. Chili and Lou went to the city, a common occurrence in the drouth of the 1950s.

Chili came back and took over the ranch in the early 1960s. He bought cows from Clyde Ikins at Kent. I pregnancy tested 205 head of early calvers. The next spring he came in and bought supplies for working the calves. A few days later he came in my office with a very serious expression on his face. The office was full of ranchers, but Chili just barged right up to me, eyeball to eyeball. He said, "You pregnancy tested 205 cows for me, didn't you?" I nodded. "I came in and bought 205 doses of blackleg vaccine, didn't I?" (It was available in 5 dose vials at that time.) Again, I nodded, trying to think of what disaster could have happened, as I had checked the cows carefully to be sure they were all early calvers. Also, I had tested them clean for brucellosis and had vaccinated for leptospirosis. These were Brangus, and I was still a little prejudiced against blacks and especially any long-eared cattle with Brahma blood because I had owned some and lost so much money on in the drouth. I tried to imagine why I was again being haunted by *ears*. It was not a bad loco year nor did he have much broomweed. Something must have caused an abortion storm. The ranchers looked from Chili to me and to each other with wide open eyes. Things got real quiet. I wanted to crawl under my desk. "Well," Chili said, "I worked those calves yesterday and I was one dose of blackleg short, and I want to know why you didn't tell me one cow was going to have twins?" This was told far and wide, at first to my embarrassment, but actually, I couldn't have had better publicity.

The Tranquilizer Gun

Soon after it began raining and the grass growing in the late fifties, ranchers began to restock as herds had been liquidated fairly drastically. Some bought good age adult cows, but this age group brought premium prices, so heifer calves or bred, yearling heifers were usually purchased. Those that were able to hold on to some cows kept their heifer calves to breed. Theoretically, it is cheaper to buy replacements rather than raise your own, but in this particular area, a cow raised on the ranch from a calf performs much better. Probably, there are a number of reasons for this. Acclimation is important, but the calf learning the poison plants from its mother is more so. Another major reason is the man selling usually retains his best stock for his own replacements. Therefore, whether anyone wants to admit it or not, the buyer is getting the second best.

Ray Roberts was the foreman of the Pruett Ranch, the Marfa division of the Catto-Gage Ranches. He was given the responsibility of calving out four hundred head of Hereford heifers. This was too many to keep up as had been customary, so they had to be calved out in a four-section pasture, about 2500 acres. He and I really had our hands full.

The successful breeding program was too successful. They had started with 500 head and left the bulls out for five months. The usual practice of breeding in big pastures using yearling bulls and feeding a conservative amount of supplement resulted in a sixty to seventy percent pregnancy in heifers, spaced out over five months of calving. In this instance 400 head became pregnant and most calved in a two month period. The pasture was triangular with the pens at a narrow point. This resulted in too great a distance to drive an animal in trouble to the pens, so they would be checked horseback, roped, tied down, and if Ray was unsuccessful in pulling the calf, he would ride to the house and call me. On a dark night we sometimes had trouble locating the heifer.

Ray was getting behind with this slow procedure so we decided on a Cap Chur gun, a so-called tranquilizer gun, and checked the heifers in a pickup. This was a good theory, but the medicine used at that time was nicotine sulfate which caused paralysis. It certainly didn't work like the advertisements or television showed. In fact, I don't know of anything that did. Sometimes, it worked too well, and the heifer died. If the dose was reduced too much, the heifer ran off and never went down. The delivery syringe would sometimes bounce off without injecting the medication in the animal. This was a major problem with the first plain needles without barbs to retain the syringe. Attempting to find the syringe in the grass and especially at night was a challenge. I'm sure we wasted much more time looking for syringes than they were worth, but remember the times. Few things were discarded even when broken. The thought was perhaps it could be repaired or a part salvaged. Each ranch had its scrap pile. Many hours were wasted looking for an object that couldn't be found or was not of any use if it could be found. The city dumps seemingly never got full; now there are not enough places to dispose of all that is discarded.

The heifer that was properly tranquilized was not without problems. Often a small assist would deliver a live vigorous calf, that was soon on its feet hunting a "lunch basket." Another heifer would come to inspect the newborn, brag to the mother, and lick the baby who would then follow her off, as the mother could not yet regain her feet and there had been no bonding. The foster mother would not have milk, but if so, Herefords would rarely allow any to nurse except their own calf. The little baby would be a leppie, a dogie, an orphan. Again, some exasperation, trying to pair them up. In retrospect it would have been better to have chalk marked them as pairs. However, marking a wet, slimy calf can be a chore. Then they could have been watched until the heifer recovered, but the few occasions this was done, the heifer jumped up and ran off and nothing was accomplished.

This sounds like the entire operation was a complete disaster. Actually, the end results were surprisingly successful. Dogie calves and full bag heifers would be placed together as pairs for adoption. A heifer would be snubbed to a post and the hind legs hobbled so she couldn't kick the calf which was held up to the udder, a teat placed in its mouth, and milk squirted in the mouth. Sometimes the use of the new fangled deodorant sprays would be used on the heifer's nose and the calf's rear end. Patience and persistence would pay off most of the time. Also it gave Ray something to do while he was resting. Ray was a very good natured, even tempered person but he couldn't see the humor when I said this.

C.C. "Coley" Means and the Angus Cows

When it finally started raining in the latter part of the 1950s, Coley Means at Chispa decided he would try Angus cattle. I don't remember him telling me why he had made such a drastic decision. This was Hereford country, and very few strayed from them. However, his father "Bug" was said to have switched to Angus in the 1940s. His uncle, Cole, and cousin, Alf Means, had kinda fooled with some Brahma bulls, messing up some of their good Hereford cows, but I think they were about the only ones, except for Jimmy Livingston and Cecil Rourk, off down by the river where no one could see them.

Good Hereford cows were hard to find after the drouth when people started restocking. He may have given up looking and decided to take second best. He received three truckloads of cows and one truckload of baby calves. He spent the whole day trying to pair them up because he wanted to put them in three different small traps. I don't remember whether these were grass traps or hay fields. The idea was to keep them handy while they recuperated from the long haul and to get them acclimated. His success rate had been poor because the calves were nursing any cow, and cows were letting any calf nurse them. He called to see if I had any suggestions. I told him that over the years I had heard Angus would do what he described. I suggested he count off the desired number of cows and an equal number of calves for each pasture. Preferably, place them with only a fence separating the groups and watch for tucked up calves hanging on the fence or around the water trough, looking like they may be a dogie. Also look for full bag cows that had not been nursed. He later told me that he only had to switch a few animals and all were doing well.

He was a good cowman. I imagine that he had more paired up than he told me about, but I guess he still had a problem. I suppose I should add that Angus cattle have now gained wide acceptance in the area. Coley kinda broke the ice and overcame the prejudice by demonstrating his success with the breed.

Cockleburs

Some years the conditions were favorable for the growth of certain weeds. It seems that if rains came when the ground temperature was just right, the seeds would germinate and certain plants would grow. Some years the cockleburs grew exceptionally well in places, so much so that it was impossible or impractical to control them. This really caused me a problem at times. I had a few instances of poisoning by the very young plants, but my main problem was mature burs in the tails of cows.

I was pregnancy palpating cows for Coley Means at Chispa on a cold, windy day. The cows had their tails full of cockleburs. It was not just 2 or 3 burs. I mean the last 8 or 10 inches of the tail was a mass of cockleburs, and cows would slap me upside the head with this club. That would smart, but the sharp spines of the burs on my cold face brought tears to my eyes. I'm afraid I said some derogatory remarks about the cows, their tails, the cockleburs, and the cold. Coley was an easy-going, good-natured man. He said, "Now Charlie, don't bad mouth my cockleburs. I sold them for more than the farmers got for their cotton." By way of explanation, his calves tails, briskets, sheath and belly had been covered with burs. The poor struggling cotton farmers in the Lobo valley were receiving very low prices. They had a good crop and raised a lot of cotton, but everyone else had also.

Dick Henderson

Dick Henderson lived at his home ranch at Ozona, Texas. He also had a ranch in the Sierra Vieja Mountains in Presidio County southwest of Valentine, Texas. Woodrow Mills ran the ranch for him, and I was the veterinarian. The ranch had belonged to Sam Bunton. Henry Wilbanks combined it with the Conring Casa Blanca and Chilicote. The three ranches combined were called Chilicote, the Spanish word for the mountain laurel bush.

I pregnancy palpated cows for him, both at this ranch and his home place at Ozona. His father ran sheep on his Pike's Peak Ranch west of Ozona and on another ranch between Fort Stockton and Sanderson. He had a little bunch, perhaps 50 or 60 head of Hereford cows. Dick had hinted to him a few times about pregnancy testing, but he made no response. They were fat and didn't have many calves so Dick decided to go ahead and check them anyway. We then went by his house and told him that we had cut out over half of them that weren't pregnant. The old gent was crowding eighty years of age. He said, "You boys leave my cows alone. My sheep make me my living and that little bunch of cows are my hobby. I don't gamble, run horses, chase women or drink whisky. I just have that little bunch of old fat cows to pamper."

Dick Henderson had a problem getting a crew of ranch hands to work cattle, trucks to haul them, and the cow buyer all synchronized for the same date at his ranch near Ozona. He called me to pregnancy test on the only day he could do so. This seemed an impossibility as it was during the pregnancy testing season, and I was going day and night. The only open date I had was about a week later than the one he wanted. He was a good friend and a valued client. I gave him the name of the rancher that I had an appointment with on the date Dick needed me. Dick called him and he agreed to release me and change his date. He and Dick were good friends, otherwise, I doubt if he would have done it. I called him to be sure of the agreement and date change and to express my appreciation.

The herd that Dick needed to be tested would take almost all day, and I had long, hard days scheduled on either side of his date. Dick's Ozona ranch was 210 miles from Marfa, and it would take a half day of driving in each direction. Therefore, I consented to fly with him. He picked me up at the Marfa airport when I came in late at night from an all day work. We left in unsettled weather. When near Fort Stockton we hit a thunderstorm. I had no idea they could be so violent. There was severe turbulence and lightning was popping in every direction. We were in it before we realized it. I couldn't tell half the time whether we were right side up, upside down, or sideways. When that storm finally turned us loose and Dick was able to get his bearings, he said we were north of Pecos 20 to 30 miles out of the way. He got back on course and landed at his lighted private strip at his ranch. I don't know if our survival was because of Dick's skill or our guardian angels working overtime. I personally asked for their help.

The cow work in Ozona was not finished until after dark, even though we had started about sun up. The days had gotten shorter, and it seems that things go slower when fingers and toes are cold. The thunderstorm we experienced had been caused by a cold front that had moved in. We had been having nice, warm, Indian summer days lately, and I had been working only in a t-shirt. This was before I started using plastic gloves, so my hands and arms were bare. I was really uncomfortable, to put it mildly, not having brought any winter clothes on the plane. Dick went to the house and brought me a nice, warm vest. I have gotten lots of mileage from that vest. I still have it and use it, even after all these years.

I had to get home for my early morning work the next day, even though it was dark and there were no lights on the runway at Marfa. Dick instructed me to call for JoAnn and her mother, Mrs. Tyler, to position their cars at either end of the runway, and when they heard the airplane engines, they were to turn on their headlights and shine them down the runway. There was only one runway, so there was no problem to decide which one. The night was exceptionally dark. The weather was clear and calm, thankfully. Dick was able to follow the Omni radio beam which led us to Marfa. We had no problem; the car headlights were turned on; and the runway was in plain view. Dick circled around and began his descent. Everything was uneventful as Dick turned on his landing lights which were very bright and shone on the runway even more clearly. We were almost on the ground when we realized that we had failed to tell them to kill their car lights at this point. I was completely blinded and thought we had had it. There was no way we could land, but Dick set it down as smooth as if he could have seen what he was doing. We transferred my equipment to JoAnn's car, and Dick took off for his ranch. I flew with Dick several other times. None were so eventful and exciting. Of course, they were never at night or in inclement weather. I made sure of that!

The only other time I can remember being banged around like we were in that turbulence was shortly after being discharged. Lynn Kern, a friend who had been a fighter pilot, asked me to go with him for a little ride in a Piper Cub. After a little sightseeing, the plane suddenly began a series a dives, stalls, turns, and I don't know what else. We finally landed and Lynn told me he was just trying to make me say "calf rope," an expression to admit defeat. I said that if I had known that was all he wanted, I would have been glad to oblige.

Chapter 8

The Veterinarian's Family Pets

Nanny Goat

I was on a call to Luther Anderson's ranch about twenty miles south of Alpine. He was a cowman, but he also kept a little bunch of Spanish goats. We were in the kitchen drinking coffee and visiting when Luther bemoaned the fact that one of his nannies had kidded a couple of nights before, giving birth to triplets. But she only had one half of an udder, having a spoiled bag. He figured she couldn't raise all three.

I talked Luther into letting me have one to take home as a pet for my daughters. I picked out a pretty, spotted female that rode in the seat of the pickup with me. Actually, she spent most of the time curled up in my lap.

Nancy and Janet fell in love with that little goat, naming her Nanny. They raised her on a bottle and nipple. Soon the little goat started following Nancy and Janet around the backyard, coming when called. She made a remarkable pet, running and playing with them. She loved to see-saw with the girls and often would do so while alone, walking up the board until it tilted down, then, turning and walking back up the other side.

Nancy was in the second grade and got permission from her second grade teacher, Mrs. Hegy, to bring Nanny to school for show-and-tell. JoAnn brought the goat and Nancy to school and then picked up the goat at morning recess. Nanny had a dog collar on and was led around with a piece of cotton rope. All the children loved petting the little goat.

When Nanny got big she would hop up on a built-in barbecue oven and then onto the cinder block fence on which she would prance around as if she was the master of all she beheld. She kept the grass fairly well mowed in the backyard, but when she got older she developed a taste for the rose bushes. This alienated

JoAnn but I thought it a little humorous until she ate the bark off my chinaberry tree that I had been nurturing, killing it. That was different. I took her back to Luther.

Zeke, Abe, and Boots

Zeke was a toy fox terrier that some call a rat terrier. He was white with big black spots and probably weighed ten or twelve pounds. He had belonged to Ira and Jean Blanton. When the drouth deepened and Ira sold all his livestock, vacated his ranch and moved to Austin, he gave Zeke away, and we ended up with him.

He had quite a personality and ruled the roost around our house. I couldn't allow him in the hospital because he would pick on all the dogs and wanted to chase all the cats. He reminded me of a lot of small men I knew who thought they could whip the world. A classmate of mine named Jack Brundrett was such a person. He had been an Army Air Corps fighter pilot in World War II. I don't know how they let him in. I would have thought he was too short, but maybe they let him bring a pillow to sit on in the cockpit. He may not have been as short as I thought. He buddied up with a six-foot-three-inch tall football player named Monte Moncrief. When seen together they looked like "Mutt and Jeff." These were two characters in a comic strip of that day. One was tall and the other short.

Jack had an older brother, Frank, who was also a veterinarian and also short. Frank had a large animal practice on the outskirts of Dallas when he first got out of college before World War II. A big German dairyman called him to help a Holstein cow that was trying to calve. The man looked down on Frank and up at that big cow and asked, "Doc, you're a pretty little fellow for that big cow. Do you think you can pull that calf?" Frank bristled up and said, "Well, if I can't and you have enough money, I'll crawl in there and ride him out!" Jack always claimed dynamite came in little packages.

Zeke would grab a hold of the hind leg of a big ole German Shepherd or Labrador and hold on with his teeth. The big dog would stop, pick up his hind, leg and shake Zeke off. I hated for Zeke to get out of the yard for I knew one of those big dogs would bite his head off someday.

Zeke would take naps on the bed with JoAnn and follow her around. He dearly loved enchiladas and spaghetti. He wasn't much on some vegetables. He would clean up meat and potatoes and urinate on the turnips. I made a rather feeble protest to my family for giving him scraps, but I never was very critical of clients about how they fed their pets or fussed at them for over-weight problems. They already had a guilt complex about it, and I figured they had the pet to enjoy. The pet also had some right to a quality of life, especially because in past years the dog food was bland and much of it wasn't all that nutritionally balanced.

Zeke was quite a stud dog and in demand as such. A litter usu-ally consisted of three pups, one of which would take after Zeke and be very small, whereas the rest would be ordinary size. When Zeke began to age, we decided to keep one of his offspring. Abe, often called Aber, was a regular size, toy fox terrier and had peculiar eyes. There was a dark circle around each eye that accen-tuated his spooky appearance and made his eyes look big as saucers when he was excited or agitated. Zeke and Aber were well-trained, house-broken, and would ask to go outside.

The Gervasis acquired one of Zeke's pups and named him Nicky, for Niccodemus, in keeping with the biblical names of our dogs. Zeke for Ezekiel and Abe for Abraham. Frank Gervasi was an accomplished artist and a remarkable one at that. He had studied art and had become good before he enlisted in the U.S. Army in World War I. He lost his right arm due to wounds. After the war he returned to his old art instructor to be taught to paint with his left hand. The instructor had immigrated from Germany and refused Mr. Gervasi because he had fought against the instructor's fatherland. He learned to paint left-handed anyway. His wife, Lynn, had immigrated from Italy where she had been decorated by the Italian dictator, Mussolini, for her work in Italian libraries. She was a librarian in New York City before the couple came to Texas. Mr. Gervasi painted an oil portrait of their dog, Nicky, and gave it to me. It continues to hang in my reception room, together with some watercolor poses of Niccodemus that Mrs. Gervasi willed to me on her death. Nicky was a dignified, well-behaved dog that was true to his bloodline. He took Mr. Gervasi for a walk each afternoon. No, I didn't have it back-wards, Nicky was the leader.

We often went rabbit hunting on a Sunday afternoon: JoAnn,

Nancy, Janet, and I with the two dogs. It was togetherness in the seat of the pickup. Zeke was alert, but Abe was the cut up. When he saw a rabbit, he would bark and run from side to side almost hysterical, his eyes big as saucers. He would jump out of the window if not restrained. He would chase a rabbit—go just a-flying with Zeke and his little short legs trailing far behind. Abe would lose sight of the fast running jack rabbit and would often continue running straight ahead long after the rabbit had turned off to one side and stopped. When he finally became exhausted, he would trot back to us.

If a rabbit had been shot and killed, Abe would run up barking, grab it, and shake it while growling. When he tired, he would return to us at a trot, proud as punch with himself. It looked as if he thought he had killed it, although he never ate any. One day, I wounded a rabbit, and Abe immediately jumped out of the window and ran towards the rabbit, getting in my way so that I could not shoot it again. When he reached the rabbit it started the characteristic cry of panic, Abe tucked his little short tail and meekly returned to us. He never barked at nor chased another rabbit.

When Zeke and Abe were still active, they disappeared. We looked high and low, drove all over town, asked everyone, and offered a reward. No dogs. There was great moaning and groaning, wailing and weeping. We had just about given up hope when they showed up one morning: lean, lank, and foot sore. We couldn't imagine what had happened. Several months later, they again disappeared. We were told they had been seen near the Tinaja stockpens on the Santa Fe Railroad, close to ten miles away and they were chasing Kerr Mitchell's heifer calves. The person that had seen them honked, and the dogs quit the calves and ran off. I drove there and looked and called, no luck.

They soon showed up, sneaking along in Joe Mitchell's pasture to the front of our house. I was so mad at them that I started throwing rocks and yelling and ran them off. I watched, and when they approached, I again ran them off. I did this twice more and they stayed away until the girls came home and called them. They shied away from me for several days, but they never ran off again.

Boots was our family cat. Not really, I don't think anyone ever owns a cat. They may hang around and accept your food and even submit to a little petting, but only on their terms. They are independent and self-centered. The only time they will come when called is when they are bribed with food. Even then it is usually only a leisurely stroll. The eating is dainty, no gobbling or gulping. They can't be medicated by hiding a pill in their food. It doesn't matter how hungry they are or how carefully it is camouflaged, they will either refuse the entire meal or eat around the pill, leaving it in the bowl. Sometimes a pleasant tasting liquid might be mixed with the food and be eaten, but don't count on it.

Boots was an alley cat. Nowadays he would be called a domestic longhair. Pretty sophisticated category for such a nondescript animal. He was gray with a white spot on his chest and four white feet, hence his name. He looked innocent enough but had a roguish personality.

I'm not sure of the circumstances surrounding Boots entry into our family. We have had so many cats that they just seem to merge together. I think he was the sorry sight that was brought to the hospital in such a mess. His rear end was plastered with diarrhea and his front end was covered with vomit. He couldn't lift his head and was too weak to give more than a faint meow.

He was obviously in the last stages of panleucopenia a highly fatal disease of cats commonly called feline distemper. He was nestled in the arms of a little girl who was crying softly. The girl's mother said the kitten was found in the front yard, a stray, and asked if there was anything that could be done, or should it be put to sleep. The little girl, Bess, looked up at me with the most sorrowful eyes that I have ever seen and silently pleaded for me to help.

I gingerly took the pitiful thing. It was so thin it didn't weigh anything, light as a feather. I carried it back to the kennel room and laid it on a towel. I fixed a heating pad to try to warm the cold little kitten, then began to clean the face with a warm wet cloth.

I started preparing a penicillin injection while Bess continued to bathe Boots. The mother said they would have to leave and that she would call later. I assured the cute little girl that I would do my best.

I attempted to inject the penicillin in the thigh, but there was only skin and bone and not much of that. The needle went clear through, and the medicine squirted out the other side. I clipped the hair on a front leg, applied a tourniquet, and tried to find the vein to give fluids but was unsuccessful because the vein was collapsed. I gave up on the vein and inserted the needle under the skin to drip some fluid subcutaneously, hoping it would be absorbed into the dehydrated body, but the circulation was so poor, I felt this was only a desperation move.

I added an antibiotic syrup to a milk formula and teased a little into the mouth with an eyedropper. I would feed a few drops of the formula every chance I got during the day and kept it up that evening 'til I went to bed. The next morning the kitten was more alert, but I was afraid this would only give the little girl false hope. I still did not think there was much possibility of survival.

That afternoon near quitting time, I still had not heard from the mother, so I asked my receptionist to phone. It was an out-of-town number, and we were told there was no such number and no one listed by that name. I'm a trusting soul and kinda hoped that the name and phone number had been recorded by mistake. I moved the kitten into the house at night where I kept it in a deep basket.

My daughters had begun helping with the kitten — feeding, bathing, and massaging. By the time I realized that the little stray had been dumped on me, my daughters had fallen in love with it and wanted to keep it. I was outwardly reluctant but secretly pleased because it was always hard for me to have to part with an animal that I had worked so hard to save. I wonder what the mother told the little girl.

This was going to be a problem. Zeke and Abe were the house dogs, and there was no way the cat could join them, for they hated cats with a passion. Therefore, this had to be an outside cat. My hospital and residence are joined under the same roof with the intervening space being a garage at that time. This garage became the cat's domain.

The kitchen door opened into the garage. Boots would lay in wait beside it, and when the dogs would be let out, he would slap them a good lick and take out running. The dogs were infuriated and pursued him as fast as they could go. He would run fast for a little ways, then slow down to let them catch up. When they got close, he would stop and turn to face them with his back humped up and his tail straight in the air. His hair would be standing on end. He would let out a loud hiss. The dogs would slam on their brakes, but usually they were too close and would slide into Boots to get cuffed soundly. They would then take off yipping. They never seemed to learn it was okay to chase a cat, they just should-n't catch it. They did learn that when the door was opened for them to go out, they would run as fast as their little, short legs would carry them to get by the place of ambush as quickly as possible.

Often my pickup would be parked in the garage, and Boots liked to lay on the fender and look through the screen door into the kitchen. Occasionally, when the dogs came by, he would jump down on the back of one of them and dig his claws in. The surprised dog would let out the most God-awful, bloodcurdling squall you ever heard. Aber, with the spooky looking eyes, had an unreal expression when that happened to him.

The backyard was enclosed by a cinder block fence. Boots would prance around on top of it and would tease the dogs by letting his tail dangle down and gently twitch it. The dogs would run back and forth, barking furiously, nearly becoming hysterical.

Boots was also quite a boxer. He would be perched on the fender of my pickup near the kitchen door. If he wasn't noticed when someone passed by, he would reach out with claws extended and grab a sleeve. When the person stopped, he would retract his claws and paw in the air. He was ready to do a little sparring. He would cock his head to one side while he feinted with the paw. If you got a little rough with him, he would sit up on his haunches, lay his ears back and get with it with both paws. If he was still losing the fight, he would grab your hand with both his paws, pull it to him, bite it, then take off running.

Boots loved to prowl around inside a covered stock trailer but would come flying out when it began to move. He disappeared one day, never to be seen again. We guessed that perhaps he had been hauled off in a trailer he could not get out of.

Our daughters, Nancy and Janet, developed bad allergies. They were tested and found to be especially sensitive to the dogs, who were then exiled to the backyard. They continued to spend the night inside in the kennel in cages reserved for them.

Zeke began to have health problems. First it was his kidneys, then his heart, next cataracts, with resulting blindness. His sense of smell and hearing remained acute and his son, Abe, guided him around. He seemed to maintain a fairly decent quality of life by taking his medication inserted in tasty tidbits.

One morning Abe was discovered dead. Quite a shock to us. He was twelve years old, but we thought of him as a pup. Zeke was pretty pitiful after that, unable to find his food unless we put it under his nose, and he would bump into objects in the yard. He just laid around most of the time grieving, I suppose, and seemed to have lost interest in living. The appetite was poor. I knew it was time to put him down. He was nineteen years old, but I couldn't do it. I took him to Dr. Jan Smith, the lady veterinarian in Alpine, who performed euthanasia in a humane and gentle manner, yet with dignity befitting the old-timer.

Many years later we had a barn cat that we called Momma Cat. She was the most prolific cat I ever saw. I'm sure she had three litters a year at least. She also would scavenge people's lunches and prowl their trailers. She disappeared, and we thought she was gone for good. One day, JoAnn looked out the window and saw her sitting on top of a swamp cooler that was her favorite perch. This cat was an ugly, long-haired, motley brown with weepy eyes. There was no doubt it was Momma Cat. She was skinny as a rail and went into the barn as soon as we fed her and never came out except when we forgot to feed and water her. She must have had a real traumatic experience during that year and a half that she was gone and didn't want to leave her sanctuary.

Chapter 9

My Prime Years

The year 1960 was memorable; lots of exciting things happened.

Mrs. Lorene Tyler, my mother-in-law, came to be my receptionist-bookkeeper. We had a mutual admiration for each other. I loved her dearly, and she looked after me, defending my property and my reputation. Ben would come storming in the office wanting to know where "that nasty ole quack was." This really upset Mrs. Tyler, and to make matters worse, he would go into the pharmacy where only prescription drugs were kept, and no one was to enter except me. There he would take down drugs from the shelves, put them back in wrong places or leave them on the counter, anything to aggravate her. "BEN GEARHART!" She was the only person I remember addressing him or referring to him as such. She knew him from just a pup. He worked in the Palace Theater as usher, ticket taker, and sold popcorn when he was in high school. Mrs. Tyler worked in her husband's (Jim Tyler) garage next door. Jane Gearhart, Ben's mother, had a beauty shop in her house that Mrs. Tyler had patronized for many years. Even with this background, I think she was intimidated by Ben.

JoAnn spent many hours in this theater as a young school girl, waiting for her mother and father to close up. Ben, and later his brother, Bill, would give her a hand full of popcorn for a penny.

*   *   *   *   *

The O.M. Franklin Serum Co. was acquired by the American Home Products Corporation which began to consolidate their stores and product line. They closed the Marfa store, which had been a combination retail and distribution center for Franklin products. Dr. A. J. Hoffman, the veterinarian who had opened the store and who had been with the company since it was started in 1917, was retired.

No one else in Marfa was interested in this business. I had originally intended to be a purist, very professional and not a pill
pusher, not even dispensing prescriptions. I soon found this to be
impractical in veterinary medicine and especially so in this isolated area, but still I only dispensed prescription items until the
hard, difficult days of the drouth. When you're hungry, you do
what you gotta do.

I visited with Dr. Hoffman and arranged to buy his fixtures and
the items that the company was discontinuing. I was also able to
purchase much of their regular stock at a discount to save them
the trouble and expense of returning it to their warehouse.

Lee Plumbley, a local contractor, converted my two-car garage
adjacent to the office into a store. The next ten years were very
profitable.

My Pickups

The Runaway

Joe and Sammie Lane were living at Charco Largo on the south
side of the Hubbard ranch that he had leased in the mid-fifties.
Joe and I had operated on some cancer-eye cows at the north end
of the ranch at a place called the Farm House. Years before there
had been a farm here, irrigated with water from San Esteban Lake.
The water ran through a tunnel about a half mile long, then in a
ditch to this place. I think the operation folded up because of the
drouth of 1917-18.

When we finished with the cows, we drove an ungraded ranch
road from there to Charco Largo. This was a shortcut in miles but
may have taken longer than going around by better roads. This
was rough, rocky and tortuous. I was following Joe as closely as
I could, but that was a problem because it was slow going, dodging the biggest rocks. The gas pedal broke and flopped to the
floor. The motor revved up and took off, a real runaway, tearing
along at a breakneck speed. It doesn't hardly seem possible that a
broken gas pedal would cause acceleration. It seems to me that
the pickup shoulda stopped. I couldn't stay on the road with all
the twists and turns, going lickety split. I took off across country
with a wild exciting ride, over rocks, sacahuiste, catclaw and cardentia. I was so busy chauffeuring that I didn't have time to

think. I finally turned off the ignition and stopped.

Joe came back, looking for me, and then he tied the thingamajig back together with a little piece of baling wire.

This was the old Chevrolet pickup that I drove during the drouth.

The Studebaker Pickups

I bought a new Studebaker pickup from Webb Brothers when it started raining and the practice picked up so that I could afford the monthly payments. The West Texas Utilities Company had discarded an old, rusty, worn-out utility bed that I cabbaged on to. Webb Brothers cleaned it up and mounted it on the pickup. A little welding, a few braces, and some light blue paint put it in pretty good shape. I could take more drugs, supplies, and equipment. It was very satisfactory. Most of the drugs at that time were relatively crude and could take more abuse than the later sophisticated ones.

My first attempt to drive this pickup was frustrating. I couldn't find the starter. Every vehicle I had ever driven had a starter pedal just above the gas pedal. This pickup didn't have one that I could locate. I thought maybe an error had been made at the factory, and I told Harold Webb to this effect. There happened to be several others present at the time. They all had a big laugh at my expense. I kinda bristled up! I couldn't see the humor. It turned out the starter was beneath the gas pedal and was activated when the gas pedal was depressed all the way to the floorboard.

I traded pickups each year for $500 difference with about 55,000 miles on the odometer. At that time, this mileage was considered to be about the maximum before repairs became a problem. My colleagues said I was a truck driver instead of a veterinarian. There may have been more truth to this than I cared to admit because I often spent more time traveling than treating. However, many times I would work all day at a single ranch.

Sometimes I would have a call waiting when I returned, to go to a place near the one I had just come from, so that I had to backtrack. Carl Williams, JoAnn's cousin, managed a two-way radio business in Alpine. I subscribed, hoping to save many miles of driving. It didn't work out for several reasons. I had trouble understanding the radio, and often I would be behind a mountain, in a canyon, or out of range so that the reception was poor or nil. But I think the worst problem was when a person contacted me and demanded that I drop everything and come immediately. Invariably, this would happen at a time that I had a pen full of cattle, and I could not leave. People didn't seem to resent not being able to contact me, but when they did and I wouldn't come, they became very agitated. A solution to the two-way radio was not long in coming.

My Last Studebaker

My first call in it was to Escondido, a ranch owned by Hayes Mitchell Sr. I had bled a bunch of cows to test for brucellosis, taking the blood from the jugular vein and collecting it in glass tubes. I was hurrying back to the hospital to test the blood because Hayes wanted to ship as soon as possible. I scooted up the Nopal road to Highway 90/67 and put on the brakes. No brakes! It was an exciting ride across the highway, through the bar ditch, up the railroad embankment, across the tracks where there was no crossing, down the other side of the railroad embankment, finally coming to rest astraddle of the Catto-Gage Ranch fence.

The glass tubes containing the blood were scattered all around the cab, and many were broken. Fortunately, there was no highway traffic or trains. I was lucky not to have turned over. All I could think of was how embarrassing it was to call Hayes and have to rework the cattle. My old pickup was still available, and I used it while this new one was patched up. The difficulty of keeping eartag number and tubes straight on the rework was more trouble than the original bleeding. Hayes was upset; I was upset; the Webb Brothers were upset; the insurance company was upset; and I suppose the Studebaker car company was also. Everyone lived over it, but there was no telling the tale and laughing. Needless to say, I always slowed down a long ways ahead when later approaching this place.

The Wreck

My practice had begun to get very busy in the summer of 1960. I started driving the ranch roads a little too fast. These were being maintained much better, which permitted faster speeds. Dumps were put in many roads to divert water out to prevent erosion. Some of these were a little high and poorly sloped. The road past the Smith house east towards Morgan Chaney's was straight and fairly level, I hit a dump too fast and lost control and rolled over.

I had always thought I could hold onto the steering wheel if I turned over, but I found out I couldn't. I was all around inside the cab with me and that two-way radio (that had broken loose) tangled up. Fortunately, the doors didn't come open, and I escaped injury except for a little skin knocked off one hand and few bruises. The pickup came to rest on its wheels facing out into the pasture. I tried to start the engine—no luck. The two-way radio wouldn't work either. I walked the two or three miles back to the Smith house. David and Gloria Pool were living there working for Gage Holland. I called JoAnn to notify Webb Brothers for a wrecker and for her to come pick me up. I called Morgan, and he came and took me to his ranch.

After we finished he took me back to the Smith house, and I met JoAnn and the wrecker.

I salvaged some of the medicines and most of the instruments and equipment. They say every cloud has a silver lining. The silver lining to this wreck was that it destroyed that aggravating two-way radio.

The Ford Pickups

I immediately began contacting utility companies in order to find a used utility bed to put on another pickup—no luck.

The Astoria Company in Astoria, Illinois, was one of the few, if not the only, company making a special veterinary bed to be mounted on a pickup. They had a demonstrator mounted on a Ford pickup that they had been driving around the country, showing it at veterinary meetings. They had a new and improved model they were going to show off the next year. They offered their old one to me at a very reasonable price if I would come get it. I was very busy, pregnancy checking cows and had a full schedule so JoAnn traveled there with our two daughters, Nancy, 8-years-old, and Janet, 6-years-old. They flew from El Paso to Dallas, then to St. Louis, where they again changed planes to Chicago. Here a small regional airline carried them to Astoria. A company car met the plane and took them to the plant. The paperwork was completed, and JoAnn gave them a certified check. JoAnn drove through Chicago, St. Louis, Kansas City, going through a bad storm between Tulsa and Oklahoma City, but they made it back to Marfa without mishap. This was a very spunky thing for her to do, and I was very proud of her, yet I had a guilty feeling.

The vet bed was guaranteed for ten years. I was still using it thirty-five years later when I retired in 1995. I moved it from pickup to pickup. It was made to be mounted on a long wheelbase Ford pickup, on which it fit nicely until the Ford Motor Company changed the design of the long wheelbase by extending its length. Pierce Motors had mounted the bed on a new pickup I had ordered. There was a twelve-inch gap between the bed and the cab. It looked terrible! Several of us were standing around looking at it, moaning and groaning. JoAnn drove up and immediately suggested putting the spare tires there. What a great idea! I had been carrying the two spare tires loose on top of the vet bed.

Mine was a fire engine type practice. The first fifteen years I went long distances to treat individual patients. When my practice became busier because of increased rainfall and better cow prices, I had a major problem attending to my practice territory. However, about that time, trailers for hauling livestock came into common usage, and I improved my hospital facilities for both horses and cattle so that more patients could be seen by their being brought to me. Nevertheless, I still had to go to many individuals, usually because the sick animal could not be loaded, or the means were not available to bring the animal to me. Large numbers were always attended to at a ranch. It always remained a practice in blood and mud, sometimes snow and ice, sometimes rain, heat or cold, but mostly dust, dirt, and manure.

Many physicians stopped making house calls except in unusual circumstances, and I believe this had much to do with clients being more willing to bring their animals to me.

Toyah Cow Work 1960

It was just getting gray in the east one day in the summer of 1960 when I pulled up to the little cafe in Toyah town about 85 miles from Marfa. I don't remember its name. If it had one, I guess it was "The Texas Cafe." If it wasn't, it should have been, because in that day and age, every Texas town had a cafe, picture show, or hotel and sometimes all three, if the town was big enough, all named "The Texas." Toyah had seen better days, having had two banks at one time. Now, it was almost a ghost town. I don't remember any occupied store buildings on the main drag along the north side of the Texas and Pacific Railroad tracks. The cafe was located on the south side near the depot on U.S. Highway 80, which was called the Bankhead Highway. (This was before Interstate 20 was built and the fancy "Asphalt Cowboy" restaurant was established.)

This cafe couldn't be dignified by calling it a restaurant. It was a little white frame building with a tin roof. The paint was peeling, and the roof was a little rusty in places. The screen door had a ragged hole, and it sagged. Some might say it was quaint, with character, while others might say it was dilapidated. I guess it all depends on a person's point of view.

The door squeaked loudly when I opened it. The men looked up to see who had disturbed their peace and quiet. I went on in and said my howdys to the three men who sat at a table draped with a blue and white checkerboard oilcloth. One was sitting on his chair backwards with his chin resting on the back of the chair. I don't know if he had experienced a bad night or was just conserving his energy in case of a hard day coming up. Another had his chin cupped in both of his hands with his elbows propped on the table, while the third fiddled with his cup of coffee. He was a fellow I knew from Balmorhea, H. McDermott. He started to get up to shake hands, but his spurs got tangled in the rungs of his chair and he almost had a wreck. I tried to give him a hand, but I hung my toe in a hole in the linoleum on the floor which had a generous amount of black showing in places where the surface had worn off. It was all I could do to regain my dignity, so we skipped the formalities and just kinda gave each other a feeble salute and let it go at that.

I climbed up astraddle of a round stool at the counter. It was kinda wobbly, and I thought it was going to throw me there for a minute. I even considered going to another, but I was determined not to let it get the best of me.

The cook brought me a cup of coffee, and I ordered breakfast. That sure was good coffee, made with water piped from the springs over close to Toyahvale. I was about ready for a second cup when a plate with three eggs, fried over easy, two big patties of sausage and a pile of hashbrowns with a couple of biscuits and cream gravy was set in front of me. Now there was a breakfast that would stick to your ribs. There was a generous amount of grease to give it flavor. That was before my heart attack. After that, I was supposed to spit out anything that tasted good. Some people would refer to this place as a greasy spoon, but it shouldn't be categorized that way because Cookie was clean.

The ranchman I was to meet showed up just as I was sopping up the last of the cream gravy, so we took out. I followed him in my new practice vehicle. It was the pickup with the special veterinary bed mounted back of the cab. It had all kinds of drawers and cubby holes for medicines and equipment, a little refrigerator on one side, and a sink with a 40-gallon water tank on the other. This was a real fancy rig for that day and age. The rancher crossed the T-P tracks with me on his heels and left town heading kinda northerly on a pretty good gravel road. We soon angled off to the northeast, winding around, taking one fork in the road, then another. I had to drop back and not follow very close because of the powdery, white dust he was kicking up. Each time I slowed down, the fine dust would envelop me, building up on the windshield so that it drifted down in ripples, looking kinda like the ocean surf rolling in waves. It would boil up in the cab and choke me. I was afraid I would lose him, but his cloud of dust always stayed in sight. I tried to look out the rear view mirror, but the back window was so dirty I couldn't see through it. The outside mirror had disintegrated a few days before when a gate post reached out and clobbered it. I really didn't need to look back there anyway, a dust cloud was all that could have been seen, and besides, I had already been there.

There wasn't much vegetation north of Toyah, a little greasewood and a few yuccas, except for the draws which had a fair amount of tobosa grass turf and some whitebrush. We finally arrived at a set of lumber pens with railroad crosstie posts that had sorta bleached out. We had come a good, long ways. I thought we must be close to the New Mexico state line. It was a nice warm day, probably 100° to 105°, maybe 110°. The cattle were a little restless, milling around, perhaps caused by hooking each other with long sharp horns. They were stirring up the dust something fierce. We couldn't see across the pen, but when pregnancy testing, I really didn't need to see, the work being done by feel. There wasn't a breath of air, still as death. I never could figure out why the wind won't give at least a little breeze on a hot day, but blows a gale on a cold one. The gyp dust eats on a person when mixed with sweat, and there was plenty of both.

We were getting along real well. The crew was a bunch of good Mexican ranch hands, but all of a sudden, there weren't any. Things came to a screeching halt. The men weren't seen running, dodging, or sneaking off, they were just gone. A few minutes later, a vehicle came into view and drove up with a couple of *chotas*. They got out and shook hands. Well, they shook hands with the ranchman. They didn't seem to be anxious to shake hands with me. I had not started using the newly developed plastic palpating gloves because they were so poorly made, especially by size (one-size-fits-all). So, I worked with bare hands and arms. The men must have been old hands, because they didn't ask any stupid questions such as if we had seen any wets around. They could tell at a glance with the pens full of cattle and only the rancher and me that there had to be some and that we needed them badly. They didn't tarry long so as to hold us up, just commented on the dry weather, hoping we weren't in for another drouth so soon after the big one. They also said how good the cattle looked. Actually they were pretty hard, but that's a polite thing to say. Then as a passing remark as they were leaving, asked to be notified when the men were no longer needed.

The men reappeared about as silently and quickly as they had disappeared, and we resumed work, finishing along in the shank of the afternoon. Actually, we had made pretty good time because we didn't have to stop and eat lunch. The *patrón* had forgot the food and water. Early that morning as he started to leave his house, his wife had called out asking if he had put the lunch and water jugs in his pickup. He had answered that, of course he had — what a stupid question. Well, as a matter of fact, he hadn't. The items were still where he had put them, in a place where they wouldn't be forgotten. The wife had prepared a good lunch with plenty of round steaks. Now some people might call this baloney, in a disparaging tone of voice, but they aren't very hungry. Well, the cowman had been concentrating on what he would do with his open cows. This is premature, because a decision can't be made until after the testing and the opens have been sorted off. Then comes the tough decisions, because many of the open cows are thin and won't dollar out at the auction and many more are young with their life ahead of them. This is one of the places that separates the men from the boys — when one tries to figure if it'll rain, whether those poor cows will put on a little weight, and what the cow market will do. Some have been known to say they had rather be lucky than smart. Usually, you have a little time to decide, unless you've already ordered trucks and they are waiting, revving up their engines and trying to get you to hurry. Trucks are always way early or way late, and you've ordered too many or not enough. If you go ahead and ship, the market will break before your cattle sell, and two weeks later you get a wet spell. If you don't sell when the market is strong, and it doesn't rain, everybody is forced to sell, and the market breaks.

There was a little daylight left, enough that they could see to sort cattle. So, I decided to leave and not wait to be showed the way back to town. I was asked if I knew the way back. Of course I didn't, with all that twisting, turning, and forks in the road, but have you ever known a man to admit he didn't know the way or to ask directions? I took off in a cloud of dust. That sounds as if I left in a hurry, but actually the powdered dirt road kicked up dust regardless of the speed. I decided my best bet was to go west to the Delaware Mountains and hit the road south to Kent that goes by the Jones boys' ranch. Actually, they were fairly old men but they had always been referred to as the Jones boys, Cal and Frank. Then I would go south by Jap Foster's place and the Drake ranch and on to Kent.

A good thing about the country is that if you want to go west, you head west. It's not like an interstate or especially a city freeway where you get in the right hand lane to turn left and left hand lane to turn right.

I wandered around a little while. I wasn't lost, just didn't know where I was or how to get to town. I could see the Delaware Mountains, and the setting sun showed me where west was. This was before people started having to lock their gates, so I was free to wander around at will.

Now I said none of these gates were locked. However, there was one particular gate that was such a challenge to open, it probably would have been easier if it had been locked. I could generally open a locked gate one way or another if it was absolutely necessary, but I guess I better not tell how.

This was a Can't Sag brand gate, identified by the hardware, because the paint with the name had long since faded out. Of course, it could have been a counterfeit, I suppose. This gate had sagged so badly that the sliding bar that was the latch was wedged and wouldn't budge.

The gate was hung by the type of hinges that have to be threaded by lifting the gate and balancing it so the two parts of the hinge are lined up just right. It's not too hard to thread one, but it is necessary to thread both at the same time. I don't know the name of this type hinge. I've heard it called a lot of names, most of which I can't mention here.

It would have been fairly easy to open if I could have lifted it off its hinges, but some devious mind had reversed the hinges so it was not possible.

I probably had been spoiled that day because all gates coming out from Toyah had been cattle guards. These are a series of bars in the ground with an empty space underneath that cattle and horses are reluctant to cross but a vehicle can drive across.

I drank a little water from a rusty tomato can with a baling wire handle that had been hanging on a water tank by a windmill. It was gyp water. There are two kinds of gyp water, bad and worse. If the water is hot, dipped out of the tank, it's worse. The fact is, it can't be drunk. The taste and odor constrict your throat and nauseate you. However, this time a little breeze came up, the windmill turned, and pumped some water from deep underground. I caught a little coming out of the pipe emptying into the tank. This is cold, and you might take on a bellyful before the realization of what you have done hits you. It begins with a burp that tastes and smells like sulfur, soon followed by a bellyache, then the diarrhea. I had been down that road before, and it makes a lasting impression. Therefore, I had sipped very discreetly, more to rinse my mouth out and wet my whistle. The only thing you can say good about gyp water is that it is wet.

I had worked up a pretty good thirst with the heat, dust, and work. We had drunk almost all my water, and I had used the last washing my hands and arms. The 40-gallon water tank in my pickup must have been low. That was more water than I had ever had in the past, having been relying on a five-gallon water can that was war surplus. I didn't think I would ever run out of water again with that big tank. Besides, my help was supposed to keep it full. I had a little trouble a short time before. A new high school boy had added gasoline to the water tank. The caps were very similar. I was upset but glad he had not put water in the gas tank. The wreck did make him a little gun shy about filling the water tank. Perhaps the help shouldn't get all the blame because I was busy, coming in late after they had left for the day and leaving early in the morning before they came to work. We had a saying in the paratroops: It don't mean a thing if you don't pull that string. This large capacity water tank didn't do much good if it wasn't filled occasionally.

This was before I started carrying emergency rations, but this and many similar instances caused me to take up the practice. I first carried pork and beans, vienna sausages, and peanut butter. I soon learned better. Others would pilfer my supplies. I finally learned I was safe with sardines and crackers.

I finally came to a camp shack and spotted two men horseback kinda circling around acting like a couple of sheep killing dogs. They finally rode on up, and I asked directions. They told me and invited me to eat first. I didn't want to be impolite, and besides, that breakfast in Toyah was about to wear off. There was a good cool spring with sweet water here at this camp shack, and I took on a pretty good fill while the wets built a fire under the beans. Now I had always believed that cooking good frijoles and making good flour tortillas was a skill Mexicans were born with, part of the genetics. I learned differently because these two were the genuine thing, being wet, I'm sure, yet those were the worst pinto beans I ever ate. I didn't say the worst beans, just the worst pinto beans. They were almost as bad as the navy beans on board a troop ship.

JoAnn told me that the navy bean and the bean in Van Camp's Pork and Beans were the same. I didn't believe her because I really liked pork and beans; you just don't want to try to find the pork. I like them hot or cold. I checked with Charlie Henderson who had been a cook on a submarine during World War II. He assured me both were the northern white bean. When I questioned this, he explained that on a troop ship the cooks didn't have the training, condiments, or time to cook them properly and asked if I had ever eaten poorly prepared pinto beans. I thought of this meal in the Delaware Mountains. The beans were half raw and unseasoned, and I think they must have imported some of the gyp water to cook them in. There were no onions or even chilies to numb the taste buds. I don't know how to describe the tortillas. They were hot off the top of that wood stove and had to be eaten quickly, because I'm sure they would have been inedible when cold. If you can imagine making some homemade glue with flour and water, then spilling some on the hot stove, you would have an idea of the taste and texture. They must have run out of coffee a week or two before and kept boiling the grounds.

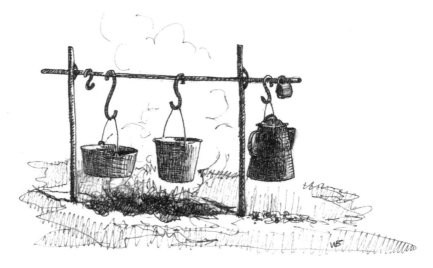

Campfire cooking.

I'm sure this is the worst meal I ever ate in West Texas. I didn't say *try to eat* because I did eat it. If the difference between a good meal and a great meal is two hours, then the 14 hours from breakfast and a hard day's work is what made this edible.

They had a little vermicelli leftovers that had been flavored with a little canned tomatoes, salt and pepper. They watered it downright smart to make it go farther, which made it difficult to eat. There were no eating utensils, which is not uncommon in a Mexican camp. You tear off a couple of pieces of tortilla, hunker down real low over the plate and shovel the food in, eating the food and the scoop together. I couldn't complain, being the guest, and I had to really stretch the truth when I told them how good it was and thanked them for their hospitality.

I began to feel ashamed that I had stayed to eat. The poor men didn't have enough for themselves, yet they had willingly and cheerfully shared what they had. I hope the *patrón* had a real good excuse for not bringing them their groceries in a timely manner.

Their directions were adequate, and I made it home without mishap about dark thirty* I had pretty well used up the day. JoAnn asked if I wanted her to fix me something to eat. I declined because those tortillas and frijoles felt like lead in my stomach.

A Complicated C-Section

A big, stout boy hauled a heifer to me that was down in the trailer saying she was trying to calve and thought he'd let me have a try at her. I had him back the trailer into my delivery room. Actually, this was a tin barn, but I was mighty proud of it, having only recently completed it. I was especially thankful of it this day, as it was cold and windy.

I washed her dirty rear end and proceeded to examine her. I couldn't figure out what I had at first, finally realizing that the uterus was ruptured and the calf outside, mixed in with the intestines. I came out, washed the blood off, sat down, lit a cigarette, took a deep puff and pondered the situation.

The fellow admitted that he had tried to help a little. After further questioning, he said that when he found her, both of the front legs of the calf were showing, but he wasn't able to locate the head. He had snubbed her to a yucca, hooked onto the calf's legs with a chain, took a wrap around the trailer hitch of the pickup and gave a little gentle pull. I knew the pull musta been *gentle* because both legs had torn off of the calf and the heifer was paralyzed.

My helper and I rolled her over on her back, tied the front legs together, and secured them to the side of the trailer. We repeated this with the hind legs. The belly was clipped and scrubbed. A midline incision was made from the breastbone to the udder after infiltrating the area with an anesthetic. The calf was no trouble to find, but it was hard to untangle from the intestines. The placenta (afterbirth) refused to release which wasn't unusual so soon after delivery, but I was particularly disappointed because of the damage and contamination. The cowboy had tried to help without benefit of soap and water.

I medicated the uterus and began suturing the laceration with

---

* This was an expression to designate a vague indefinite hour. It may be as early as thirty minutes after dark, but more likely much later.

both hands, but was unable to finish because the udder had prevented my making the abdominal incision far enough. I continued to suture one-handed with the catgut on a loopuyt needle. This seems rather simple writing about it, but it was slow and laborious, standing on my head and trying to keep the guts out of the way while suturing. It seems like they were taking a life of their own, trying to make my job harder. The frequent sticking the needle in the end of my fingers added to my frustration. Sulmet solution was poured into the peritoneal cavity before closing the abdominal wall.

The kid had the audacity to complain that fall because the heifer didn't get pregnant.

This laceration had been lengthwise whereas the tear usually occurred in front of the cervix in a transverse plane when the uterus ruptured and the calf was in the peritoneal cavity. The cervix had not completely dilated in these cases, and I was able to anchor the uterine edge of the laceration to a fold in the cervix. This wasn't very sophisticated suturing, but the results were always satisfactory.

Horses and Colic

Jess Fisher was raised near Ft. Davis. The family ranch became part of the Eppenauer ranch. Jess was living at Sanderson working for the railroad but still kept a horse or two in his backyard. A mare developed severe colic, and her abdomen was distended. I passed a stomach tube and drained an enormous amount of fluid from her stomach. It ran across his yard and out into the alley. I couldn't believe the amount. When the flow stopped, I sucked on the tube to see if it would start again. A hot pepper taste burned my mouth. I pumped in water and drained it back a few times in an attempt to clean it. Then I pumped in mineral oil and gave another intravenous injection for pain. Jess said the back gate was open, but the mare was in the pen so he hadn't really thought much about it. We went into the alley and followed her tracks about three-quarters of a block and found a 55-gallon barrel being used for a garbage can. In the can were many chili peppers. The mare had eaten some, then tanked up on water to put out the fire.

Jess frequently helped the Sanderson area ranchers work their stock. He was especially good horseback. A rancher, who raised very good horses, gave a good young colt to Jess. He halter broke him, fed, and groomed him, resulting in an outstanding individual. Jess took him to the Denver stock show, and a man offered him $5,000. This was an enormous sum at that time, and especially to Jess. Jess was so proud of this colt that he finally refused the offer and took him home. He said he had always wanted an outstanding horse, and now that he had one, he couldn't part with him. Soon after returning to Sanderson the colt got the colic. I was called. It is 115 miles and takes two hours to get there. When I arrived Jess told me the colt was well, and he didn't need me. I returned to Marfa and on arrival my wife said Jess had called, and the colt was bad again. Intermittent pain is not uncommon in horse colic. The colt was dead when I got back, and I thought I was going to have to bury Jess.

Snow and −15° F

It was January 10, 1962, according to my records. I had been up late the night before. A snowstorm had hit during the night, and the bottom had dropped out of the thermometer. Although, I didn't have an outside thermometer at that time, and it was probably a good thing.

The phone rang bright and early. The sun wasn't up yet, but it was fairly bright with a full moon shining on the snow. Guy Lee and his son, Jerry, were living at the Crawford Ranch, a part of the Catto-Gage Ranches near Marathon, and calving out Hereford heifers in a relatively small pasture between their house and the railroad. They had just checked the heifers and found one trying to calve with only a foot showing. They had roped her and tied her down but were unable to find the other leg.

I really hated to crawl out of that nice, warm bed. I felt like I had just climbed in it. I put the coffee pot on, dressed and staggered out into the hospital which was attached to the residence. I began cleaning the calving equipment that I had used the night before. I was tired then, but now I wished that I had washed it before the blood and juices had dried so hard.

My pickup had been in the garage, but it wouldn't start. I should have tried before I washed my equipment. I was to learn later that I should have had starter fluid on hand. Others have told me a little ether in the carburetor would have done the job, but I have never tried it. Chicken, I guess, because Bill Gearhart once came in with his eyelashes and eyebrows burned off from its use.

The pickup started just before the battery gave its last gasp, and I pulled around to the hospital to load up. I filled a thermos with coffee to drink on the fifty-six mile drive to the ranch. I had drained the water tank in my vet bed, because during the previous winter the water had frozen and broke it. The man who crawled inside and welded the galvanized metal in the cramped quarters had moaned and groaned, using strong language. He told me what I could do with it if I allowed it to freeze again. Therefore, I filled a five-gallon, war surplus water can with hot water and put it in the cab.

A client and friend, Rust Largent, had reassured me of my opinion that cold weather could be tolerated better if a heater in the pickup was not used because the body could acclimate to the cold better. I wasn't going to test the theory on a morning like this and left the motor running with the heater going full blast while I loaded.

The snow was only a couple of inches deep as I started off. This may sound like I was accustomed to snow. Actually I thought this was bad at the time and felt sorry for a cute little Mexican boy carrying a can of kerosene with a potato in the spout as he hot footed it across the street from Colomo's Handy Store. I guess this is a poor expression to use for this little fellow walking briskly in the snow. I doubt his feet were warm, much less hot.

When I got to Altuda about halfway between Alpine and Marathon, I got into some real snow. There wasn't a traffic problem. In fact, there never was on this stretch of road, especially this time of day. Somebody had been by and cut some ruts. I don't know enough about snow to know whether this is good or bad. I thought it was good at the time. I managed to keep going in spite of the fact that I didn't put tire chains on. I just didn't want to get out there and wallow around in the snow.

The weather was calm, clear, and cold. The snow covering everything and smoke curling up from the chimneys in Marathon looked so peaceful. I didn't see why I should have to go and disturb it. I finally reached the ranch, and after saying my howdys, we drove out to the heifer. They said they thought their main problem was because of her violent straining. I clipped the hair over her tail head and disinfected with tincture of phenylmercuric nitrate, then attempted to load a syringe with procaine, a local anesthetic to give a spinal. Both bottles of procaine had frozen and broken. This was going to make my job harder.

I prepared suture material, a three-eighths inch umbilical tape threaded on a large curved needle. I placed this along with scissors and a needle holder in a tray, put in Quseptic disinfectant, and added water from my can.

I washed the cow's rear end. Guy said, "Doc, we've already been in several times without washing, why worry?" I answered that she probably had enough contamination and didn't need any more. However, my arm was so cold when I washed it, I decided they were probably right.

I sure did hate to lie down in about eight inches of snow, but I did and went to work. True to form she strained. Some heifers that have been in labor a little while develop diarrhea. She was no exception. This was one of the times I wished the Good Lord had arranged the anatomy a little differently. Each time I attempted to extract the lost leg, I released the pressure on the urethra and a great gush of urine would scald me. Insult to injury or injury to insult? If there was anything good about the whole thing, it was because the heifer had not lost all her natural lubricant. I wallowed around in the nasty mess in the snow, finally getting a hold on the leg and maneuvering it out and straightening the head just as the heifer gave a big push and the calf popped out. I wanted to kiss the lively little booger, but not bad enough to do so.

I tried to look humble as I grinned up at father and son heaping praise on me, but I reveled in it, making all the effort worthwhile. Suddenly, everything went to pot. The heifer struggled violently, the rope on her legs came untied and the entire uterus came out, a complete uterine prolapse. Now I really had problems. Both of them had their hands full, wrestling the heifer back down and holding her. I tried to wash the uterus, but the water kept freezing. I finally replaced the uterus and got up to get medication and the suture material, but it was frozen solid in the tray. I was forced to prepare new suture. I turned suddenly at my companions' yelling; the blooming thing was out again! I don't remember doing so, but I was accused of using an expletive. The procedure seemed longer and more difficult this time, but it was eventually accomplished and the sutures applied. I had not added water to the tray this time.

We turned our attention to the calf. What had been a live vigorous calf was now a cold, stiff, lifeless form, frozen in the snow. We couldn't even move him. We were disappointed, cold, and tired. We drove to the house to warm up and drink some coffee. The outside thermometer by the kitchen door read 15° F. below zero.

I peeled off my nasty coveralls on the small back porch. I struggled to get it off over my boots and nearly fell down as I was hobbled by the thing wadded around my ankles. I managed to hop over to a little wooden bench where I sat while I pulled off my boots and kicked off the filthy garment.

A veterinarian's wife is a very special person who cleans up after a large animal practitioner, and JoAnn was really exceptional. I'm sure there were many times she wanted to just throw the clothes away, but I don't remember her ever complaining (loud enough for me to hear, but I think there was a time or two when she gave a little sigh as she surveyed a mess.)

Maisie, Guy's wife, was a delightful and talented lady. She began fixing us something to eat while we drank coffee and bellied up to the stove to thaw out. Soon she fed us bacon and eggs, hot biscuits and cream gravy with a side dish of that good fried deer meat.

Ahhh! There's nothing like good food, a warm stove, and good companionship to change your whole outlook on life. This was one of my more memorable moments, and I have been fortunate to have experienced many. My father said he felt sorry for people that have never had some of the real joys of this life:

1. Really cold and feel a warm fire.
2. Really hungry and savor a good meal.
3. Really thirsty and enjoy a glass of cool water.
4. So sleepy it hurts, then be allowed to sleep.
5. So tired you can't put one foot in front of the other, then to sit or lie down.
6. Really sweaty and dirty and take a bath.
7. Boots or shoes that are killing you and being able to take them off.

Trouble with Blood Samples

J.M. "Manny" Fowlkes had a ranch near Hot Wells. This is about 10 miles south of Allamore on the Southern Pacific Railroad. Dry weather, which has been known to occur, had forced the sale of some of his cows. Brucellosis testing was required. These were Brahma, crossbred cows with lots of spirit. The work was in a set of old, dilapidated railroad pens. Lots of sagging gates, splinters on the boards, some of which were broken and must be repaired, often with baling wire. It was an especially hot, dusty, July day and I was using the tailgate of a pickup for a table. There were about 200 cows and the work was disgustingly slow. We pretty well used up the day. These pens were about 95 miles from Marfa so it was late when I got back.

Next morning I began centrifuging the blood to separate the serum which was the portion used in the test. I spent all day and was unsuccessful. The sun and heat had cooked the blood and it would not separate. I had no choice but to call and explain the situation and ask to re-bleed.

This time I obtained two number-two wash tubs and filled them with ice in which to place the blood. Of course, the cattle were more difficult to work. It was hotter and dustier, and I would get my paperwork wet with melted ice. Still, we were able to finish in the one day. The next day, my efforts to separate the blood were again futile. The blood had chilled too quickly and congealed so that it would not separate. I worked with it several days, used a stirring rod repeatedly, and centrifuged again and again.

I finally had to bow my neck and call Manny again, as bad as I hated to do so. He just laughed at my embarrassment and made another appointment. This time I rigged up a shade, placed a blanket and cardboard on the hot tailgate, placed the ice in the vicinity of the blood tubes, but not too close, to protect the tubes. The poor old pens barely survived. Success this time, and all were negative to the test and could be shipped. Fortunately, they had been sold by the head and not by the pound, as all our chousing had caused considerable weight loss. Manny accepted it all like a gentleman. I learned a valuable lesson and never lost blood from weather conditions again.

Dry Spell at the Six Bar Ranch

We were at the Six Bar Ranch drinking coffee, having finished our work. Rocky Reagan, Jr. was the manager and Mike Capron, his foreman. Rocky's father, Rocky Sr., was visiting from his place near Corpus Christi. The Six Bar Ranch had been bought by a man from Corpus after Billy Crews went broke during the drouth of the fifties.

This was the mid-sixties, and this area was experiencing another dry spell. We were discussing what would be needed to break this spell. Rocky Sr. spoke up and said he didn't know about this country, but that if it ever got this dry where he came from, it would take a ten-inch rain and drizzle 'til it dried up.

Rust Largent

Rust Largent was a breeder of fine, registered Herefords. He had the McCabe ranch leased and was breeding heifers here to bulls he had selected for throwing small calves. He was feeding range cubes daily and began to notice evidence that some heifers were aborting. Many more were observed the next few days, and I was consulted. The bulls were home raised, as well as the heifers, but a neighboring ranch was buying thin bulls at an auction ring and pasturing them for a weight gain. These bulls were crossbred Brahma that continually jumped the fence into Rust's pasture and kept Rust busy throwing them back where they belonged.

I strongly suspected trichomoniasis from the visiting bulls. I took cervical smears from several cows and carried the specimens back to the hospital but could detect nothing. I consulted Dr. Gibbens at Auburn who suggested that I take my microscope and heated incubator box that I used to fertility test bulls and set up next to the chute and transfer specimens immediately from the heifer to the slide and examine it under the microscope. The trich were seen and diagnosis confirmed.

Rust didn't want to take any chances getting this in his herds, and he didn't want to sell them to endanger his reputation. He sent them all to slaughter. He visited with the neighbor who also sent all the bulls to slaughter, as he didn't want them on his ranch. The neighbor came out all right by having a weight gain plus an increase in price, but Rust took a terrible beating.

Trailers to haul horses were rare in the 1940s and '50s. The few I knew of belonged to rodeo contestants to haul their horses. They were too expensive to haul saddle horses around over rough ranch roads. Pickup racks were used. This was a metal frame that slid into the back of a pickup. A horse or cow would be brought up a loading ramp to the level of the pickup, loaded, and the gate closed. Some of these racks had a wooden floor, so the animals could get a better foothold. These were mostly used to carry animals a distance, as horses were usually ridden instead of hauled.

My first loading chute was designed expressly to accommodate these pickup racks. Often a ranch would have a loading chute such as mine or maybe just a framework where the rack was kept when not in use. It could be slipped in and out of the pickup with relative ease. It really wasn't very easy, just better than picking it up off the ground. Some would slide the rack part way out of the truck and cock it so that it stood up on end. A pickup could be backed up to it so that it could then be tilted and scooted into the bed of the pickup. The tailgate would be closed to hold it in.

Rust had a rather small ranch for this area when he first came, about 10 sections of the old Skinner place. He also had several leases. These were ranches and pastures owned by others that he rented for a designated time. He hauled sacks of cake around to feed the cattle. When he found one that needed doctoring, he would go get his saddlehorse. This was a remarkable horse in that he would jump in the back of a pickup when the tailgate was lowered, stay in when it was raised, and jump out when it was again lowered. No rack needed.

When Rust came to this country, I was driving an old beat-up, worn out Chevrolet pickup that the practice had inherited from the Coffield-Gearhart Ranch when I was still working for Dr. Ben Gearhart. I had purchased it with the practice and had continued to drive it long after it was worn out. My father-in-law, Jim Tyler, had a garage and was able to keep the old thing running. At the time, I believed that a heater in the truck was unnecessary. I could get acclimated to the cold while driving in the pickup, and I would not suffer so much when I had to get out at a ranch and work in the weather. Most people questioned my sanity, but Rust agreed with me saying he never bought a pickup with a heater. This caused me to respect him, because one of the most important criteria of a smart man is one that agrees with you. Now, I know Rust was an authority on the subject because he had ranched near Clayton in the northeast corner of New Mexico. This was only a short distance from Amarillo, Texas, which had the dubious distinction of being just a little colder than the North Pole. My classmate, Dr. Dee Ray Jenkins, said the reputation was unfounded, that he had practiced in and around that area for a hundred years and hadn't frozen to death a single time.

A few years ago there was big push for dehorned cattle. There is still a strong argument against horns on cattle. There are definite disadvantages to horns on cattle such as working them through a squeeze chute, injuries to each other from fighting, a horse gored and a ranch hand injured either by the cow or the cow making the cowboy hurt himself trying to get away.

Rust contended that when the horns were cut off or bred off, the cow lost her brains. Anatomically, the brains aren't in the horns, but you wouldn't know it the way that cows act sometimes. They have a tendency to ball up when being driven horseback, get their head on the wrong end when trying to put them through the gate, have trouble establishing their pecking order because they can't whip one another. Many people believe the maternal instinct is greater in a horned cow. Predator defense is a somewhat controversial issue. Some people don't think the horns make any difference when a cow is defending her calf, but I personally believe it is important. I know the lack of handle bars to tie and stabilize a cow's head when I am involved in eye, ear, nose, mouth, or throat treatment was a distinct disadvantage to me.

Rust was a strong believer that a heifer should not miss her two-year-old lactation. If she didn't become pregnant as a yearling, she was sold. If she lost her calf at calving, she was given another calf. If a dogie was not available, he would teach a calf to nurse two cows. This takes skill and patience which few possess. He was a master. His contention was to prevent two conditions: one, that the udder would be infiltrated with fatty tissue displacing the milk producing glandular tissue; second, the body would grow larger. He believed, and many agree, that the larger body needs more nutrition to maintain itself. Also the smaller animal can climb higher in the hills and travel farther to water and graze.

Rust's brother, David, who came with him to the area, went to

Arizona during the drouth of the fifties. He came back when it started raining and the grass grew, but another dry spell caused him to move to the Montana-Wyoming country. These trying periods caused many changes, and David had all the hot, dry weather that he thought he needed. David was one of the first to breed the big Hereford after the short, squatty type was discredited. He sent some of his big bulls down to Rust's Point of Rocks Ranch. Rust was impressed, but not favorably. He thought David had gone overboard and began to modify his own breeding program, but in the other direction, a smaller, but not the low-slung, blocky animal that had gotten us into trouble with dwarfism. His aim was first, fertility; second, conformation; third, a small size; and somewhere in between, he wanted the genetics that resulted in a cow that would wean a calf weighing at least 60% of the cow's weight. He was successful to a greater extent than he had originally hoped for and produced a miniature that is considered an exotic and is bringing comparable prices to other exotics.

Rust's original goal was to produce a cow that would raise and sell more beef per acreage, and the calf would gain profitably and cut out a more desirable size piece of meat for the modern consumer. His sales to Canadians as well as to many in various parts of the United States has shown a widespread interest in the original, miniature Herefords. He is still working to improve on what he has already produced.

Sanderson Flood in 1965

The Sanderson flood of 1965 was caused to large extent by big rains, not only in Sanderson and the immediate vicinity, but also on the watershed that drained into Sanderson Canyon.

Jack Shely had a ranch at Tesnus on the Southern Pacific Railroad about 30 miles west of Sanderson on Maxon Creek that emptied into Sanderson Canyon. I was at the ranch to castrate horses. After we finished and were watching them as they recovered from the anesthesia, the subject of the flood came up. When the horses were all on their feet, Jack took me in his Jeep to see a big hill, 150 or 200 feet high. I was told that before the flood this hill was covered with vegetation—yuccas, sotol, quailbushes, and grass. Now it was a bare rock. We speculated that it must have been a terrible downpour. The bottom really must have dropped out.

My father told me that he had stopped in Dudley Harrison's service station in Sanderson about this time, and the men were laughing about one of them, an old worn-out cowboy who was pumping gas into a tourist's car. A fellow had been looking at the barren rocky hills around town and asked the old cowboy how much rain they got around here. The answer was about ten inches. The stranger said, "That isn't much is it?" The old gent got kinda huffy and said in a rather harsh voice, "You'd thunk it was a hellava rain if you wuz here the day it falls."

One Memorable Postmortem Event

A number of animals both domestic and wild were being found dead near the scenic loop in the Davis Mountains, obviously having been shot. Four two-year-old heifers were dead near the loop road on the Barrel Springs Ranch leased by Hayes Mitchell, Sr. Hayes had hopes that the bullets could be retrieved so that the rifle could be determined if the culprit were apprehended. The heifers had undergone considerable decomposition, and the odor was sickening. I made an initial incision, and the gas and juices were nauseating. I got rid of my breakfast, then got down to serious hacking and whittling. I tried to stay upwind to the smells, but they would follow like smoke at a campfire. I would cut a little while and vomit a little while. Hayes would call encouragement from a safe distance. Maybe not entirely safe, as he got a little green around the gills a few times and would think of something that needed looking at behind a bush. If he was gagging, he was doing it much more discreetly than I. I eventually got so weak from the dry heaves, I wanted to give up. I really wanted to stop before I started cutting, the odor was so bad. It reminded me of seasickness on my first island excursion during World War II.

Hayes finally had compassion on me and called off the enterprise. I had thoroughly mutilated all four carcasses. I discovered a lot of tissue damage and found a few bullet fragments but nothing that would be of any value to identify the gun used. Shortly thereafter, the shooter was caught, prosecuted and convicted. The penalty was not as severe as most of us thought the deed deserved, but the publicity was a deterrent, as most of the poaching on the loop stopped for a long while.

Grass Seed

One year, I think it was the mid-seventies, there was an especially good stand of blue gramma grass. Previous years of good rainfall at the proper time had sprouted new grass, and much of the bare area that had been caused by the drouth of the fifties had healed. The amount of rainfall is important, but also the time of the year, temperature, and frequency of the rain determine whether the grass comes or weeds grow. We are fortunate most years in that the rains are grass rains. There have been years when tumbleweeds or annual broomweed were so dense they starved out the grass in places. A time or two it was conyza or pepperweed that took over.

This particular year the blue gramma was thick, loaded with seeds and almost no other plants to contaminate the harvest. Contractors came with combines and bought the seed in a number of places. It looked like an excellent opportunity to supplement the ranch income. After the combine passed, Dick Swartz raked the places and gathered and stacked the stems and leaves discarded by the combine. Dick routinely harvested the bar ditches for grass hay; therefore, he possessed the equipment and know-how to do this harvest.

The end result was disappointing. Cattle congregated on these cut over areas because the coarse material was out of the way, and they could eat the low, tender part. They ate this area right into the ground. After a cow work one day, Dick took me to the area south of Carpenter Mountain to view this. The cattle were still there after no grass could be seen, yet where the combine had not worked, the grass was still plentiful. The next year he showed me this area, and it was still bare. I knew of several other areas that had the same result, but the flat in the lower pasture of the Clay Mitchell ranch was damaged even worse. This flat in 1996 is still relatively barren compared to the way it was before the combining. It looked this way after the drouth of the fifties, and I keep hoping it will eventually hair over[*].

Preston Johnson

Preston Johnson had a little place down Limpia a little ways

---

[*] The grass will grow again.

from Fort Davis. It was on a side draw that was actually a meadow, or *vega*, sort of sub-irrigated. Preston said it used to be a permanent spring with running water. He originally had some apple and other fruit trees, a truck garden, and put up hay. It was a pretty good living until the spring dried up. The apple market went to pot about the same time the trees started dying, and the whole way of life became more complicated. A person could get along pretty well with a plow horse, saddle horse and wagon, or buggy horse. Sometimes one horse would fill the bill for all of these purposes. A milk cow or two for milk, cream, butter, and cottage cheese for your own use and maybe a little extra to sell, chickens for eggs and meat, one or more hogs. But then came automobiles, telephones, radios, washing machines. Homemade clothes looked country. All this and much more required money, and more of it. Preston's little outfit wouldn't support this high living so he had to scrounge around for extra income. He cowboyed here and there, took odd jobs and had a little grocery store that his wife took care of. The grocery was a pretty good little business until the biggest customers started going to Marfa and Alpine to buy from wholesale houses, and the better automobiles allowed others to shop the fancy foodmarts. That generally left him with the nickel and dime trade on credit.

When phenothiazine drench for stomach worms in sheep was developed, Preston did a lot of drenching, and he was good at it. Fortunately, this medicine didn't burn him like it did so many people. The drouth decimated the sheep population and ruined this business. The first time I remember working with him was at Dick Swartz's Merrill Ranch. An old cow got down in the chute, and I jumped in to tail her up. Preston said, "Doc, you let that big stout Mexican do that!" José Escovedo was big, and he was strong. He lifted that cow up with no problem. I don't know whether Preston had said that to save my back or because he knew I couldn't, and he wanted someone that could to have room and for me to get out of the way.

The Inconsiderate Cow

A few years later, Preston Johnson was working for Dude Sproul, and a heifer had a uterine prolapse. The whole plumbing had followed the calf out and immediately was covered with manure. Preston tied her down to prevent further injury and called me. The thing was a swollen mass when I got there, and I told Preston I thought he ought to call a veterinarian. He didn't think this wisecrack was very funny because I was the only veterinarian in 200 miles, and he was worried about the heifer. I gave her a spinal, and we tied her hind legs backward and her tail out of the way. I had given her oxytocin and ergonovine immediately on arrival. These are like antibiotics — they are wonder drugs, when they work, but you wonder if they are going to. When effective, the uterus shrinks marvelously. Many veterinarians claim (I really don't doubt them) that they had good results covering the swollen uterus with sugar to draw the swelling out, but I tried it a number of times and never could tell that it helped me. I have noticed over the years that I have had poor results with some treatments other veterinarians used, and a few have not reported good results with some of mine.

The heifer was in pretty good condition when I started: bright eyes and normal respiration. Preston poured my disinfectant solution while I washed the uterus. I placed it on a tow sack and worked sulfathiazole powder in the caruncles which had not come as clean as I would have liked. Preston offered to assist, but there isn't room for two to work. Besides, I rarely allowed anyone to spell me because the tissue is very friable and easily ruptured. A finger penetrates it with the greatest of ease. The injections had not been effective in causing the uterus to shrink, but gradual, steady pressure did so. Sometimes as the last is going back in, it goes with a rush and a slurp sound. It almost sucks you inside. There is a wonderful sense of satisfaction and accomplishment. I stood up to admire my handiwork and receive Preston's praise. The cow was dead! What a disappointment! Preston began to fuss and fume, ridicule her for being so inconsiderate as to die after all we had done for her. I couldn't help but laugh. Sometimes one has to laugh to keep from crying.

Kick in the Chest

H.E. "Dude" Sproul had a set of pens and a shed on the hill behind Jim Espy's house on the outskirts of Ft. Davis. Like most of the older pens, it wasn't much punkin. We rigged up a makeshift crowd pen and short crowd chute and tied a headgate on the front. Big, growthy, Charolais, two-year-old heifers were being pregnancy tested. They weren't sticking their necks in the headgate so I got in among them, doing the rectal palpation from behind, of course, testing with one hand and chalking with the other. I frequently tested some of the contrary, spoiled individuals that would not feed into the chutes this way, so it was no big deal. I was getting along fairly well when one was a little goosey. She jumped up in the air and kicked me in the chest with both hind feet. Anatomically, a cow cannot do this, but I guess this dumb heifer couldn't read. I was laid out on the ground and couldn't catch my breath. The heifers were milling around, trampling on me. Preston Johnson and Graviel took the pen apart and got the heifers off me. They asked me if I was all right. I don't know why we say this when someone is obviously injured. On the other hand, we'll answer we're O.K. with our dying breath! Of course, I wasn't all right. I was dern near dead. I still couldn't catch my breath and thought I was going to die and was afraid I wouldn't.

This is the only time I can remember that I was unable to finish my work. My chest hurt so bad that several days later I went to Dr. Stover. He listened to my chest, felt my ribs, and asked if I had spit up blood. He said I probably had broken ribs, but they were in alignment, and there was no need to x-ray or tape my chest, just take care of myself while they healed. My coughs were pretty feeble for a long while, but the pain stopped long before the hoof prints on my chest disappeared.

Cold and Colder Weather

Frozen ground

I was pregnancy checking cows for Clyde Ikins on the east side of the Garren Ranch. A norther had blown in the day before, bringing a pretty good rain. It had been enough to make the pens a little boggy as evidenced by deep cattle tracks in what had been mud. There had been a hard freeze during the night that had frozen the ground so that the place where I was standing by the chute was hard as cement and as cold as the ice that it was. The temperature stayed below freezing all day.

I was still wearing cowboy boots with the thin leather soles. I might as well have been standing barefooted on a block of ice. Perhaps if I could have walked a little it may not have been so bad, but everyone else was doing at least some walking, yet they were complaining, that is, all except the boss, Clyde Ikins. I guess this is the penalty a boss and a veterinarian suffer — they are not afforded the luxury of griping.

I don't want to leave the impression that others complaining of the conditions bothered me. Actually, it helped. There have been a few times I worked with a group of strong, silent types. That was terrible. Misery loves company, and I would wonder if I was the only one that was miserable.

My feet almost thawed out at the campfire when we stopped at noon. However, it seemed like the cold ground was worse when we went back to work. I sure was glad to see the last of those cows about sundown. My feet still hurt when I think about that day.

Several years later a cowboy from Montana told me about felt-lined rubber boots and gave me the address where I could order them. It almost made me mad to learn of the years I had suffered when, in fact, there was a remedy.

Black Ice

My first experience with black ice was my worst and perhaps the worst I ever had with ice on the highway. I had been called to Sanderson about 115 miles from Marfa. I was driving a Ford pickup with the veterinary utility bed mounted on it. I was traveling along near Altuda, the pass in the mountains between Alpine and Marathon. It was cloudy but daylight, and no other vehicles were on the highway, which was not unusual early in the morning.

I was probably going the speed limit of 70 miles per hour as I am sure it was before the oil crisis of the 1970s when the speed limit was lowered to 55 nationwide. The highway was level and straight. Suddenly, the rear end of my vehicle began to sway and weave. My first thought was a low or flat tire, and I began to apply the brakes. That was a mistake. I began to spin completely out of control. I had the sensation that the truck was actually accelerating. I twisted the steering wheel first one way and then the other, with no effect. I finally came to a stop out in the middle of the highway facing back the way I had come. I have no idea how far I skidded—it seemed like a long time and a long way.

I opened the door and stepped out on the pavement, and my feet went out from under me. It was quite a shock. I couldn't get up, no toe hold. Eventually, I was able to pull myself up by grasping the door, seat, or anything I could get ahold of.

I had put the gears in neutral and left the engine running. Now I tried to drive it off the highway, but no traction. The heat of the engine eventually melted the thin sheet of ice under the pickup, and the tires took hold. The bar ditch was shallow and covered with grass so that when I finally did move, I went down in it and turned around. I should have headed back to Marfa, I suppose, but perhaps the Sanderson call was an emergency. I don't remember, anyway, I thought that the ice probably extended only a short distance.

I managed to drive down the bar ditch most of the way to Marathon. When I had to get on the pavement I was able to keep the right hand tires on the shoulder that was not so slippery. There were periodic stretches of ice almost all the way to Sanderson. It seemed as if it took me forever to get there as I crept along. Most ice on the highway is white or at least opaque and can be seen. I suppose black ice is called such because it is completely transparent, and only the black pavement can be seen.

Ice on the Highway

The weather had been fairly nice in Marfa when I left early one morning, pulling my portable squeeze chute on the way to a cow work north of Pyote, Texas. I was on the old Highway 80 before Interstate 20 was built. It had only the two lanes. Shortly after I passed Barstow, I hit an ice storm that had covered the pavement. Fortunately, I had plenty of time to slow down and was just creeping along.

I had never realized how much slope there was on the banked curves of the older highways. When the highway turned to the right I would slip off onto the gravel shoulder and get traction so there was no problem, but one relatively sharp turn to the left was sloped so that I slipped into the left-hand lane. It was really exciting as I faced the oncoming traffic. I was not spinning, and the chute was straight behind me, but I had no control as I slid in front of a car and onto the shoulder. The driver gave me a greeting with his horn, because I'm sure I gave him a thrill. My ears burned, so I suspect that perhaps he may have said unkind words in my direction.

There was a good, wide, gravel shoulder that I drove on until the pavement leveled out. When I could see no one coming, I eased back across the highway. From then on, I kept the tires on my right side on the gravel for traction. It really helped for my pickup to have a power-trac rear end.

Call to Dell City in the Snow

About 1974 or '75 we had a 3 or 4 inch snowfall in Marfa. I was standing by the front door of the hospital enjoying the scenery and congratulating myself that I didn't have to go out and work in that today. About the time I was engrossed in the reverie, the phone rang!

A phone call from Dell City—now the term *dell* conjures up thoughts of a small, secluded, wooded valley and *city*, a town of considerable size teeming with activity. Neither of these word pictures was appropriate for Dell City, which was a small community out in flat country with hardly a tree.

There was a great deal of anxiety in the voice telling of the fine stallion that was the boss man's pride and joy. The boss had ridden him a couple of days before, and he had been fine—the horse, that is; the boss was in a bad mood, giving everybody a bad time. Now that the horse was sick, there would be hell to pay. He said the horse didn't come to his morning feed and was found about 100 yards from the pens. He was locked up like he had the lockjaw, stiff, sweating, wouldn't move, eat or drink. While trying to get him to walk, the horse urinated coffee. I told him it sounded like Monday morning disease. He said, "But Doc, it's Tuesday!" I told him the condition had a lot of names. That was just one of the more common ones.

He asked if it was serious, to which I replied, "It doesn't get much worse when the condition is as bad as you describe." He asked if I could save him. I said that I had done so in a few cases as bad as this. I didn't tell him there was a possibility these cases survived in spite of what I did, rather than because of it. But I had poured so much medicine into the horse, surely it helped. He asked me to come. I told him the weather was bad here, and I thought he should get a vet out of El Paso, which was closer anyway. He gave me a long song-and-dance ending up by buttering me up with wild tales of how good a vet I was, that everybody said so. Well, all that praise went to my head, so I got directions and started loading my pickup. JoAnn thought I had lost my mind, but I assured her the snow probably only went west to the Ben Avant hill about 8 miles.

I put everything in my pickup cab that was loose plus an extra thermos of coffee and realized there wasn't room for me to get in, so I put a few items on top of the vet box because the rest of it was full. I left after topping off both gas tanks.

The further I went, the deeper the snow, but enough traffic had traveled the highway to cut good ruts, so it wasn't too bad. Highway 54 north out of Van Horn was still pretty good about twenty miles to the old Daugherty Figure 2 headquarters. A couple of cattle trucks had been out that morning. I speculated that they had made a dry run (no cattle). From there on, I was on my own in about five inches of snow. Nothing had marred the beauty of the scenery, and there was nothing to disturb the peacefulness of the moment except the pounding of my heart and my labored breathing of anxiety. I had enjoyed the view early that morning. Now I was experiencing a little more enjoyment than I really wanted. I began to question my hasty decision to make the trip. I guess that if there was a good thing about it all, it was a dry snow, fluffy powder and crispy cold, but no wind—still as death—now that's not a good thought!

I got on up the road and thought about turning in at the Six Bar Ranch to pester Mike Capron and see if there was any other life on the planet, but decided it was only a short ways up to the junction with Highway 62/180. It would have been cleared because it is the main east-west road from El Paso to Carlsbad Caverns and Carlsbad, New Mexico. Well, somebody was smarter than me, because the highway had been closed to traffic. Therefore, I got to enjoy some more solitude and pristine beauty. The new-fangled, new and improved, transistor radios that replaced the old vacuum tube-type don't receive past city limits, so I was undisturbed.

I arrived at the Salt Flat store and post office (it was closed) and turned off on a county road. The series of rights and lefts, east and west directions, that had been given me were followed without having to watch out for heavy traffic. I finally arrived at the ranch. There was a small but fancy sign that identified the place as the Salt Flat division of the Figure 2 Ranch. The long, low, adobe house with a shed and pens built-on, about like I thought that Mr. Daugherty may have had on this end of his ranch many years ago. The new owner had preserved this old building.

The man that had called met me as I drove up. He was dressed appropriately in insulated coveralls, cap with ear flaps, and rubber boots. The snowfall seemed to have been rather uniform in depth, except perhaps it was somewhat wetter here, piling up on fence posts. We said our howdys, and I put on my uniform that matched his. I was a slow learner, but I had eventually acquired clothing to fit the occasion.

We found the horse as had been described. I had been hoping he had exaggerated. I began treatments with stomach tube and intramuscular medications, but giving the intravenous fluids was the time consuming therapy. I would warm these fluids in my pickup cab using the heater, but by the time it was carried to the horse and it ran down the rubber tube, it had become cold, so must be administered relatively slowly. I had a little problem with it freezing in the tube. This is one of the joys of large animal practice out in the good, clean, fresh air.

We entertained ourselves by discussing the disease, the symptoms, and the various degrees of severity, from the mild stiffness called tying-up to this severe form with myoglobinuria, usually called azoturia. The causes ranged from the completely unknown pasture cases to the severe, exertional rhabdomyolysis. The typical, or textbook case, of "Monday morning" is the animal on good feed with regular exercise, a day or two of rest on full feed, then forced to return quickly to strenuous work.

I finally gave all my fluids and put a blanket on him and was carrying the empty jugs back to the pickup when I noticed goldenrod in the path we had beaten out in the snow. I pointed this out to the caretaker who said there was a lot of this plant, and he had heard that it was toxic but nothing ever ate it. That's true under ordinary circumstances, but during and following a snowstorm, it seems to be readily consumed by both horses and cattle. The symptoms in a horse are identical to azoturia but less chance of survival. I was depressed because I had missed my diagnosis and because of the extremely poor chance that the horse would live. This made the 150 miles back to Marfa seem like a mighty long trip.

Lost in the Snow Storm

Maureen Godbold called me to her Clay Mitchell Ranch about midnight one time. Her Mexican ranch hand, Merced Ramirez, was having trouble trying to deliver a calf. I examined the two-year-old, first-calf heifer. The calf was still alive and much too big to be delivered, so I decided a caesarean section was necessary. We laid her on the side, clipped the hair, scrubbed, and had made the initial incision when it began to snow. The further we progressed, the harder it snowed. Maureen was very spunky as always and stayed with us the whole time, but there wasn't anything we could do but try to hurry.

It was a very wet snow, big soupy flakes that landed on my old dirty Stetson. The temperature was mild, and the snow would melt and run off my hat brim and into the incision. I tried to take my hat off, but it was snowing so hard it would get in my eyes and I couldn't see. It seemed as if it took me longer to suture this than at any other time. Finally, I finished, milked her and gave the baby calf his first colostrum. This is very important to their health, especially when a caesarean is performed. Their maternal instinct is not as strong, and often there is a problem pairing them up.

I left and started driving the three miles to the highway. I couldn't see the road, but part of it was right beside a fence. I made the mistake of trying to follow the road and losing it in the snowstorm after it turned away from the fence. I wandered around for hours in that heavy snow storm. I thought there wouldn't be much problem because the pasture was only a mile wide, and I would simply go straight, hit a fence and follow it either to the highway cattle guard or the house. However, I wasn't able to go straight. I would circle around a yucca or sacahuiste but couldn't line up with anything to go straight. Fortunately, I had started with a full gas tank, and I did not get stuck. The fence finally appeared, and I followed it to a gate on the highway. It was only a wire gap, and usually I hated wire gaps, but not this one at this time. The cars on the highway were a welcome sight.

The Ranchwomen

The ranchwomen were truly remarkable. Many of them were good cowhands and worked along side of us. All were good cooks who fed us a banquet at each meal. Some would cowboy until mealtime, then fix the groceries and often return to the work. Some would travel long distances over poor roads and in adverse weather to bring us our meal. Although these women worked hard, I never heard any complain. All were gracious ladies that were treated with respect. Never any vulgarity nor innuendoes.

Many played an important part in my practice. There were so many, in fact, that I am reluctant to single out any one of them. Many have been mentioned in the course of telling an episode and others when writing of a man or family. However, there were others that don't fit in to those categories.

Lee Bennett was a Marfa High School history teacher, a very capable and remarkable lady. She was always cheerful and smiling, enthusiastic, optimistic, and encouraging. She built self-confidence and self-esteem in her students and an interest in history that was contagious, even to the parents, especially me.

She and Mrs. Kathryn Queenie Steen, a high school math teacher, co-sponsored the Marfa Chapter of the Junior Historians. Mrs. Bennett frequently made assignments to the students that would include original research into local history, much of which included interviews with old timers, who have since died, therefore, preserving history that probably would have been lost.

Lee was a special inspiration to my daughters, Nancy and Janet. She and Queenie spent many hours helping their students fine tune their research papers. Students learned as much about creating a well-written composition as learning how to research. When Marfa High School students were asked to present their papers at the state convention, these two ladies spent much time helping them become comfortable speaking to a large group.

Both of these ladies were ranchwomen, mighty good cow hands and excellent cooks—a fact I can vouch for because of the many times they fed me at cow works.

There were three young girls that were as spunky as they come: Sally Roberts, Ann Holland Daugherty, and Jettie Steen Whitlock. These three not only knew how to work, but they got right down in the chute wading in the muck and mire—actually getting their chest right up against the rear of a cow with a hand on either side of the chute to pull while pushing the cow forward.

When a person looked at those cute girls at other times, it was difficult to imagine them doing this strenuous, unpleasant work. They weren't harassed to do this, they just knew what needed to be done and did it. This wasn't a one-time occurrence. It was done anytime an ole cow would balk.

Barbara Saunders owned a ranch, raising registered Hereford cattle and registered racing quarterhorses. She did all the many aspects of operating and working this outfit, besides taking an active part in several organizations. One of these was The West of the Pecos Cattlewomen, a group of very special ranchwomen, organized to promote beef and dedicated to the advancement of the cattle industry. It was nicknamed "The Cow Belles."

Lee Ann Tate was another small, slender woman who was a good cowhand and a good cook.

Dr. Bonsma's Demonstration

Dr. Jan Bonsma was a Dutchman from the Republic of South Africa. He had gained an enviable reputation as a judge of livestock and as an animal husbandry man. He was especially adept at visual evaluation of pregnancy, fertility, and mothering capabilities. The Highland Hereford Association was a very active and progressive group of cattlemen. When Dr. Bonsma visited in the United States in the late 1950s or early 1960s, these men invited him to come give a demonstration.

Joe Lane had an excellent herd of registered Hereford cattle and kept a complete set of records. This was no small chore in the days before computers. He could tell you if ole Nellie's grandmother raised good bulls and sorry heifers or vice versa, just to give an idea of what he had in his little black book, which incidentally wasn't so little. Joe had leased the Hubbard ranch south of Marfa and ran his registered herd on the north end with the working pens at the place called the farmhouse. It is now the Bill Hubbard ranch. Joe had gone to considerable effort to assemble a variety of subjects. Some had never calved, some had missed a calf, some that were poor milkers, some heavy milkers, easy keepers, and as it turned out, there were all stages of pregnancy. In all there were about forty head of selected cases. All needed to be gentle so that after I pregnancy palpated without revealing my findings, the cow would be turned into a pen where Dr. Bonsma would evaluate her and give his reasons while pointing out each feature. One of the most impressive eyeball determinations to me was an uncanny accuracy, not only of the pregnancy, but of the stage of the gestation. He explained and pointed out a hairline on the side. If there was no distinct hairline, the cow would be open, a small hairline high up would be a very early pregnancy, and as the pregnancy progressed, the hairline would become lower (the lower the line the more advanced the pregnancy). His other determinations were equally impressive, as Joe would read the cow's history after each explanation. I was not able to fully grasp this portion of the demonstration, partially because I was at a distance palpating the next cow, but also I had difficulty understanding his accent. One of the features that he stressed and impressed on all of us was that a bull should look like a bull, masculine, and a cow should be like a cow, feminine, and neither should look like a show steer, which is blocky.

I began a critical evaluation of his pregnancy determination by the hairline but found that it did not hold true in most cases. We were disappointed. I was and am still perplexed why Joe's cows that day were so close to the pattern yet other cattle varied so much that the criteria was completely useless in pregnancy determination. We learned later that American cattle were constant in being inconsistent in this respect. Was it the different breeding or climate conditions that caused this variation from South African cattle?

Pine Country of New Mexico

My first pregnancy testing of cattle on a ranch in New Mexico was with Joe Lane at the Drag A Ranch near Datil, New Mexico. I guess it is peculiar, but I cannot remember the percentage of pregnancies here. This was in pine and piñon tree country, and if my memory serves me correctly, this type country always produced poor calf crops. Perhaps this ranch and these cattle were an exception to the rule. The cows bred up well in areas where there was open grassland. It was the forests where I found the problem. This was blamed on the combination of the shade and the pine needles that covered the ground, which reduced the ability of the grass to grow. Also, when snow covered the ground, often cattle would eat pine needles which were known to cause abortions.

This was beautiful country with the sights and smells. The weather was perfect, and I thoroughly enjoyed myself working with a good crew of men and good cattle. I had ridden up with Joe and the good company may have made a good trip even better. I felt a little guilty sending a statement for my services.

A.R. Eppenauer, Sr. and the $5,000 Chickens

Many of us referred to Mr. A.R. Eppenauer, Sr. behind his back as "Mr. Ep," but I never heard anyone call him that to his face, certainly not me. He wasn't the kind of man one got too friendly or familiar with. Most of us held him in a little awe. He would often sing the Marine Corps hymn when I was present and he had taken a little nip. I often wanted to ask if he had been in the Corps perhaps in World War I or, if he was singing it for my benefit because I had been a Marine in World War II.

He always had an old, English bulldog for a companion. This breed of dog was the Marine Corps mascot. His latest dog was named Mr. Ep, and I wondered if it had anything to do with our nickname for him. His dogs were always very dignified, reserved, and well behaved, and would ride in the seat beside Mr. Eppenauer looking all around to see if all was in order. The dog was always well cared for and treated with kindness and attention. I'm not sure I can say affection, but perhaps I should only say he really liked that ole dog. But he wasn't a complete fool about him like Dr. Ben Gearhart was about his English bulldogs, Sissy and later Nikki.

As I said, Mr. Ep's dog, Mr. Ep, was treated with respect, and I was shocked one day when I arrived at his office to find the dog being severely reprimanded and lying cowed in a corner looking contrite. I had never heard Mr. Eppenauer speak harshly to his dog and asked what had provoked this outburst and was told the dog had just killed five thousand dollars worth of chickens. I questioned this statement as no dog could possibly kill that amount of chickens. He told me that a poor transient-type employee had a small daughter who had been born with her urinary bladder outside her abdomen. He had sent the little girl for surgical repair together with her family to Rochester, Minnesota. The operation had been successful, and when the family returned, they gave him their five chickens as a token of appreciation, because that was all they possessed besides the broken down car that had been the cause of their layover in Marfa to begin with. The surgery and the trip had cost five thousand dollars, and the dog had just killed all the chickens.

Mr. Eppenauer happened to be at the garage in town when the family had limped in with the car that was only barely running. He had given the man a job and a place for them to live until they could save enough to afford to have the car fixed. The man had a big ole kid about 12- or 14-years-old, perhaps a little older, that helped cleaning the pens and troughs. His father called him "Boy," not "John Boy," "Joe Boy," or "Jack Boy," just "Boy."

Texas Veterinary Medical Diagnostic Laboratory

The establishment of the Texas Veterinary Medical Diagnostic Laboratory at College Station, Texas, with its excellent staff of consultants, specialists, and technicians was of immense value to me in the diagnosis and treatment of problem cases. The following was the first case that I submitted and was the first submittal they received, resulting in it being assigned Accession #0001.

About the first of September, 1969, I was called to look at some horses in Fort Davis. There were several dead horses, several sick ones, and others that appeared to be unaffected. Two of the dead horses belonged to a prominent rancher in Marfa and were valuable, so an effort was made to determine the cause of death. Specimens were sent to the newly established Texas Veterinary Medical Diagnostic Laboratory at College Station, Texas. Extensive tests were performed, resulting in a tentative diagnosis of mycotoxin poison from moldy feed.

The feed company wanted a specimen of the feed sent to a laboratory in Lubbock. The available sweet feed was bright, clean, and odor-free. The lab got abundant growth but none of which proved to be toxic.

The caretaker of the horses had a good reputation. However, he had been out of town for a few days and had a Mexican to feed and clean the pens. This man also was well thought of, trustworthy, energetic, and completely dependable so that no one questioned his integrity.

About a year and a half later, a cowboy and I were visiting while waiting on a truck. He seemed a little uneasy, so I asked what was bugging him. He finally told me that he had been in a beer joint hoisting a few with a man that had fed the horses that day. He confided this story. It was the policy to add fresh feed when it got a little low in the 55-gallon barrel. The loose upper portion had been fed, so he decided to clean out the barrel. He dug out the caked portion that the horses seemed to eat with relish. He then washed, dried and filled the barrel with fresh feed. The horses that received mostly the caked portion died, those that received a mixture were sick, but the ones that got only fresh feed were unaffected. Both labs received only the fresh feed.

I was always amazed at what the lab was able to do with samples that I collected in the field under poor conditions and shipped long distances from my isolated area. The laboratory increased my usefulness to the public, and the cheerfulness, enthusiasm, and thoroughness with which they performed their duties made the association a pleasure.

Venezuelan Equine Encephalomyelitis

Fritz Kahl was from Iowa and came to Marfa during World War II. He was an instructor at the Marfa Army Air Base for bomber pilots. He married Georgia Lee Jones, a local girl, and remained in the area after the war.

I wasn't an airplane enthusiast, and we often harassed each other. He said it was foolish to jump out of a perfectly good airplane. I told him that he had been brainwashed by the U.S. Army Air Corps because they wanted him to bring that high priced plane back home.

Now the U.S. Marine Corps taught us in the Paratroops the truth: it was dangerous when an airplane and the ground got together, whether it was intentional or accidental. Planes were only good to get you where you wanted to go and high enough to jump, and then you're supposed to get out and walk. My jump-master, a Marine sergeant, told us this, so I knew it was right. Anyone who has been through Marine Boot Camp can vouch for the fact that sergeants are the closest thing to God that there is on earth.

In 1971, a disease known as Venezuelan Equine Encephalomyelitis (VEE), a type of sleeping sickness of horses and man, escaped from its native habitat and migrated north, finally reaching Texas in the lower valley. It started traveling up the Rio Grande, killing lots of horses and also some people. The powers that be decreed that all horses along the border should be vaccinated yesterday. The death reports were spooky, and everybody with a horse wanted to be first. Fritz and I got our heads together and figured out a route that we thought would make a pretty good dent in numbers while pacifying some of the most vocal ranchers. I consented to fly with Fritz, or he consented to fly me. I don't know which was making the greater concession. The vaccine was an experimental, modified live virus and was rationed out by the government men. The first day that I was given a batch, we took off from the Marfa Airport bright and early. Fritz wouldn't let me have a parachute. We headed for the Petan Ranch where Jim Phillips had assured us there was a good landing strip. Now his definition of good and mine weren't exactly the same. Fritz came down nice and easy, and we were taxiing along at a pretty good clip when we hit a washout! I knew I should have jumped out! I don't know how Fritz managed to control that plane, but he was just cool as a cucumber and calmly chauffeured us along just like that was a normal, natural landing. I've heard it said any landing you can walk away from is a good one. My legs were a little rubbery, but I could walk. Jim met us in his pickup, and we transferred my things. He and I went to the flat corrals and vaccinated horses while Fritz stayed with the plane. He didn't volunteer any information, and I wasn't too inquisitive. But, I think he was patching up the plane with baling wire and throwing rocks in chuck-holes. When I got back, he assured me it would fly, and sure enough it did.

Fritz flew us to the Brite Ranch where he landed on a ranch road. Jim White had about the same opinion of airplanes as I did and wouldn't let one land on the ranch, much less ruin good grass by making a landing strip. Fritz dodged a few mesquite trees and set the plane down pretty as you please in a road. It seemed to me we could have picked a much better place to land on this big beautiful ranch, but this was close to the pens where the horses were congregated. He went with us to do the paperwork while I vaccinated. Fritz not only knew how to write, but you could actually read his writing. That can be both an advantage and a disadvantage. If a mistake is made, it can be discovered, whereas if it can't be read they might give you the benefit of the doubt. Some of the horse descriptions got us into trouble on the blood bays, sorrels, chestnuts, grullas, zebra duns and buckskins. Everything was a quarter horse if they had ever been in the same pasture with one, including the genuine Mexican plugs. I certainly wouldn't insinuate such a beast was on Jim White's outfit. Fritz didn't know how to spell some of the names, and if he asked, he would get ten different spellings, so he wasn't a bit better off. Then there were the colorful names of some of the more ornery horses that Fritz didn't think would be in good taste to send to the hallowed halls of Washington D.C.

You don't ordinarily think of ranch work as being graceful, but there are several things that are, when done skillfully. One of these is the overhand roping of a horse in a remuda where the loop is laid down right over the horse's head. Little Jim did this with as smooth a motion as I've ever seen.

We flew on to the JD Ranch near Kent. The landing here wasn't nearly so exciting but much more to my liking. It was a good paved strip because the owners came from San Antonio in a plane. Fritz went with us while we vaccinated not only the JD horses but also those from Berry Hart, the Nunn Ranch and Clyde Ikins, all of which had been brought here. He had to leave us then, as it was getting late in the evening, and the Marfa Airport runways didn't have lights at that time. JoAnn had driven my pickup to meet us at the JD Ranch, and she and I went on to the Reynolds Brothers' X Ranch and the Rube Evans' Billingsley, vaccinating by moonlight.

JoAnn drove me much of the time during the next three weeks. We usually got home pretty late at night. JoAnn bathed and slept while I telephoned ranchers to arrange for vaccinations for both my assistant, Dr. Elmer Herndon, and myself. Every effort was made to vaccinate as many horses as possible by scheduling so that little backtracking was necessary. The ranchers were very cooperative by talking to me at odd hours, gathering horses, and working out schedules that sometimes had to be changed several times.

I was usually on the phone until the last possible minute. Then I would wake JoAnn and would bathe while she fixed breakfast. We would meet Dr. Herndon at the pickup point to get our vaccine. I would give him his schedule and directions to any ranches that he was not familiar with. We would hit the road. I slept while JoAnn drove. JoAnn was the bookkeeper and filled out the required forms describing each individual horse while I vaccinated. Like most of the things that the government has anything to do with, the paperwork is the most important part and also the most time consuming. It was a very hectic time.

One night I finished with phone calls early enough so that I could get a little sack time. When I climbed in bed, it woke JoAnn, and she asked if I had bathed. I admitted that I had not because I was tired and had been in the habit of bathing in the morning. "You're not getting in bed with me! I know where you have been and what you've been doing all day!" I filled the bath tub with good hot water and climbed in and went to sleep there. Soon JoAnn woke me and said to get outa the tub and go to bed. "Leave me alone. I'm sleeping just fine," I answered.

Dr. Gearhart had been inactive in practice since selling out in 1953 but volunteered to help in this emergency. His services were especially appreciated by me as he took some territory that was my responsibility but was a problem to cover, being few horses in widely scattered, rough country especially the area under the rim. (The area south and west of the Sierra Vieja Mountains from Chispa to the river.) He vaccinated all the horses in the area but was unable to reach the Evans Means Ranch because the road had been washed out. He drove to the Miller Ranch at the mouth of the Viejo Pass, borrowed a horse there, and rode through the pass to the place called the Viejo Ranch. He vaccinated the few horses readily available there and made arrangements to return at a certain date when Evans would have had an opportunity to gather the remainder of his horses. Ben observed that the old man had very few groceries on hand and appeared to be thin and malnourished. I never saw him look any other way, as he was lean and wiry. This is a nice way to describe a dried up little runt. When Dr. Ben returned, he took two gunny sacks of food. Ben talked a rough, tough way, but he was a big softy.

The government vaccine had not been approved by the FDA. There was considerable paperwork required, including a waiver to be signed by each horse's owner who must be informed of the experimental status, and they had to agree to report any ill effects of it. The vaccine was furnished gratis and veterinarians were remunerated for its administration by the U.S. Department of Agriculture.

Every equine was to be vaccinated so no animal would remain that could act as a reservoir of the virus. Therefore, every effort was made to gather every horse, mule and burro. Most ranch horses that could not be used were disposed of, but when a good, honest, hardworking saddle horse or especially a kid horse was no longer useable, it would be turned out to pasture. Therefore, when the horses were gathered, many from the backside, some very old cripples showed up. I arrived at one ranch to find a dead horse with the others that had been penned the day before. The stress of the roundup had proved too much for the old-timer. After we finished, I reminded the rancher to report any ill effects. He said he already had the dead horse to report. I reminded him the horse was dead and had not been vaccinated, so his death could not be blamed on the vaccine. He thought a moment and said, "Well, I'll be doggoned, that's right!"

Jim's Cow

There was a set of antique cattle working pens between the Brite Ranch headquarters and the place called the farm. These pens were torn down when Mac White built the excellent pipe, "Jim pens." It is a shame they were lost to posterity. Not many of the younger generation would believe a description of them. We were trying to operate on cancer eye cows. Now a cow with a sore eye has a short fuse, and we really weren't doing much to placate them. We spent more time patching on those pens than we did working on the cows. I use the term "we" a little loosely because Big Jim White and I didn't have our own hammer. We were harassing his sons Jimmy, Beau, and Mac, telling them what to do. The lumber was too old and cracked to hold nails, so a generous amount of baling wire was used. A lot of modern day practices have their drawbacks. One of the worst is the use of twine instead of baling wire on bales of hay and the next is putting feed in paper sacks instead of tow sacks. I thought for awhile I would have to quit practicing before my time, because I didn't think I could do without those two items.

One of the more aggressive cows came over, under or through the fence to see us. We were not certain of her intentions, but the way she was bellowing, shaking her head and pawing the ground led us to believe that she had malice aforethought. We piled into the cab of my pickup, including the cow. This was more togetherness than I wanted, because I was on the bottom, then Jimmy, Beau and Mac with the cow on top. This may sound impossible to look at those boys now, but at that time they were not yet full-grown, still lank and agile. The cow was mature with well developed horns, but she was kinda lean and mean. She had raised a good calf, and some cows turn to milk, that is, they'll raise a good calf and sacrifice their own condition.

We didn't suffer any physical damage by our little get together in the pickup, but our dignity was badly bruised. The cow didn't act like she was hurt, and I doubt if we even hurt her feelings by our comments on her ancestry, morals, appearance, and disposition. Big Jim just sat quietly on his horse and said, "Now, you boys don't chouse my cow." I think he was confused on who was the chousor and who was the chousee.

Charlie Gregory and the Old Mule

Charlie Gregory ranched about eight or ten miles west of Sanderson on the south side of the Southern Pacific Railroad. The house was near Emerson, a siding. Close by, my parents had lived and ranched in 1924 after abandoning their ranch in Mexico during one the many military misunderstandings that occurred there shortly before I was born. Charlie had come out of Mexico where he had been ranching when the foot-and-mouth disease quarantine caught him. When the quarantine was lifted and he was able to sell out, he did so and bought this ranch about the mid 1960s.

In the early 1970s, he had an old mule that he had ridden in Mexico and was now retired. The mule was 36 years old and stove up with arthritis and could barely get around. Charlie had called me to drive a hundred plus miles from Marfa just to put him down. Now some might have thought Charlie was a sentimental old fool, but he and the mule had been through a lot together. He had his Mexican ranch hand to toodle the old timer slowly to the gravesite away from the house and we went to join them. I gave the mule an intravenous and he went to sleep. Charlie held his head and talked to him, while I continued with a massive dose of Chloropent, a Fort Dodge Labs product containing chloral hydrate, magnesium sulfate and pentobarbital. I gave this long after I could no longer distinguish respiration or a heartbeat.

Charlie said his goodbyes to the mule, and we went to the house. We drank coffee while Charlie reminisced about some exciting adventures he and the mule had experienced in Mexico. I am sad that I didn't write down the things old-timers told me that I have since forgotten. I guess they are lost forever. Although some of the things that were told are probably better not having been written and recorded. I don't intend to write all of mine. I think of what my father told me once when I asked why the Mexican general gave him the gold and silver mounted spurs and why he had to leave Mexico. His answer was, "Son, there are some things that is better you do not know." That satisfied me at the time, but now it increases my curiosity.

Just as Charlie and I walked out the door to take my leave, the old mule walked up. I was dumbfounded and terribly embarrassed. Charlie said he was going to town, that he couldn't go through that again. He asked that I shoot him after he was asleep. I did and left never seeing Charlie again as he died soon afterwards of a heart attack.

John P. Searls, MD, Tetanus Vaccinations

John P. Searls, MD, who most people called Dr. John, was a local physician. He had a nice little hospital in Marfa that was acceptable at that time. I think the medical profession and the health care system as a whole lost a lot with the passing of these general practitioners and their modest facilities.

Dr. John had been an optometrist before going to med school and almost anyone that came into his office wearing glasses would get an eye exam also, if they stood still for it.

He would lecture on the dangers of smoking, going into great and gory detail, then when he finished and felt he had done his medical duty, he would bum a cigarette and smoke with the patient while examining or visiting about other things. A pure case of do what I say, not what I do.

He delivered both my daughters in his hospital, impressing JoAnn and me with his skill and expediency. JoAnn was threatened with a miscarriage during her second pregnancy. I requested everything possible be done to save the baby. Dr. John would not give any medication, only bed rest. He advised us that in almost every instance of so-called heroic measures to prevent miscarriage there was regret because the baby was deformed. His explanation was that a miscarriage was the natural termination of a poorly developing fetus.

The first dog I had with a perineal hernia broke his sutures and re-herniated. Dr. John invited me to bring it to him and he would show me his method. He ended up doing the entire operation while I watched and he explained. He was a good teacher because I operated on quite a few, all being successful. This was a common problem in the early days of my practice, because of the high incidence of constipation in dogs.

A horse was admitted to my hospital with tetanus. I was reminded that I had not had a tetanus toxoid booster vaccination in several years. I questioned my employees and learned they had never been vaccinated to their knowledge.

I never permitted my lay employees to give injections to dogs, cats or horses because these animals are very susceptible to infections. They were allowed to give injections to cattle after being subjected to detailed instructions as to sanitation. Cattle are more resistant to infections.

Glass syringes were still being used that required washing with soap and water, thorough rinsing, first with tap water, then with distilled water. They were sterilized in an autoclave which is steam under pressure. The two parts, barrels and plungers, were sterilized separately, then had to be assembled carefully to match because they were ground to fit perfectly. This had to be done carefully to prevent contamination after sterilization, and I personally performed this step.

My help at this time consisted of a young man, Tootie Garlick, and two high school boys, Glen Ceniceros and Carlos Carrasco. They didn't mind seeing me give injections or giving cattle their shots, but they were deathly afraid of a needle for themselves.

I called Dr. Searls for an appointment and suggested a prank. I had trouble getting them to go, but I finally herded them into Dr. John's office. He began to rummage through a drawer full of syringe barrels, plungers and needles laying loose. He would attempt to fit a plunger into a barrel after wiping it on his pants leg. Occasionally he would shake some debris from a barrel. Once in a while he would lick a plunger to make it slippery. My crew became more nervous by the minute. After several syringes were put together, he scrounged around for needles. He would rub the ends for sharpness and burrs. Occasionally he touched up a point on a whet rock. My boys almost went into shock when he blew through the needles to see if they were stopped up.

All this time he talked to them, which was disconcerting because of his speech impediment. At times he stuttered badly. Although they were staring at what he was doing, I doubt if they heard a word he said. I had quite a problem preventing them from stampeding. He left the room and made them promise not to run off after he had gone to all that trouble. He came back in a few minutes with filled syringes in an old chipped porcelain tray. I am certain that it was clean and sterile, but it sure looked like the devil. I had retired one that looked just like it recently when I converted to stainless steel.

The setup sure looked bad to them. They whispered to each other and insisted that I go first. I toyed with them a little while saying that I didn't think I really needed one at that time. They started for the door, and I realized I had pushed my teasing a little too far, so I rolled up my sleeve. Dr. John swabbed it with alcohol. I had intended to squall when he gave the shot, but by the looks on their faces and their body attitude, I decided I had better not.

I was afraid they were going to back out until they saw me grinning. They took their injections with their eyes closed and faces screwed up, biting their lips. I didn't get much work out of them the next few days with them holding their arms with sleeves rolled up, comparing each other's injection sites, and coming to me every few minutes to see if I thought the places were infected. They got their revenge on me claiming to be sick and unable to do this or that.

Some Airplane Trips

Bryant Harris

Bryant Harris had a ranch near Marfa and another near Magdelena, New Mexico. Robert Humphries and I flew to the

New Mexico ranch with him. Robert went to inspect his cattle for the Marfa Production Credit Association (M.P.C.A.). I don't remember why I went, surely not just for the ride. We buzzed the ranch house so that his cowboy would come to pick us up. We landed on a graded county road, a couple of miles from the house. Bryant landed smoothly and turned the plane around at the mail-box which was mounted atop a big juniper post. The tail of the plane hit the post and warped it considerably—the plane, that is; it didn't hurt the juniper post.

There was a large pile of ice at each water trough. Bryant said that the size of the pile was used to show the severity of the winter because it was broken and thrown to one side to allow the cattle access to the water . He also stated that almost every spring the tumbleweeds came as soon as it warmed up because of the moisture provided by snowfall, giving the cattle an early nutritional boost.

After looking at the cattle and when we were ready to leave, I wasn't too enthusiastic about riding in that plane but we were 400-500 miles from Marfa and probably 40 or 50 miles from the closest town, Magdelena. A little far to walk and hitchhiking was pretty poor on a road where a vehicle didn't come along but every day or two. Bryant assured us the plane would fly and was safe, but still we flew over Magdelena and through a relatively low pass in the mountains to Socorro, New Mexico on the Rio Grande River instead of the more direct route over the high mountains. We followed the Rio Grande down to El Paso where we stopped for repairs. No other excitement.

Hayes Mitchell Jr.

Hayes Mitchell Jr. had some calves pastured on Moody Bennett's Green River Ranch on the banks of the silvery Rio Grande up the river from Porvenir and Pilares, about 50 miles up river from Candelaria and some 70-80 miles upriver from Presidio. They had pneumonia, which is fairly common in shipped-in cattle, especially if they have just been weaned. Most of the time pneumonia is diagnosed and treated by the ranchers, but sometimes an outbreak may not have typical symptoms or not respond to the usual medication. Then, a veterinarian may be called for an examination and sometimes a postmortem, in which case a lung specimen is obtained to be sent to a laboratory for bacterial isolation and antibiotic sensitivity testing.

The ranch was nearly one hundred miles from Marfa, with a big part of the road dirt and somewhat slow travel. A call to the ranch by pickup usually ruined a whole day. Hayes had an airplane and we flew. This was not only faster travel, but a more direct route could be taken over the Sierra Vieja Mountains. As we neared the top, Hayes asked me to keep my eyes on the ground. It sloped up, and we came very close to the ground which caused me a little concern, then suddenly, the world dropped out from under us, giving a very weird sensation. We had crossed the rim, and I estimated there was at least a 1000-foot, sheer drop. On the return trip we approached this bluff from the lower side. There was an optical illusion, and I knew we were going to hit. Hayes assured me we were high enough to clear the rim, but I still raised up as much as the seat belt would permit, to try to help the plane go high enough. Hayes was a good pilot and never had a wreck, although rumor had it that he tore up a yucca with the propeller of his plane on one occasion.

A few years later a big Air Force bomber, a B-52 I think, was flying night practice runs under this rim to evade radar. There was a relatively low place in the rim over the Brite Ranch cienaga pasture where the planes were supposed to cross the mountains. One night a plane hit the bluff. When the black box was recovered it revealed that the crew had overridden the computer that controlled the auto pilot.

Muffin

Morgan and Frances Chaney lived on the San Francisco Ranch during the winter, and in the summer, at their historic and picturesque colonial farmhouse overlooking the harbor at New London, Connecticut. The ranch was close to 100 miles from my office. It was 56 miles to Marathon from Marfa, another 7 miles south on the Big Bend National Park highway, then some 25 to 30 miles of primitive dirt road. It took almost the entire day to make the trip by pickup. Of course, I always had to eat with them, Frances being an excellent cook, and drink a few cups of coffee with Morgan while we told stories and solved the problems of the world. If my schedule was tight, Fritz Kahl or Ray Hegy would fly me to the ranch, if I didn't need too much equipment and the stay would not be too long.

The Chaneys had numerous animals, but the real apple of their eye was Muffin, a little nondescript, shaggy female terrier. When Muffin was ailing, she got attention one way or another, and quickly.

Muffin was prone to sore throats. Poor little dog. She wouldn't eat, just lie around with her neck stretched out and look so sad and pitiful. I would fly down and pick her up and take her to my hospital. Aureomycin capsules were the wonder drug at the time, and I always had her up and going in a couple of days. I usually kept her another three days to make certain she wouldn't relapse. I wanted to leave a supply for the Chaneys to administer, but they would rather I came. It was quite a sight to see their reunion. The little dog rode the airplane like a real trooper, nestled in my arms. She was a lot more relaxed than I was.

A few times, Fritz provided air ambulance service, making the trip as pilot and Muffin as co-pilot. Muffin was a good traveler and also a good patient, in demeanor as well as response to medication. She sure made me look good.

The Cotton Gin Scales

Sometime in the sixties, cotton farming began to lose favor in the Balmorhea-Saragosa-Verhalen-Pecos valley. Part of it may have been caused by low prices for the cotton. I think more was caused by increased cost of labor and farm machinery, but also the underground water table was dropping, and the quality of the water was deteriorating. However, the crowning blow was the energy crisis of the early seventies, resulting in a jump in the cost of pumping.

A number of the cotton gins were folding up and the equipment moved. Truman Foster was driving by one of these gins when it began to hail stones the size of hen eggs. He whipped in right quick under the canopy that covered the scales. However, the scales had been moved, leaving an open pit. Truman drove off into that gaping hole. The story I heard was that the pickup was wrinkled up pretty good. Truman sustained little physical damage to his person, but his ego and dignity took a terrible beating. I asked him about the incident, but he didn't want to talk about it.

Horse Castration

When I first came to the area, there was not much demand for me to castrate horses. Most ranchers either did it themselves, or had an employee or sometimes a friend do the job. The animal was thrown and tied, cowboy style.

Frank Warren was a big man, probably six feet five or six inches tall weighing perhaps 250 pounds. He was the manager of the Allison Ranch in the Glass Mountains between Fort Stockton and Marathon.

When I began castrating horses for the ranch, Frank would put wild young broncs in a round pen one at a time, run them around a couple of times and rope both the fore feet, called forefooting. In the same fluid motion he would wind the rope around his rear and jerk the feet from under the colt, causing him to fall on his side. Frank was so strong and skillful that the colt usually hit the ground so hard it knocked the breath out. One of his men would quickly grab the head and twist it backwards while another man pulled the tail between the hind legs and up the flank. Frank would take a loop of the rope that was on the forelegs, pass it back between those legs, loop it over the upper hind leg at the pastern, and pull that leg up between the forelegs and tie them together. This was common procedure, but neither I, nor anyone else I ever watched, could do it with the speed and apparent ease that Frank did. The graceful action of Frank was something to behold, a real thing of beauty.

I usually had the colt castrated, and he was untied before he fully caught his breath. He would get up a little shakily and step gingerly about, looking at us out of the corner of his eye.

A few others forefooted their broncs, but most roped them around the neck, then several men got ahold of the rope and pulled until the colt choked down and fell. Some had a big heavy post in the middle of a round pen. As soon as the horse was roped, a few wraps were taken on the post. The colt was then choused, so that it ran around, tightening the rope and choking itself down.

I thought if I could castrate standing it might drum up some business, but few horses were halter broke before the deed was done. The thinking was not to waste time and effort on a horse that might be lost because of the operation, either from bleeding, infection, or crippling. All were a good deal more common that was generally admitted.

A fairly gentle horse was dropped off at my place to be castrated. Dan Perry, a Negro, very skillful with horses, had come to work with Mr. Eppenauer's horses. When their arrangement didn't work out, I was able to hire him. I mentioned to Dan that I sure would like to see if I could cut that horse standing, as the owner had kinda jokingly requested. Dan assured me he could restrain him for me. The result was so successful and satisfying that I adopted the practice when Dan could help me. He showed me just how much pressure to use with the twitch, and later I would apply the twitch and then let someone hold it for me. Dan also showed me how to fasten the twitch to the halter so that I could castrate standing without assistance in selected cases.

The word got around pretty fast that I could castrate standing without the danger of injury to the horse. Therefore, many began to halter break colts and have me castrate them. This not only helped to build my practice, but it was terrific for my ego. I guess I am somewhat of a ham because I thoroughly enjoyed the comments and awe expressed by the bystanders. I suppose embarrassing incidents, the humbling experience that bruises one's ego, are character builders, but I would prefer not to have so much character.

Mr. Hubert Honaker, from over near Balmorhea, had witnessed my standing castrations and told a number of friends and acquaintances who were doubting Thomases. He arranged to have a horse and a large audience to witness my expertise.

The horse was a big, stout, ill-tempered, three-coming-four-year-old stud that I should not have attempted to tackle. However, I had driven seventy miles, and a large group of men had gone to some trouble to come see the show. Well, they got their money's worth, but not quite as planned. I let my ego overwhelm my judgement. I had a difficult time getting close enough to grasp the testicles and then got kicked down twice without ever making an incision. I gave up, threw, and tied him. I learned a valuable lesson: to use discretion in choosing a procedure for certain patients.

I was never kicked a good solid lick that would break a leg. Most of the kicks I was able to dodge completely or escape with only a brush-type sideswipe. The Honaker episode was the only time I was laid out on the ground until several years later during the fall of the year I turned 40. I don't remember the occasion, but a group of ole rusty cowboys happened to be there. This horse was on a farm at Lobo and was a gentle, good-natured horse, just touchy about his testicles. I had been kicked down a couple of times in the previous month, so I was being careful. The first testicle was removed uneventfully, but the second incision caused a violent reaction, and down I went. I was rolled in a ball in a pile of dry tumbleweeds up against a fence. I had my head under me, so I couldn't get up, and my neck was bent in such an angle, I couldn't call for help. The men were laughing uproariously, thinking it was the funniest thing they had ever seen. I almost suffocated before they finally untangled me. My pride was badly damaged. It was hard to look professional in that position. I would not let that horse get the best of me. I finished the job while silently telling him what I would do to him if he kicked me again. I sure wasn't going to allow him to tell any offspring about the time he disgraced the vet.

I swore I would never castrate another horse standing. That third time in less than a month convinced me I had lost my reflexes. Several times I was sorely tempted to show off, reasoning that it may have been caused by fatigue, but I resisted.

Bob War

This is properly spelled *barbed wire* and some folks call it that, but generally they aren't the ones out there with it. These people are likely to use little colorful expressions when cussing or discussing it. This is something a rancher can't live with and sure enough can't live without.

My father told me when the family first started fencing their country, the horses didn't know what barbed wire was and that they were slow learners. Screwworms in wire cuts just about ate them alive. So, they took it up in the horse pasture and strung up slick wire, more properly called smooth wire. Dad said this was even worse because the horses didn't respect it, yet it cut like a knife. They had to go back to the barbed wire.

I wonder how many hours I have spent suturing wire cuts, but I guess I really don't want to know. Some of the cuts were in places that were accessible, but most were situated so that one had to be a contortionist.

I knew a fellow who lived in Presidio. He was a pretty good roper and had some good horses. They were forever getting cut on wire. He got disgusted, having to haul a horse sixty miles to me every few days, so he decided to build himself a set of pipe pens so that no way could a horse get cut.

Lo and behold! The very first night his horses were put in that pen, one did what seemed the impossible. He laid open a place on his shoulder like you wouldn't believe. Took me close to two hours to patch him up. The man never did figure out how he did it.

Horses have the most delicate skin and almost anything can cut it. There were times I think, when the wire reached out and snagged a colt when he came close—he didn't even have to touch it. It seems like a young colt, before he is castrated, has the least respect for it. I don't know for sure if he just runs into it on purpose or if he just doesn't care. Of course, sometimes another horse runs him into it.

I guess a horse is pretty smart, all right. Otherwise, why would he stand up against a fence and paw it until he dern near cuts his leg off. Maybe he knows that's the way to get out of being ridden. I have harangued the horse pretty bad, but I loved the beast, and it was sad to see one hurt.

And the Rains Came

The rains came, but they were a mixed blessing! There was plentiful rainfall in the years 1971-1975 beginning, during, or shortly before, the VEE epidemic. The rain caused a bountiful crop of mosquitoes that made the epidemic more exciting because they are the principal carrier of the virus.

The water caused a problem in my travels from ranch to ranch. Often it would be necessary to wait for the high water in an arroyo or draw to run down so it could be crossed. Bridges were very rare on ranch roads, and even those were very small. Many of the state roads and almost all the farm-to-market (ranch-to-market) roads had dips for water crossings, and some had cement slabs.

A rock would be placed at the water's edge to determine if the water was rising or falling. I would occasionally tie a rope to my pickup and the other end around my chest, then wade a suspicious place. Sometimes it was to determine the depth but more often to check for potholes or large rocks, because there had been problems with these hazards. I have found some the hard way and fallen.

At this altitude the rain is cold, and often the water would have some hail in it. I would nearly freeze. There have been a number of times where I found myself in an awkward, unprofessional situation, and almost always there was an audience to be highly amused. I guess floundering around in the water trying to regain my feet, while hanging onto the rope attempting to pull myself out was pretty humorous. As often was the case, it was caused by a lapse of judgement.

I have been stuck in mud, and for some reason it always seemed to have happened at an inopportune time. There were times I took a circuitous route around an obstacle, and at other times a rancher has helped me with his four-wheel drive vehicle. One time at the Brite Ranch when I was stuck, I walked to the house. Mac White brought me back, then got in my truck and calmly drove it out. Was I embarrassed!

Some ranchers had problems with too much water too quickly. Water gaps and even some rather extensive sections of fences were washed out, causing not only the expense and labor of repairs but the headache of mixing of herds. The water overflowing some draws and flats irrigated them and filled dirt tanks, but in some cases the dirt tank dam was washed out, ruining it.

As I said, the rains were a mixed blessing. It grew some grass okay and maybe some years the grass produced enough seed that it was harvested by combines, but it also grew some weeds. The Mexicans call these plants *hierbas*. They are more properly forbs, I guess, but this term was rarely, if ever, used among the ranchers and cowboys. However, it was thrown around quite freely by visiting agronomists.

East of the Davis Mountains in the area from Balmorhea north to and past Toyah during this time, there was the most bountiful growth of filaree and yellow top that I ever saw. These are both excellent for grazing, and the cattle got hog fat. These weeds were so lush that it was impossible to put enough cattle to properly utilize them because of the limited stock water.

West of the mountains there were good weeds such as some

types of mustard, some peavines, tallow weed and bladder pod, but it also grew toxic weeds, causing the worst problems with them I ever saw. The psilostrophe (paperflower) and senecio (groundsel) were plentiful, but the bumper crop of loco was our main concern. All three astragalas gave us a fit, but the one we called purple loco was the worst overall, although garbancillo was close behind. The red stemmed peavine, if eaten in moderation, was beneficial, but in places it was lush and consumed in excess, causing problems. The southern part of the area was heavily infested with desert baileya and desert spike, two plants that rarely caused trouble, but this period was an exception. These poison plants caused a severe financial loss to many of the ranchers and a real headache to me. I was terribly frustrated because of my limited ability to be helpful.

Joe Lane had so many succulent weeds on his ranch south of Alpine that he was having a major problem with foamy bloat in his cattle. Many died. At first he tried calling me for help, but they would die before I got there. He would try to pass a stomach tube to relieve the gas, but the frothy, foamy material would not come through the tube, even if they lived long enough for the procedure to be tried.

The emergency treatment of "sticking" had to be resorted to. This is done by jabbing a knife into the highest point of the left flank. Ordinarily, one could insert the knife and twist it sideways, and the gas would escape. One could more properly use a bloat instrument (trocar), which is composed of two parts, a solid central part with a sharp point to penetrate (this would be extracted leaving a cannula) and a hollow tube which should allow the gas to escape. However, both of these methods were unsuccessful because the froth was so thick it would not come. Therefore, the knife had to be pulled downward to make a large hole. The rumen contents would be under pressure and would blow out with force. The operator had to be nimble to prevent his being sprayed. This large wound would result in peritonitis if not treated and sutured, which was no small chore and usually had to be done by a veterinarian.

Joe made the statement that he had hoped for a good spring like this all this life and now that it happened, it was so good he couldn't stand it, being worse than a drouth.

Mutilations

I began hearing of so-called mutilations by the media in early 1975. I didn't take these reports seriously, having doubts as to the accuracy of them. I assumed them to be either pranks or poorly diagnosed death losses and played up by sensationalism.

March 17, 1975. I was called to the M.A. Grisham Ranch by the manager, Jack Burchard. The location of a dead cow was 50-60 feet from an ungraded, infrequently used ranch road. Jack was feeding range cubes and would count the cattle so that he could feed the allotted amount to the number that came to feed. Also, he could determine if any were missing and check on them to see if they were in trouble. He was short a cow and while looking for her, he found this cow.

She was a horned cow and was lying directly on her back with both the hind legs and the forelegs flexed. Her head and neck were straight. The entire chin including the lip had been removed back almost to the throat, exposing the jaw bones. The tongue had been removed completely back to the base apparently through the intermandibular space. No other parts had been removed. The edges of the cut skin were remarkably smooth. It would have been tedious to make such precise incisions with a scalpel. There was no blood on the ground, not any evidence of seepage of blood or serum from the cut surface. An incision into the jugular vein and the brachial vein revealed them full of clotted blood. The remarkable things about this case were the position, the precise incisions, the lack of bleeding, the tissues that were missing (lip and chin, tongue) and the fact that exposed flesh, eyes, and rear end had not been eaten by varmints, although there were coyote tracks around the carcass. Even the buzzards had not bothered it. The animal was badly decomposed, bloated, with a strong odor so that a postmortem was not attempted.

March 31, 1975. A 300-pound Charolais calf was found approximately one mile west from the previous cow. This calf was on her side, decomposition odors suggested she had been dead a couple of days. The left ear had been removed, as well as the left eyeball and eyelid, and the tongue back to the prominence. A 9½ by 12-inch elliptical area of skin had been removed from just anterior to the umbilicus to just anterior to the udder with the udder undermined and the mammary gland tissue removed. The vulva and anus had been removed symmetrically. Coyote tracks were near this area, and some flesh, showed a little evidence that the coyote may have gnawed on the flesh, but little if any was missing. The uterus and ovaries were still present but the urinary bladder was missing and presumed to have been taken with the vulva and vagina. The remarkable things about this case were the tissues that were missing, the precise incisions, the lack of blood on the ground and seepage from the cut surfaces. All incisions were symmetrical and precise with the flesh showing to have been chewed on a little but none missing.

Early in the morning of May 23, 1975. A Hereford cow two years of age was found near the road leading from the highway to the JD Ranch Headquarters approximately 5 miles south of Kent. No decomposition was noted, but rigor mortis was present. She was on her side. The skin area including the following tissues had been removed: the mammary gland (udder), rectum, vulva with the entire vagina, cervix, uterus, ovaries, and bladder. Also some skin had been removed from the inside of the left thigh together with some flesh. The remarkable things were the precise incisions, the lack of blood on the ground or seepage from the cut surface. The incisions were symmetrical. Buzzards, coyotes and small animals were plentiful in the area, yet there was evidence of only one small varmint gnawing on the carcass. The remains completely decomposed without ever showing any evidence that anything had fed on it.

One of the more remarkable facts of all cases was the absence of any disturbance of the surrounding ground. No kicking, struggling, or drag marks were present. This was in contrast to some copy cat mutilations which showed considerable disturbed ground, and seepage from the cut surface. Buzzards and varmints would feed on these, yet they did not feed on the mystery mutilations.

There were numerous other cases that were reported to me, but we could see no advantage to my going to view or postmortem. One obvious copycat mutilation was viewed by me. The cow had been roped and choked down from horseback as evidenced by marks on the ground and rope marks on the neck. The perpetrator was apprehended and confessed.

At the height of the trouble, Eddie Orth told me that his brother ranched in the foothills of the front range in Colorado. There had been large numbers of mutilations in the vicinity on all species, not just cattle. Helicopters were seen frequently and heard often at night. He reported that several ranchers had begun shooting at them, and the mutilations stopped. I shared this information with the ranchers in that area. They reported they had seen a few helicopters flying low and heard others. None admitted to firing at these helicopters, but the mutilations stopped abruptly.

There are a number of questions regarding this episode but no satisfactory answers. Specimens from the JD Ranch cow were obtained and sent to the Texas Veterinary Diagnostic Laboratory for examination. No toxic substances or any pathological condition was found.

Another peculiar thing about the entire episode was that there was little or no interest shown by the authorities. They kept trying to tell us the missing tissue was caused by varmints feeding on the carcasses. They might convince some city slicker, desk jockey of this, but it was foolish to try to tell it to a bunch of old ranchers, ranch hands, and Mexicans who had spent their lives in the country with animals. Actually, I had seen a dead cow or two myself. However, it is difficult for me to be too harsh on the disbelievers because of my early reservations before I personally saw and examined these animals.

Horse Gore at the X Ranch

About 1978 Mike Williams, foreman for the X Ranch at Kent, Texas, brought in a horse from the Rock Pile division. Cowboys had been taking the bulls up after the breeding season. One particularly old, cranky one didn't want to leave his harem, and one of the men had pushed his horse between them. The bull had especially long, sharp horns with which he gored the horse. Mike said he was watching at the time, hollering to be careful. He said it looked to him as if the bull stuck a horn all the way to the hilt in that horse's rear end and lifted him three feet off the ground.

The bull returned to his cows apparently satisfied he had made his point, literally and figuratively. The horse stood, quivering and bleeding. The rider dismounted, unsaddled, and stepped back, half expecting the horse to drop dead. The horse broke out in a cold sweat and continued to shake. Someone brought a couple of blankets from the house and covered him. He soon seemed to ease in pain but continued to bleed, so they loaded him in a covered trailer and drove the sixty miles to my hospital.

I administered intravenous cortisone-type steroid for shock and an analgesic for pain, then began an I.V. drip of lactated ringer's solution while I cleaned up the wound, which was to the left side of the anus.

I evacuated the rectum of feces and examined it to determine if it had been penetrated and was relieved to discover it had not. I loaded a 60cc syringe with a mixture of penicillin, dihydrostreptomycin, and neomycin, three antibiotics that I had found to be particularly valuable in deep wounds of horses. I attached an insemination pipette to the syringe and began to infuse the antibiotics as I explored the large wound with my hand encased in a surgical glove. I discovered a bleeding artery as it pulsated in time with the heartbeat. It was about four inches into the wound, and I continued to feel and infuse along the tract as it extended beside the rectum. I stopped about eight inches deep as the channel had become too narrow for my hand. I deposited the remainder of the antibiotic and withdrew my hand. I threaded a 3-0 loopuyt suture needle with catgut and began a one-handed attempt to obliterate the defect with special emphasis on the region of the bleeder until the blood stopped. I now re-entered the rectum and was satisfied I had not incorporated any of it in my sutures. I felt that my efforts were reasonably satisfactory. The blood loss had been substantial but not critical, and because blood transfusions were no small chore in horses, I did not give any blood but gave several liters of lactated ringer's intravenously.

Tetanus antitoxin was administered and a generous dosage of penicillin and dihydrostreptomycin was begun. He was placed on a bland, mostly bran diet to produce soft stools. The horse was hospitalized a few days and then was released when we felt he was out of danger. I was told he made an uneventful recovery but was always a little shy around bulls.

The Easter Eggs

I was called to the Crawford Mitchell Ranch, being told that a ranch hand was having trouble with a heifer calving. When I arrived, Chon told me that he was pulling gently on the calf, and it suddenly came in two. The head, front legs and chest had come on out, but the hips and hind legs were still inside the heifer. If he was going to tell me about how gentle the pull had been, it seems like he would have waited until after dark so that I could not see the marks on the ground where the heifer had skidded along and the tires of the Jeep had spun. Come to think of it, that might be the reason so many of my obstetrical calls were at night.

At times like this, I was faced with a dilemma. I hated to act as if I was so stupid that I could not see that he had tied on the calf and dragged the heifer around until the calf finally tore. On the other hand, the man was already ashamed of himself, and anything that was said would cause further embarrassment to the point where he might not call for help at all the next time and just let her die. I didn't need to alienate a client. I looked at the ground, then at him, and raised my eyebrows. He got the message.

I clipped the hair over the heifer's tailhead, disinfected the area with tincture of phenylmercuric nitrate and injected procaine hydrochloride for an epidural nerve block, that we usually called a spinal, to prevent her straining against my manipulations. I cleaned her rear and pumped in some Lubrivet, a commercial lubricant, which was much more satisfactory than soapy water or mineral oil I had been using. I explored and assessed the situation. I poked around in my obstetrical kit and retrieved a wire saw. This woven steel wire will cut both soft tissue and bone. In this case, I threaded it over the top of the hips at the midline of the fetus and dropped the handle between its hind legs. I then withdrew my hand and arm and ran them under its belly and between the hind legs to grasp the handle and pull. I now had both handles out the back end of the cow and the flexible wire saw around the pelvis of the calf. A back-and-forth motion soon had the hind end split into two pieces. The hind quarters were then delivered one at a time, relatively easily.

I then attempted to extract the placenta. It didn't come. The complex nature of the attachments often just take their own sweet time to separate. (I never have understood this expression as it usually refers to something taking an agonizingly long time, there being nothing sweet about it.) I inserted some uterine boluses to help control infection. One of Chon's small boys was watching intently as I put the blue Nolvasan, red sulfa urea, yellow Furacin and the white neomycin inside. I told him to remember where the Easter eggs were hidden so that he would know where to look. He didn't comment, but his eyes got very large.

A few sutures were placed to prevent her turning wrong side out (prolapse). An antibiotic was injected and a hormone to aid in expulsion of the placenta. She couldn't get up, caused by calving paralysis, so I tied a short rope around the hocks to hobble her to prevent the splits which could cause permanent injury. I instructed him to attempt to keep her upright and turn her twice a day.

Cold and Hot Hands

I palpated Limousin cows at the Bryant Harris Ranch near Valentine for Eddie Orth on one occasion. I was distressed because my findings did not fit his insemination dates. I would call the stage of pregnancy in days and he would compare it with his artificial insemination (A.I.) dates. The purpose was to determine whether the pregnancy was from the A.I. procedure or from a clean-up bull. The cows were kept from the bull for 30 days after insemination.

A definite determination could be made when the calf was born. Calculation was made on a gestation period of 283-285 days. This particular day, the embryo would feel too small for the insemination date and too large for the possible bull date. The discrepancy was not only a blow to my ego but also caused me to question my skill or my criteria. This was very frustrating, because I had palpated this herd for several years and had never had this problem before.

That afternoon I went to Bill Sohl's ranch near Alpine to perform the same service on Charolais, except these had been hand bred instead of A.I. bred. That is, the bull was placed with a cow in heat for a natural service then separated and the date recorded. The results here were uncanny. I was not off more than two days in any cow of a total of 28 head.

I was very perplexed — one of my worst and one of my best occurred on the same day. I made several inquiries regarding the different size embryos, wondering if differences as to breeds, type of breeding and ranch conditions could explain it. No one thought so. Most said I had a cold hand that morning and a hot hand that afternoon.

The Newcomer's Bull

Sid Harkins ranched north of Sanderson on the Corder Ranch and several leased ranches. He married the daughter of one of the old-timers, Monte Corder. Sid was an excellent rancher, both as an animal husbandryman and as a businessman.

He sold a bull to a neighbor who was a newcomer, having recently inherited a ranch in the vicinity. Sid told the fellow that the bull was in a certain pen and that he was gentle. He said that he could not be there at the time the buyer wanted to pick up the bull and asked if he could load it by himself. When the young man answered in the affirmative, Sid told him that he would pay for a fertility test at my place. The fellow arrived with a steer. I told him it was a steer and no need to test. He insisted that I do so, that he had just bought him, paying a good price. I put the steer in a chute and thoroughly examined him, showing that he did not have any testicles and pointed out the testicles of a bull in one of my pens that were very noticeable, even from a distance. The man was very upset, and I was bothered somewhat because Sid was a very reputable person. I could not understand this thing happening. I called Sid on the telephone and was fortunate to catch him because he was on the go during the daytime and difficult to reach except at night. I explained the situation. Sid was pretty bewildered, saying there was a sorry milk pen steer calf that had been put with the bull for company. He thought surely the guy could tell the difference. However, they were both black.

I loaded the steer in his trailer, and he left in a huff. Perhaps I had not been very diplomatic in handling the situation. I never saw him again. Later, I ran into Sid in a cafe in Sanderson and asked about the fellow. Sid just shook his head and wouldn't tell me any details, as there were several people present.

The Carpets Versus the Rancher's Boots

Sid Harkins had a few good years, back-to-back good rains, good grass and good livestock prices. His wife had been harassing him for several years to build a new house on the ranch. They were living in the original ranch house that Sid thought was vintage, old and comfortable, but his wife wanted a new house. Sid couldn't think of a legitimate reason not to build the new house, therefore, he agreed and was well-pleased with the result.

I was pregnancy testing some juicy[*] cows at the headquarter pens. We stopped for a water break, and Sid wanted to show me his new house. When we started in the back door, I stopped and started to take off my boots. Sid said not to bother, that it was to live in, not show off. I went ahead and took off my boots anyway and was glad that I had because new beautiful carpets had recently been installed. I told Sid that he had better start taking off his boots to protect the carpet because shampooing was expensive. Sid insisted he would never do that. About a year later I was there, and he stopped at the back door and took off his boots. I harassed him, reminding him that he said he would never do that. He frowned at me and gave a disgusted grunt, but no comment.

Grass Fires

Grass fires were numerous when I first came to the area. The rains were good, and grass was plentiful. Because the moisture content of the grass was high, the fires seemed to be easily controlled.

Most of the grass fires that I was aware of were started by trains, mainly caused by their hot boxes. Before trains had roller bearings, the wheel turned directly on the axle, being encased in a box containing waste, a shredded cotton material which was kept well oiled by periodic additions of heavy grade oil.

When these boxes were neglected by allowing the waste to deteriorate or by failing to add oil in a timely manner, the friction would cause hot boxes. These would become red hot and throw sparks and molten metal. These could be seen in the daytime, but at night they were highly visible, looking like sparklers. I saw spectacular sights on a few occasions when several hot boxes occurred at the same time on a train during a dark night. Hot boxes were not common, and it was rare to see more than one on a train.

I don't know the routine for maintenance of these boxes, but a careful watch was made for trouble. The brakeman and conductor riding in the caboose would watch from the back while the

---

[*] These cows had been eating green grass and their bowel movements were soft, very soft.

engineer and fireman would watch from the front. The men at depots and workers of the track crew also kept a lookout. If a boxcar developed a hot box, it would be left at a convenient siding.

The oil-burning, steam locomotives would develop soot embers in the smokestack if it was not cleaned regularly. These would build up in size and become red hot. Sometimes on a grade when the engine was laboring, there would be a spectacular display on a dark night as a shower of these would be blown out. The sight would resemble roman candle fireworks. I was told this was much more common when coal was burned and even more when wood was the fuel.

Although these sights were pretty, they were viewed with apprehension because they were certain to cause a grass fire in many cases.

Most of these fires were accessible by pickups, sprayers, and men with water and tow sacks. They could be readily contained if discovered soon and the wind was not too strong. I was told that in some instances the railroad companies compensated ranchers for the loss of grass and fences.

So far as I knew or heard, the fires caused by lightning the first few years that I was in the area were extinguished by the rain that followed.

*   *   *   *   *

The first years after our marriage, JoAnn and I often drove out on a highway to watch a rain. There wasn't much in the way of entertainment, and rain was an oddity in the 1950s. Money was about as scarce as rain during the drouth years, and this was inexpensive, besides being a welcome sight.

One evening just after dark there was a terrific lightning display north of Marfa in the Mimms pasture just past the municipal airport. It was the most spectacular display of that kind that I ever saw. Lightning would hit yuccas which would explode in a ball of fire and burn for a short time. There was no grass to burn due to the drouth, so there was no danger of a grass fire. Some of these hit only 50 yards or less from us as we stopped on the highway to watch the show, under the mistaken idea that we were safe in the car.

The first big fire that I saw was set by lightning in the high mountains on the X Ranch, southeast of the headquarters where Mr. John Reynolds lived. Conditions were dry. Grass, brush, and trees were plentiful up high and burned furiously. It had been a dry lightning storm with no rain.

Mr. John would not let his cowboys go up high to fight the fire and discouraged others from doing so because the terrain was so high and rough cattle could not graze it, so that it was of no value. Besides, not enough men and equipment could get there to be successful. The neighbors and others that came to fight the fire were plumb put out at Mr. John. They fought the fire about two weeks, not making any progress on it, being successful only in tearing up some equipment and exhausting the men that were fighting on foot with tow sacks and shovels. The women also were give out from bringing food, water, socks, and other clothing.

It was soon learned not to wear any polyester clothing because it burned readily. Eventually, everyone realized that Mr. John was correct and gave up, letting it burn itself out. They kept a watchful eye on it and would fight it when it came down to where it was accessible.

Two other big fires were fought, one on the north side of Livermore and another on Brooks Mountain. After that, few fires were fought in the high rough country, but the firefighters would wait until the fire came down. A notable exception was a very bad fire in the Chinati Mountains in 1998 caused by a so-called, controlled burn that got out of control in a high wind.

*   *   *   *   *

There was a particularly bad fire in the Marathon area in the early 1990s. A very strong west wind broke electric power line poles, and the electric sparks started a fire near Altuda. The wind was so strong and the grass so dry it traveled almost to Marathon, a distance of ten miles, in about an hour. Cattle were caught, but I didn't hear of any that were killed. Some had their teats scorched, a condition similar to sunburn, chapped teats from snow reflecting sun rays.

*   *   *   *   *

I was returning from Van Horn one day and saw a small grass fire in the tobosa grass next to the railroad. I grabbed my shovel and a couple of sacks, climbed the fence and soon had the fire out. Occasionally, someone on the highway would stop, but I would tell them I had it under control. I got back in my pickup very pleased with myself and drove up the highway a short distance and saw another. When this one was out, I drove a little farther and saw another. By the time I got this third one out, I could see that the first had started again, probably from some dry cow chips that are bad about smoldering and flaring up again by a little breeze. Then the second fire had flared up. Now when cars stopped I couldn't ask them to help. Besides, I had ruined all my sacks and towels and only had the shovel to fight with. I sent word to Valentine by way of these people who stopped to tell someone I needed help. It was about ten miles up the road, but no one came.

I went back and forth on those three fires until it got dark, and I was able to see the glow of a smoldering cow chip and bury it. The only reason I was able to whip these fires was because there was so little wind and the fire area was so small on all three. The turf not being very thick helped. I was finally satisfied all three were completely out. I was hot, thirsty, exhausted and mad as hell because no one from Valentine had come to help.

When I neared Valentine, I discovered why no one had come. A very large fire was burning on the outskirts of town, threatening to burn some houses. The railroad had set a total of five fires with a hot box. I did not stop. My muscles were sore, and I coughed up smoke for several days. I felt sorry for these people and regretted the many harsh things I had thought because they hadn't come to help me. I promised myself that was the last grass fire that I would fight, rationalizing that my services were more valuable to the public as a veterinarian than as a firefighter.

However, as has happened so many times that I have said I would do or not do certain things, I ate my words in this regard. A year or two later, I was returning to Marfa on the Ruidosa Road when I saw lightning strike a yucca which burned intensely. I stopped to watch, and the adjacent grass caught fire. There was a wire gap gate close by on this Clay Mitchell Ranch, and I thought I would run over there and put that fire out before it spread. The ranch was owned by Maurine Godbold who was a valued client and a good friend. I stopped up wind from the fire and started beating on the edge of it. The way it acted one would think I was fanning it and herding it. I was trying desperately to try to keep the fire from getting into some rocky hills nearby where it would be hard to fight.

Buddy Eppenauer was taking his father, Mr. Ep, who had suffered a stroke, for a car ride. Buddy turned around and sped back to town to sound the alarm. The Marfa Volunteer Fire Department had a special grass fire truck that they used in these situations. The truck pulled up behind me and stopped near my truck. Then I saw a tongue of the fire that had circled around behind me and was very close to my truck. If the firemen had been a few minutes later, I would have lost my truck.

Several vehicles were burned in the area over the years. No one to my knowledge lost their life, but several were burned. Bill Cowden on his ranch near Kent was on a bulldozer attempting to clear a fire lane when the fire engulfed him. He was fortunate to have survived although his face was badly burned.

*　　*　　*　　*　　*

Over the years, many miles of fences were lost, much in terrain where replacement was difficult. The last few years, steel posts have been used in places where cedar posts were burned. These tee posts are about the same price as the cedar, but they won't burn and are easier to install. Digging a post hole isn't necessary. They are hammered in with a steel post driver.

Grass lost from fires caused by the railroad was sometimes compensated by the railroad company, but lightning fires were just part of the cost of ranching.

High Lonesome

Maureen Godbold called me one day in the fall from the Clay Mitchell Ranch saying that her ranch hand, Merced Ramirez, had seen a cow trying to calve. She was lying down at the foot of a hill that I called High Lonesome. There are lots of places in this beautiful country that are called High Lonesome and always with justification, but this high basalt mesa was my own special place.

A few years before, I had been hunting in the Crosson Hills and spotted a big, buck, mule deer lying down under a cedar tree on top of a basalt mesa that was isolated from the rest of the Crosson Hills. I had been searching the area with field glasses.

I looked at the deer, then studied the intervening terrain. I was on the edge of a twenty-foot high rock bluff, then the ground had a steep slope downward about fifty yards away. The hillside was covered with all kinds of interesting vegetation such as sotol, algarita and largancilla-type catclaw. There was about three hundred yards of flat land to the base of the hill the deer was on, which had about the same type obstacle course up to its top.

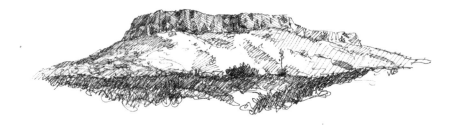

High Lonesome - basalt mesa.

I looked back at the deer and estimated the size of his horns. I know deer are supposed to have antlers, but west of the Pecos they are called horns. I decided I just had to pay him a visit. I tried not to make too big of a racket as I eased down, snagging my clothes on the catclaw and stumbling on rocks. I don't know why those big rocks have to turn under a person's weight. It was a relief to get down on level ground and slip around among the cardentia, yucca, and sacahuiste to the foot of the big hill. The rifle sure got heavy as I struggled up.

I finally topped out and peeked over the edge with my rifle at the ready. I didn't see him. I was hoping he might be in a little swag out of sight so I eased along, hunkered down. I had circled around to be down wind so he couldn't smell or hear me. It wasn't a very big area on top, maybe two or three acres. He just wasn't there. I don't know if he was bashful or just got tired of waiting for me. I sat down on the stump of a gnarled, dead cedar, leaned my rifle on a rock, lit a cigarette and scanned the countryside. I watched a herd of antelope grazing in the pasture below and fat Hereford cows scattered around in the tall gramma grass, a windmill turning lazily in the distance, and smoke curling up from the bunkhouse at the headquarters. I was kinda glad the deer hadn't been there; I mighta shot him, then had to clean him, and try to get him down. I looked off in the distance to Capote and Chinati Mountains to the west and south, southeast to Cienaga and San Jacinto Mountains, Mitchell and Crosson Mesas, then east to Goat and Cathedral. I turned and looked at Paisano Peak and Haystacks. When I glanced to the north towards Old Blue and Livermore, I saw that old buck slipping up the hillside that I had just left. That smart rascal. That's how he had gotten old.

I shifted my position to move off a stubby limb that was poking me, and I noticed the big black jagged rocks with the little diamonds embedded in them, sparkling in the sun and the colorful moss growing on their north side. There are some folks that would try to tell me that the sparkles were quartz or calcite or some such thing not nearly so exotic and that the moss is properly lichen, which, of course, it is, but I like moss better. They probably wouldn't have been able to see that Indian peeking around the trunk of that crooked, dead, cedar tree on the edge of the bluff. Maybe think that arrow laying there on the ground was a dead limb or that bear over yonder was a dead yucca. Now, wouldn't that be sad?

This place was high up over the countryside, maybe not as high or as lonesome as some other places called High Lonesome, but it was special to me. It was not a bad kind of lonesome, but a relaxing and peaceful kind that gives a person a chance to enjoy the real pleasures of life as you watch that eagle soaring overhead. The silence was complete, calming and soothing, only broken occasionally by the far off bawl of a cow calling her calf. I have prowled around some to unwind from a sometimes hectic practice and hide from the telephone, ending up in isolated places that I thought no other person had ever been, not even an Indian, only to look around and see a rusty sardine can that breaks the enchantment. This place did not have any such object to spoil it.

I always thought I would climb back up there someday to experience the view with the peace and quiet. I even drove to the base one time, but when I looked up at that high, steep hillside, I just sat there in my pickup to bask in my memories.

After Maureen's phone call, I put a couple of jugs of warm water in my pickup and drove to the ranch past the headquarters and through the gate into the Crosson pasture and up towards the hills. I circled around a washout in the road and took off across the pasture, dodging rocks, palmilla-type yuccas, a dagger or two, some sacahuiste and patches of largancilla-type catclaw. I arrived at the appointed place, but no Merced and no cow. I climbed up on top of the VetBed of my pickup with my field glasses and looked all around, and still couldn't see hide nor hair, of either. I climbed down, got back in the cab, and circled around the hill. There was the cow, lying down, with a calf's leg sticking out.

I got my rope and started toward the cow, and guess what? The stinking rascal started wobbling up the hill. I ran after her, and she gathered a little speed, just enough to stay out of range of my rope. She wasn't moving very fast, but you can rest assured I wasn't either, as I stumbled over rocks, up the steep hillside.

I finally caught up close enough to throw a loop, and I lucked out. She stuck her head in it. I took a dally on a palma, a dagger-type yucca, and she pulled back and choked down. When she fell, I hurried over and moved the rope so that it was around her horns. I took up the slack and snubbed her a little closer. I went back down the hill to get my equipment. I looked at my clumsy calf puller, then up to where the cow was, and decided I would give it a try without it.

I wrapped an OB chain around my neck and hooked a couple of handles in my belt. I stuffed a bottle of soap in one pocket and a bottle of disinfectant in another. I stuck a big needle, threaded with umbilical tape through the flap of my shirt pocket, then I put a needle holder and a pair of scissors in my hip pocket. I hung a bucket in the crook of my arm and got hold of a gallon jug of water in one hand and a jug of obstetrical lubricant in the other. I took a deep breath and started back up the hill. Without the adrenaline flowing, it was a lot farther and steeper. I began to think that hill was growing.

I finally got back up to the cow and realized she had squatted down like a frog with her rear end up against a big rock. I grabbed her tail to pull her over on her side, but she didn't budge. I strained and grunted. My goodness, she was a big ole fat cow and didn't have any business having trouble calving, besides being so inconsiderate as to climb a hill to do it. It was against all the laws of nature. I guess she didn't know that or maybe just didn't care. I finally flopped her over, and she struggled, ending up with her rear in a sotol. This was physically accessible, but I was not going to work through those saw-like leaves. She was lying on her side this time, and I hobbled her by tying her hind legs together with my tail rope. This time I grasped the hind legs and flopped her over. Her rear end was clear now, but pointed down. I was going to have to work against gravity. I washed my hands and her rear, smeared lubricant on both, wallowed out a little nest in the rocks, dug my toes in, and went to work.

A little pink nose was peeking out beside the leg with the nostrils working. No sight of the other leg. I couldn't get in past the head and leg. No room for my arm, so I had to stuff his head back inside. I always hated to do this to make room, because sometimes they would turn their head back over their shoulder to see what's behind them, and then I have ole billy hell trying to get it straight.

This is one of the many times I had wished that my arms were about a foot longer. I strained to get a little deeper, made harder by her straining against me. Sure was hard on hernias and hemorrhoids.

Finally, I hooked a finger around the crook of his elbow. That sharp rock gouging me in the ribs was just going to have to watch out for itself, 'cause I wasn't about to turn loose of that leg. By squirming and twisting my fingers, holding my breath and distorting my face, trying to hold my mouth just right as my eyeballs were about to pop out, I managed to straighten the leg and bring it out.

Now where did that head go? There, tucked down under his chest with his neck bowed. I guess he was ashamed to have caused me all this trouble. Well, I hooked a finger in the corner of his mouth and eased it around between the cow's labor contractions. Ohhhhhh! That hurt when my hand was mashed between the calf's head and the cow's pelvis bone. I had tried to wear a ring in my earlier days and had nearly got a finger torn off when a similar situation occurred. The head finally popped out, and I was looking eyeball to eyeball with those big black eyes in the white face. He winked and wiggled his pink nose. I said, "Howdy," but he didn't say anything. I pulled one leg at a time to get the elbows over the brim of the pelvis. Come on now, cow, push! You had been straining all the time. Now that I need you, don't quit on me. I put obstetrical chains on the legs and hooked the handles on. They look sorta like hay hooks. I put both my feet against her rump and pulled for all I was worth. She was a grown, mature cow and should have plenty of room, having previously had several calves. I sure didn't want to go back down the hill to get my calf puller. Maybe I wasn't grunting loud enough. She hunched up and started pushing, and I figured it's now or never and gave it my best shot.

I hadn't been very enthusiastic about striking that pose with my feet up and head downhill. The calf slid out, and I fell back with that slimy calf on top of me. I was wedged between some rocks and in my awkward position, I couldn't get up, so I had to submit to his showering me with kisses of gratitude. I thought I had it made. He was blinking his eyes, shaking his head and snorting, but his rear end wouldn't come. A hip lock! I finally managed to get to my feet and jiggled the calf up and down, back and forth, side to side, twisting and turning. Believe me, prayer really works. The little fellow came out, but I had fooled around too long. He wasn't breathing.

I pulled some secretions out of his mouth and poked my fingers in his nostrils, beat on his chest, and rubbed his back. No response. I hadn't realized how big the calf was until I tried to lift him up to sling the juices out. I couldn't do it. Perhaps his slick hind legs and the rocks rolling under my feet made the chore harder. Either way, I decided I didn't really need to do that. I kneeled down, put my mouth over one nostril and blew while holding the other nostril and his mouth closed. I could feel his chest expand. I did this a few more times, and he started gasping. I rared back on my haunches, grinned at the calf, and started spitting. I retrieved my shirt and wiped my mouth on the sleeve, lit a cigarette, and admired my handiwork.

Little Lazarus soon started struggling to get up. I dragged him around to the dinners and helped him get latched on. While he nursed, getting a belly full of colostrum, I put a couple of sutures in the cow's rear end to prevent a prolapse.

I untied the rope I had her hobbled with, then took the rope off her horns. I massaged where the rope had been and behind her ears, bragging on what a fine baby calf she had. I slapped her on the side to encourage her to get up. She was laid out flat, and she just dog paddled in the air. I took ahold of her tail and pulled her up to a normal position. I wondered how Merced was going to feed and water her up here. She looked around at me as I scrunched her calf up towards her head. She didn't pay that calf no nevermind. She just bunched and struggled up and stood there a minute, spraddled out to get her sea legs, then staggered off down the hillside. Do you know what that dumb cow did? She went and laid downright beside my truck! I was so mad I wanted to bite myself. I hauled off and kicked a big rock! That was a mistake with that ingrown nail on the big toe. And I'll bet it didn't hurt that cow a bit.

I looked over at the baby calf that was struggling to stand. Big ole black eyes asking for a little help. I put one hand under his rump and the other under his neck, and with a little help, he stood wobbly-legged. He went to nuzzling me like I was his momma. There I was stuck up on that hillside with a newborn calf and all my calving equipment. I kept trying to tell that baby where his mother was, but he continued to follow me. So I gathered up my tools and started down the hill, hoping he would follow. He stopped and bawled at me. I coaxed a little, but he had stalled out, and his bawls just sounded more plaintive.

I stumbled back down the hill, only falling twice. The jugs were plastic so they survived. Only the glass bottle of liquid soap in my pocket broke. I dropped my stuff on the open panel shelf of my pickup and looked at the cow who was calmly chewing her cud. I gave her a little verbal abuse, but the toe still hurt so I resisted a temptation that crossed my mind.

About that time, Merced drove up and started telling me his troubles about why he was late. I really wasn't very sympathetic to his problems. I pointed up to the calf and assured him he wasn't going to miss out on all the fun.

For some reason ole High Lonesome didn't hold the enchantment that it used to have for me. In retrospect, I think maybe lonesome might not be an accurate description of my feelings up there on top. *Solitude* may be a better word. I think *lonesome* denotes a sad, depressed feeling, whereas solitude to me is a more relaxed, tranquil state of mind.

Poochie Quigg

Poochie Quigg was a legend in his own time. I don't know if Poochie was his proper name or a nickname. Some parents have been known to bestow some rather colorful names on a newborn, innocent babe. Of course, he may have earned his name, if it was a nickname, which could add a whole new chapter to the legend.

Poochie took over management of Bobby French's Chilicote Ranch west of Valentine in the Sierra Vieja Mountains around the middle of the 1970s. I had heard some tales about him but had never met the man until I was first called after he took over there. I anticipated our meeting with a little apprehension because I really didn't know how we would get along together. I was running around like a chicken with its head cut off trying to get as many cattle worked in as short a length of time as possible. Ranchers shipped in the fall and were anxious to get their cows checked, sorted, and put to pasture as soon as possible to keep from eating out their holding traps near the working pens.

Some outfits would dilly dally around, short-handed, and it would take forever to get the job done. This wasn't the case with Poochie at the Casa Blanca pens. Everything was always well-organized, and the work went relatively smoothly. Now, I say, relatively, because it was about as well as can be done with an old, sorry, worn-out, squeeze chute. The rest of the pens were in good shape. Poochie kept them repaired by scrounging boards and nails, but the squeeze chute was another matter. It had welds on top of welds and was mostly held together with baling wire, chains, and a come-a-long, which is a ratchet type puller and a big improvement over a block and tackle.

All these make-shift repairs worked fairly well, but there just wasn't any substitute for the headgate, which is the front end of a squeeze chute to catch and stabilize the head. This was important here because a decree had come down from on high that each cow was to have a Temple tag inserted in one or both ears according to a prescribed code. The Temple tag is a small plastic tag that is inserted into a hole made in the ear with a punch kinda like a leather punch.

Different colored tags positioned differently in the ear were to give a record of the cow's sex life without having to resort to a written page in a notebook. The theory is great. I don't know how successful it was on this ranch.

I carried a front headgate and its frame on top of the veterinary bed of my pickup for use when and where it was needed. It was pretty heavy, and I usually left it in place up there because putting it up and taking it down was sure difficult for one person. The first years of my practice, I carried a Turner headgate which was really gosh-awful heavy, but hell for stout. Later, I would carry a

WW headgate. Often, we would secure one of these to Poochie's squeeze chute.

Along late in the 1970s, we were experiencing a dry spell in the fall. It was so dry that fall that water had only a 50% relative humidity. Poochie had delivered his calves about a week before and had a problem sorting and weighing them. Because the dust was so bad, the cattle couldn't be seen well enough to separate the steers from the heifers or to distinguish the sizes, the calves having been sold on a sliding scale, that is, a different price per pound for different weights.

I had been going from one ranch to another, day after day, for two months, breathing dust and dirt. My eyes were swollen from rubbing rocks out of them. I really enjoyed the practice of veterinary medicine and the fellowship of the cowboys, but I was beginning to dread the dusty pens. The day before my appointment with Poochie, there was a great big, beautiful cloud built up in the west and someone told me it was raining cats and dogs in the Valentine area. From all appearances, it was covering a wide area. I was elated and anticipated a nice work with no dust.

The dirt road from the paved highway to the pens was mostly over a gravel type soil but the tobosa grass flat near Wildhorse Draw was pure dirt that had become very slick mud. A good deal of slipping and sliding, mudslinging, and chauffeuring was experienced. When I got to the pens, lo and behold, the pens were a lake.

Poochie had wet the pens down with a hose for three days. One of the *gentes* (men) said he had drained a water storage tank. Poochie really looked crestfallen. He had worked so hard to prepare the pens for a decent work, and a two-inch rain had fallen the day before. The problem was compounded by rainwater running down a slope into the pens. There was no dust, but the cows running and kicking up mud and crud was worse. Most places, the mud and water was knee deep, too shallow to swim and too deep to wade.

We were almost exhausted and had lost our sense of humor when Poochie's wife, Jan, drove up with lunch. She was always smiling and laughing, soon getting us in a good humor so we could enjoy the meal. We laughed and told of seeing a big catfish chased by an alligator.

Copperheads

Jess Fisher left his job with the railroad and went to work on the Michigan Flat Ranch east of Van Horn. He lost two or three horses from snakebite and called me on one. The horse was dead when I got there. Jess and I wondered why they had died so quickly, and I guessed it was caused by the Mojave rattler. Most rattlesnakes have a hemotoxin (blood poison) in their venom that is very dangerous, but most cases survive with treatment. However, a Mojave produces a neurotoxin (nerve poison) that usually causes death fairly quickly, and victims rarely respond even when treatment is initiated soon after the bite. Jess insisted they were being bitten by copperheads. I assured Jess this was not the case, for two reasons: one, they are found only around wet areas such as springs and *ciénagas* and the only water on this dry rocky part of the ranch was in the cement water troughs; and, the copperhead toxin is reputed to be one of the least toxic of the poisonous snakes. I had just finished my lecture, when a snake crawled in front of us on the old, dry, rocky road. We stopped and examined the snake. It was a copperhead! Do you suppose those dry land copperheads were more poisonous because the venom was concentrated from dehydration?

I was told years later I had been misinformed. Copperheads are as toxic as any rattlesnake.

Ken Rolston and the New Mexico Snowstorm

Ken Rolston was a lawyer in Houston, but was raised (some say reared, either way, he grew up) in the Mason-Llano area of the Hill Country in central Texas. Working with horses, cows, sheep, and goats, he knew what hard work was before he went off to college and got educated. He practiced law in the city, but he longed for ranch life. He managed to acquire several ranches in the Marfa-Valentine area where we became acquainted.

Later Ken bought two ranches in New Mexico: the Slash Ranch near Beaverhead and the Luera Ranch about 25 miles north of there in the Luera Mountains. The ranch kinda overflowed out onto the southern edge of the Plains of San Augustin.

Now, to make a short story long, I oughta tell you where these were located. They were out west of Socorro and on past

Magdelena. A little farther on, a dirt country road turned off south to the ranches. The pavement continued on west through Datil and Pie Town to Arizona.

Pie Town was a quaint little place sitting on the edge of the Cibolo National Forest and astride the Continental Divide. I was told that a combination cafe and filling station had been built out in the middle of nowhere hoping to scrape out a living, serving the rural area of large ranches and the lumbering industry.

The pies in the little cafe were excellent. Cowboys, lumber-jacks, and truck drivers were starved for this type fare. It was said that men would travel miles to eat there. Actually, if a person went there he would have to go miles in that sparsely settled area. A community grew up, gradually becoming a little town, famous for the pies which resulted in its name.

A tale was told about a long-haul, truck driver who stopped here and ordered a cup of coffee and pie. The waitress asked, "You mean a piece a pie?"

"No, a whole pie."

"Well, okay, how do you want it cut?"

He asked, "What do you mean?"

She answered, "I can cut it in 4 pieces, 6 pieces, or even 10 pieces."

"Oh my goodness! Not 10 pieces. Nobody can eat 10 pieces of pie."

The town of Beaverhead wasn't any town a'tall. It was only a forest ranger station high up in the mountains. Because it was the only habitation (except for a few widely scattered ranches) in the area, it was a well known place to those living in central western New Mexico.

The entire area of both ranches was not only high in elevation but surrounded by even higher mountains. My usual traveling route was by way of Dusty and Winston from Truth or Consequences. Several years previously, the town of Hot Springs had changed its name for a television program, hoping to get a little publicity. Actually, all they got was a headache, with all the changes and the long, clumsy name.

For several years I had driven to the ranches in my practice pickup which was well-equipped and gave me freedom of movement. One year Ken insisted on taking me in his airplane, but I refused since I never liked to go with someone else in their vehicle. I rarely had everything I needed and was forced to move at their discretion. I assumed that he would make arrangements with another veterinarian, but at last he relented and allowed me to drive.

I always enjoyed working in this country. The men were good cowboys who knew their job and were hard workers. They were friendly and seemed to like their work. The wives would show up with hot food, and the noon meal was kinda like a picnic. The weather had always been pleasant, and the day's work was usually relatively short. I never had to go to work before sunup and was finished well before dark.

The short workdays resulted in a longer time away from Marfa. It took two days traveling, one each way. I generally was gone seven or eight days to do maybe three days of the usual time it took to pregnancy test an equal number of cows. However, this work came at a time in the fall when I was really tired from a heavy work schedule, and the rest was welcome.

The beautiful scenery of mountains and pine forest was a pleasure to look at and a change from my area. It was different, but maybe not quite as pretty. Of course, I may have been prejudiced.

The last day of this work, the cowboy checking the teeth for age was finding a high percentage of old cows that supposedly had lost their front teeth, called "smooth mouth" or "gummers." Many of these were not pregnant, and all were marked to ship. Often, an open, young cow might be kept to give her another chance.

This situation was particularly depressing because this herd had been cleaned up (old cows and poor doers had been shipped) the year before, and young replacements had been purchased in Colorado.

I was concentrating only on the state of pregnancy because I could see little of the animal besides the rear end in the type of squeeze chute we were using.

After eating and while the cowboys were resting, Ken and I were looking over the cattle we had worked. We both commented that although the old cows were in poor flesh, most seemed to be young by the body conformation and shape of the mouth. These cattle were Angus, so that without horns their age was not obvious.

When we began work again, I started examining the gums of cows that were being called old. I found that they were indeed smooth, but the middle incisor teeth that are supposed to erupt at 24 months of age were barely discernable by a bulge in the gums with an occasional pearl just peeking out. This delayed dentition was probably caused by the calves nursing these young cows that had been on poor pastures.

The cows had not been marked as to whether they were pregnant—only as being a shipper. Therefore, they had to be reworked.

Snow began to fall which wet their hair. Keeper cows were being branded, so the wet hair added to our frustration because it made them more difficult to brand and usually causes a blotch.

The longer it snowed the heavier it became, and there was at least an inch on the ground by the time we finished. I left as soon as possible and went back to the Slash Ranch for my clothes. I had left them there because I had originally intended to go there, shower, spend the night, and leave for Marfa the next morning. There were no facilities for me at the Luera, and I had been driving between the two ranches each day.

The road out from Beaverhead to Winston was over a high mountain pass. The snow was deep and I barely made it with tire chains and positive traction rear end on my pickup.

Ken and his men had to stay at the pens to sort cattle, because trucks were on the way to haul the open, shipper cows to town to be sold. Some of the men drove keeper cows to pasture. The snow became so deep the trucks couldn't get to the ranch. The snow continued for several days and became very deep.

I understood that the keeper cows were successfully driven horseback into some sheltered areas in the Luera Mountains and survived the snowstorm but the selling cows were in bad trouble, being caught out on the flat with no protection and very little hay. I was never told how severe the losses were. Most ranchers don't talk much about their bad luck. Ken was not able to leave the ranch for two weeks. He never pressured me to fly with him again.

Horse Gore at Chinati

Jack Wood was running the Dipper Ranch for L.R. French. They were using Longhorn bulls on heifer yearlings for ease of calving. This worked pretty well until some of the bulls got older and cranky, especially those that didn't see a person often. Jack was in the rough, mountainous, Chinati pasture of the ranch picking up the bulls, as the breeding season was over. One bull didn't want to leave his harem, so Jack was harassing him when he got mad and hooked at Jack and his horse. The long horn barely missed Jack's leg but didn't miss the horse's belly. Jack said it looked like the horn went up to the hilt. That seemed to satisfy the bull, and he ran off.

The horse stood, trembling, with a cold sweat and the nostrils flared. Jack pulled off the saddle and walked to his pickup. He drove to the house and called me. I thought the horse would be dead by the time I got there, but I loaded my pickup and went.

We were able to drive up to the horse. A little gut was poking out, but no feces could be seen. I gave an intravenous dose of analgesic and a type of cortisone for shock, then started a continuous flow of lactated ringer's. I scrubbed and searched the wound, finally deciding I would do more harm than good by puddling guts anymore. I infused penicillin and dihydrostreptomycin in the abdominal cavity, sutured the peritoneum, the muscles, then the skin. I gave all the fluids I had, and by that time the horse's condition had stabilized. He looked pretty good, so Jack loaded him in a trailer and took him to the house. He made an uneventful recovery, to my amazement.

A few days later, Jack got his rifle and looked up the bull who trotted docilely to the pens and was loaded on a truck to town. Jack was after blood and was a little disappointed that the bull hadn't acted up.

Blue Norther

One day in October, 1981, Kiki Aguirre, his brother, Lourdes, and I were pregnancy testing (we hadn't gotten high toned yet to call it palpating) and vaccinating cows on the McCabe Ranch belonging to W.B. Blakemore II, called Bill, who was operating as Alpha Twenty-One Corporation.

It was a nice warm morning; there was no wind; the sun was shining brightly; and we were in shirt sleeves. The cattle were working smoothly, and we were enjoying ourselves, laughing and telling each other stories, and commenting how great it was to be alive.

Kiki looked up north and asked me what it was he saw. It was a blue haze coming over the Davis Mountains and approaching fast. Kiki knew that was a Blue Norther. He just didn't want to accept the fact. We were in shock a moment, and a cow got upside down in the chute. We struggled frantically, trying to get her out before she died and that norther hit. We were successful in getting the cow straight but not before the norther caught us. We nearly froze before we could get enough sweaters, jackets, and coats on. You can't believe how our dispositions changed. Everything went to pot.

Removing Porcupine Quills

A veterinarian from western Montana wrote an article in one of the scientific journals describing a new technique for the removal of porcupine quills from a dog. He claimed it was simple, quick, and easy.

This chore had always been an unpleasant task for me. Invariably, it was a late night procedure because the porcupine is primarily a nocturnal creature, or so it seems, because that's when most of the dogs were presented to me. When the poor ole dog got a snoot full of quills, he would begin the most bloodcurdling howling. There is no way a person can sleep and ignore the problem.

A few dogs will quit a porcupine when they get a few of the long tail quills in their nose. Many just become infuriated and continue to harass the animal until their head is a solid mass of quills, not only the face and neck but also inside the mouth.

The big, long, tail and back quills are not too hard to remove, but the real problems are the little ones from the porcupine's sides and belly. It's especially hard to locate them in a fuzzy-faced dog. It seems that many can only be located by feel. The back end of a quill is sharp also; therefore, the ends of the fingers are continually pricked, which doesn't do a lot for one's disposition.

A lot of people believe a quill is easier to pull out if the end is cut off. Their reasoning is that the inside of the quill is a vacuum. I disagree because I tried it a few times when only a few large quills were in the dog's nose, and I sure couldn't tell it made any difference. I think the difficulty is that the end penetrating the skin has multiple small barbs. Also I would challenge anyone to cut every quill, many of which are very small. I have attempted several times to count them in a dog that had a snoot full but was never successful, losing count and losing interest.

Along about midnight the doorbell rang, and someone beat on the door. Here was this guy with a dog on a leash, which he was holding way out at arms length, trying to keep the dog from nuzzling his leg.

I took one look at the dog and figured this was the perfect place for the new technique. I managed to give a big dose of tranquilizer injection in a hind leg without getting jabbed but three times. While this was taking effect I read and reread the published directions to be sure I understood them correctly and studied the subject.

He was a shaggy dog with long upper lip hair and chin whiskers. It would have been a chore to remove them the old hunt-grasp-and-pull-with-forceps way. This was a classical case with the entire face and neck covered and the mouth so full the dog couldn't close it. I mean there were quills through the tongue, in the gums and roof of the mouth with the inside of the cheeks a solid mass. The dog must have killed that porcupine.

The odor was pretty rank. I don't know if this was the musk, urine or feces of the varmint or the dog or both, it surely was more than pure dog.

I started my preparations. This was before my heart attack, and we still cooked with good ole hog lard. I carefully heated a batch just right and started applying it to the dog. I would put a layer on, then let it cool to solidify, then apply some more. I kept repeating this process until I figured I had built up just the right thickness. I then poured apple cider vinegar over it, waited exactly the time recommended and poured another generous helping of vinegar—enough so that it ran off freely. I then timed it again by the clock.

The vinegar was to completely solidify the lard and the mask could be peeled off, bringing all the quills with it without damaging the hair or skin.

You can't imagine the mess! I couldn't scrape it off. I couldn't wash it off. I couldn't find the quills to pull them out. I had lard all over the dog, my hands, clothes, instruments and table. Disaster!

I thought I would never clean up this and I was right, I never did. After profound apologies to the owner and finally getting enough off my hands to write, I sat down and wrote a scorching letter to the author of that article.

However, after I had vented my feelings, but before I mailed it, I decided I would not give the rascal the satisfaction of knowing I was a sucker and had fallen for his joke. It made me shy of trying new and radical procedures for awhile.

The dog and I both survived the ordeal, but neither of us were ever the same afterwards.

I still kinda get my feathers ruffled when I think about it.

Lorena Ann Kelly and Shannon

Lorena Ann "Rena Ann" Kelly had a most remarkable dog, a female pit bull terrier named Shannon. She was brindle with a white spot. She was an excellent specimen, although a little stout. If she had been a male, I would have said fat. Her face, though, was one only a doting owner and a dedicated veterinarian could love.

Her ears had been trimmed. Had they ever been trimmed! They were not only trimmed, they were completely obliterated. Pit bulls were supposedly originally bred to be fought in a pit. Therefore, their ears were trimmed to restrict the opportunity for an opponent to get a mouth full. The ears are carefully measured by the surgeon and the incisions made. The two pieces cut off are compared to see if they are equal in length. If not, a little is taken off the longer ear. Again they are compared. If it is discovered that too much was removed, then the other ear is re-trimmed. A careful comparison may reveal they are still unequal. This is very similar to cutting the leg off a table or chair to steady it. Now, I never had this happen to me, and if I had I wouldn't admit it. Well, in this particular case there must have been a problem, but they were eventually made to match: there was nothing left at all.

I don't know that I ever heard how Rena Ann ended up with this dog except that she is such a compassionate, tender-hearted person that I suspect she took pity on the poor creature.

The first time I saw Shannon I didn't know how to react. I couldn't determine whether the appearance was fearsome, laughable or to be pitied. I soon learned it was none of the above. The personality was so delightful that the appearance was overlooked. She kinda reminded me of a big ole horse-faced boy I knew once whose face would stop a clock, but his heart was as big as all get out. You soon forgot what he looked like.

Shannon always came into the office eagerly, pushed open the little swinging door, and walked into the exam room. She would rear up on her hind legs, put her paws on the table edge, and look at me, waiting to be helped onto the table.

She developed a lesion on her thigh and another on her chest. We knew these were skin tumors, but we hoped they might possibly be infections and respond to medication. They didn't though, so surgery was decided on. She was placed on the surgical table, Rompun and Ketaset were administered. Rena Ann was there to comfort and console her. Apnea and fibrillation set in, much to my dismay. Apnea is respiratory arrest and fibrillation is an irregular, non-functioning heartbeat. This was a rare reaction in my practice, but it would have to happen to a favored patient in the presence of a favored client. I immediately started artificial respiration and cardiac massage. I couldn't look directly at Rena Ann, but I did sneak a peek now and then out of the corner of my eye. She showed no panic and uttered no hysterical sounds but seemed to be calm and confident that I could resuscitate Shannon. It must have been close to an hour, but finally she stabilized. I proceeded with the surgery with fear and trembling.

After Shannon recovered, was alert and on her feet, I confessed to Rena Ann my anxiety, and she told me of hers. Her self-control had been amazing. A very remarkable lady.

F1 Tiger Stripe

Joe Lane was a dyed-in-the-wool Hereford man. He had a fine herd of some of the best registered cattle and was very active in the Highland Hereford Association. L. R. "Bobby" French had bought a lot of country in the area and was running Hereford-Brahma crossbreds. They were mostly half blood and were brindle (striped), long-eared, long-headed and long-legged.

Joe was managing all his ranches for him. We were at the U Ranch near Balmorhea looking at some of the cattle while waiting on trucks. Joe and I hadn't said much, just looking and keeping our thoughts to ourselves. Suddenly, Joe asked me if I knew who the smartest man in the world was. I admitted that I didn't. He then told me it was the man that started calling his cattle, F1 Tiger Stripe. Everyone wants an F1 Tiger Stripe cow, but nobody wants an old brindle crossbred.

Braford Bull

I was operating on a crossbred Brahma bull. Well, actually it was a Braford. Technically, this is 3/8 Brahma and 5/8 Hereford. The breeders don't like for their cattle to be called crossbreeds. I had the bull up on my surgical table in my large animal operating room. These are awfully high class sounding names for my facilities. Actually, it was a tin barn, and the table was a squeeze chute Keezy Kimball had made. An animal was caught in the chute and could be laid over on its side by converting it to a table by adding a little here and subtracting a little there, then cranking up a winch. It really wasn't very fancy, but it was excellent facilities for its day and I was mighty proud of it.

These bulls have a tendency to develop a prolapse of the prepuce which is often injured and infected, necessitating surgical removal, called circumcision. Jim White came in while I was operating and started watching. Soon he walked all the way around studying the subject. It had been rumored that Jim was partial to Herefords. Actually, Jim was a registered Hereford breeder and didn't have anything good to say about any other breed, especially those with Brahma blood. He finally commented that I should be working further back. I asked what he meant by that remark. He said, "You'll help that rancher a whole lot more if you will go ahead and castrate that sorry excuse for a bull."

The Pregnancy Testing Horse

Jim White had his own outfit and was the manager of the Brite Ranch. Together, this amounted to a large number of cattle. The fees for pregnancy testing them would have been substantial. I had a veterinarian with me now, so that I could take on more work. When I was so busy in the sixties and seventies, there was a possibility that Jim had become discouraged trying to get an appointment with me, but I did not know or at least I couldn't remember having ever been too busy for him. He was a friend, and we could have worked something out, I'm sure.

Now that I had the time, I began to hint that his cows needed me. I very subtly tried to convince him I should pregnancy test his cows. Maybe I wasn't too subtle. One day I was bending his ear trying to tell him all the money I could make him by finding and culling the open cows. He wrinkled up his forehead and told me about his ole cutting horse. He claimed he could wander through the cow herd, and that horse would pick out a cow and take her to the pens. The herd was being held kinda loose outside the pens by several cowboys. Jim said that horse could determine an open cow. He didn't know if it was by sight, sound or smell. He swore by that horse. I kept thinking that horse would wear out, but I did before he did. However, in his later years, I checked some yearling heifers and some old cows. I don't know if the horse was losing his touch or if he felt these were below his dignity.

Bodie's Teeth

We were working cows through the chute at the Y6 pens. Sometimes we would be short handed; this was one of those times. Bodie Means would put cows into the crowd pen from a larger pen. Then he would fill the crowd chute while Alf, his father, prodded them forward and scotched them so they couldn't back up. I was giving them moral support while I waited to pregnancy test. After the crowd chute was full, Bodie would half climb and half jump out and lope up to the front to work the head gate.

These were crossbred Brahma cows that had long legs and a short fuse. There was one cranky, silly cow that refused to cooperate. She refused to go into the chute. Bodie would whack her with a black plastic pipe when she turned towards him, trying to run over him. Then when she headed in the right direction he would really lay it to her, smacking her on the rump. The plastic pipe does not bruise, but stings and makes a loud noise. It is one of the more humane, yet effective tools to convince a cow to see it your way. After making about a dozen circles around that little pen, Bodie had her going just right and was close behind, giving her encouragement when she jumped up with her rear end and kicked Bodie in the mouth.

The blow caved in Bodie's front teeth. He looked kinda like some roadkill. I tried to get him to nicker like a horse or whimper like a dog so I could treat him. He finally made some kind of noise that was inhuman that I interpreted as being animal, and I gave him a pain killer. Alf hauled him to El Paso, and the dentist tried all sorts of things to try to save those teeth, but I think he finally had to trade them in on some store-bought ones.

Jon Means

The deer hunters on Jon Means' Moon Ranch were complaining that there weren't any deer. They had been hunting several days and hadn't seen any. Jon and his men were gathering a pasture of cattle, and a big buck mule deer jumped up. Jon bailed after him, taking down his rope as he ran. Jon rode good horses and was a good rider and roper. He caught up with the deer and roped him. He and his hands loaded the deer in a trailer and hauled him to the deer hunters in their camp. There weren't any more complaints about there being no deer at the ranch.

I was told that Duncan and Joe Kingston's daddy, W.L. Kingston, Sr. (I think), was the old gent that settled the country just west of San Solomon Springs. Balmorhea and Toyahvale didn't exist then, to my knowledge. In the 1880s before the country was fenced, Mr. Kingston would drive his cows with their calves to Toyah to the Texas and Pacific Railroad, ship the calves and drive the cows back home. One year had been pretty hard, and when Mr. Kingston turned his cows loose on their home range, they all went back to Toyah looking for their calves. He went and got them after they had quit bawling and took them back home. He said he didn't have hardly any calves the next spring. The fellow telling me this yarn was saying that a good way to pregnancy test is: any cow that hangs around the shipping pens wanting their calf is open.

I told Jon Means about this one day while we were checking his cows. A few years later, Jon said that this didn't work. I gave this some thought. I wonder if those black Angus cows of Jon's just didn't have the maternal instinct of the old Longhorn, or perhaps Jon had fooled around and bred up his cows to where the calves were so big that the cows were glad to get rid of them. There is always the possibility that the story I had heard was a windy. I wouldn't think so, but I have known men that would tell a lie when the truth would have made a better story.

I always enjoyed working for Jon, especially pregnancy palpating. His cows were always well bred-up and were a good set of Angus cows. These cows caused me to change my opinion of the breed. Jon had two excellent sets of pipe working pens, one at the Moon Ranch and another at Ridgewell.

Alejandro and his son, Sergio, were full-time employees, living at Chispa, and another son, Efrin, frequently helped. There was also a son, Art, who lived at the Moon Ranch where José Lujan also lived. All were excellent, hard-working, good-natured ranch hands who were a pleasure to work with.

Jon's wife, Jackie, always fed us a great meal at the Moon Ranch in the cook shack. This terminology really didn't do this place justice, because it was the nicest place solely for preparing and eating meals on a ranch that I can recall. His mother, Barbara, who lived at Chispa, usually hauled us our noon day meal when we worked at Ridgewell. She was truly a gracious lady and a wonderful cook.

Lizzie Means

Lizzie Means, the daughter of Jon and Jackie Means of the Moon Ranch, was one of the most remarkable girls I knew, and this is saying a lot in an area with so many. She would ride horseback to gather cattle, work in the pens punching the cows, and work scotch pipes in the chute.

One day when she was about twelve years of age, I noticed that she was not working, but standing close behind me watching as I pregnancy palpated cows. She had an intense expression on her face instead of the wrinkled up frown so many exhibited when watching me do this somewhat indelicate procedure.

I playfully asked if she would like to feel the calf, expecting a violent shake of her head as she turned away. I was flabbergasted when her eyes brightened and a big smile came on her face as she nodded vigorously. I was taken aback and really didn't know what to do. I looked around for Jon to ask him if it was all right, but he was on the other side of the pens weighing calves. Finally, I pulled a long plastic exam glove from a package and helped her put it on. She didn't hesitate but eagerly put her hand and arm in the cow's rectum. A little questioning look came on her face, and I asked her to pat downward. Suddenly, her face lit up with a big smile and her eyes danced. "I felt it; the leg moved!"

Mrs. Ron "Janet" Helm

Janet was a pretty, blond, slender, little thing who looked too delicate for ranch work, but don't let looks fool you. She could, and did, work longer and harder than many men. She was a fine lady and a remarkable ranchwoman.

I was never at the pens during a calf branding but was told she did her part. I sure can vouch for her actions during the times I was there inspecting calves for shipment, palpating cows, and vaccinating heifer calves for brucellosis. I have seen her go horseback to gather the cattle, help sort the calves and weigh them on the cattle scales, then help load them on trucks.

She would work the cows through the chute, encouraging them to move forward and placing a scotch bar to keep them in place. She would load syringes and vaccinate the cows that I pregnancy tested.

Along about noon she would go to the bunkhouse that also served as a hunting lodge. There she prepared the noon meal, most of which she had cooked the night before and had brought from the house. It was quite amazing how she could serve such a meal under those conditions. She would clean up and straighten things while the men loafed and visited. She would go back to the pens and work all afternoon, then go horseback to help take the cattle back to the pasture.

She always had a smile and a cheerful word. I don't remember her ever being upset, and believe me, there were plenty of things to try one's patience working with a bunch of crossbred cows.

Lou Cowden Edwards was usually at the same work, doing the same thing. She was also a slender, attractive woman about the same age. When we were working Lou and Tim's cattle of the ranch of her parents, Bill and Mary Cowden, Lou would often stop working and prepare the noon meal. While working Bill's cattle, Mary would feed us a banquet at their ranch house.

I had the greatest admiration for these ladies for they were true ladies, although they worked as hard as men and in some ways harder.

Sue (Keeling) and Dan C. "Topper" Frank Jr.

Topper and Sue lived up in the Diablo Mountains north of Allamore on the Circle Ranch where they raised fine Hereford cattle and pretty good boys, Dan III and Scott. I don't think many people knew Topper's proper name was Dan. To most people Dan was either his father or his son. He was Topper.

Sue had been raised on this ranch by her parents, Mr. and Mrs. Scott Keeling. The ranch was in Hudspeth County pretty near the Culberson County line. Topper had been raised or at least went to school and slept in Marfa. He went to school with my daughter, Nancy. He spent much of his time with his dad on ranches. I had known him since he was a pup. He would often help me with C-sections on cattle at night when he came in from the ranch. My hospital was on the highway, and if the lights were on, he would stop.

They had a pretty good crop of big, beautiful mule deer up in the Diablos, but when the mountain lions, more properly cougars, proliferated in the 1980s, they thinned out the deer badly.

The Diablos were the last place in Texas that the desert bighorn sheep had survived until the 1950s. I don't think anything ever got the blame for their extinction officially, but I personally think the introduction of domestic sheep into the area, bringing blue-tongue disease and stomach worms did them in. I'm sure some were killed by hunters, but I never heard of it. Not even a rumor. Their habitat was in such rough rocky cliffs that the casual hunter was not likely to even see one without an expert guide, much less

325

get close enough for a shot. Come to think about it, the severe drouth of the fifties may have been the crowning blow. Well, this was one of the first places that the Texas Wildlife Department reintroduced the big sheep. There had been no domestic sheep in the area for forty or so years so the country was clean again and the bighorn sheep have done well.

The only one of these new sheep raised in the wild to be killed was a big ram. The hunter had been chosen by lottery and Topper had been the guide.

The ranch also had antelope down in the gentle, rolling foothills, but the coyotes were working on them pretty bad. The only wildlife to do well that were not predators were the prairie dogs. These upset Topper considerably because they devastated the vegetation in the prime grassland of the overflow draws by their large towns, as a community of the animal is called. The holes caused many a fall when a horse stepped in one of their burrows. Rattlesnakes lived in the burrows with the dogs, and I was told the dogs would contribute one of their own to the snake occasionally in exchange for it keeping out bothersome varmints like badgers.

Sue was more than the typical ranchwoman. Oh, she took care of the house and the men folk all right, but she was much more. She helped with the cow works and was the school bus driver. The boys went to school in a little one room school house in Allamore. The school may have had more than one room—well, I know it did because the outhouses were in separate buildings: the girls' on one side of the school and the boys' on the other side.

The drive was twice a day, about twelve or fifteen miles over dirt ranch roads which were not too bad, considering everything, although they were a little hard on vehicles. The trip was usually made somewhat faster than the usual one a rancher made to town because there were no stores, beauty shops, or cafes in the little town. I use the word *town* pretty loosely, but there was a sign on the Interstate 10 highway with the name on it pointing to this wide place in the road.

It was a good little school because the boys had no problem at the New Mexico Military Institute. Of course, I strongly believe that Sue may have given them a little tutoring at home on the side. I know they had a good education in ranch life and work because I've spent many hours with them working cattle. They knew how to work.

The whole family participated in the cow works. Sue would go horseback with the rest of them packing a pistol by her side, probably for rattlesnakes and varmints.

The times that I was there to pregnancy test, there was always a big crew, plenty of help. Of course, there were hired hands, but a bunch were friends that came for the camaraderie and the good feed that Sue always prepared. This was one of the places where the term, *cook shack,* was a misnomer. It wasn't a fancy place, but it was substantial and comfortable, far from being a shack. I always ate more than I should have, but I wasn't alone — everyone else did, too.

The work was well organized. The calves were cut off and the steers shipped. The cows worked through the chute smoothly. The cows were well bred up which made my work easier. They were sorted as they came out, going into an alley that led to several pens to put the different categories. Last, I worked on the cancer eye cows that were being kept and ended up the work vaccinating the heifer calves with brucellosis calfhood vaccine. Then I went by the cook shack for a piece of meat and some bread to eat on the 100 mile trip back to Marfa.

The biggest mountain lion that I ever declawed belonged to the two boys, Dan and Scott. It was still fairly young but grown like a weed and played pretty rough with the boys. This turned out to be major surgery. I've amputated lots of dogs' legs that weren't as big as each toe. I thought for a while that I had bitten off more than I could chew. Both the lion and I survived.

They would take the lion to various places, always attracting lots of attention. The boys would lead it around like a dog. It wore a collar, and a length of chain was used for a leash. The lion had gotten big, perhaps it was full grown. It ran around the house loose, often laying up in a tree on a big limb. There was a bench or log under the tree. I always found some other place to sit.

One time, Dan and Scott were sent on an errand. I guess it was something they wanted to do, because I have never known boys to hurry on an errand otherwise. Of course, it may not have been an errand. Anyway, they were running, perhaps a foot race. The lion was lying behind a wall, and when they came by, he jumped on them. Quite a wrassling match took place. I was pretty nervous. He had been declawed but still had the teeth. The boys were laughing and rough housing, but the lion had gotten entirely too big for this type of fun and games to my way of thinking. Sue showed remarkable restraint by allowing the boys to enjoy this cat.

Topper's Lion Hunts

Topper named his dogs, Dawg, much to his wife's displeasure until he began hunting lions about the mid-1980s. Previous to that time, he assured me there were no lions in the Sierra Diablo Mountains because the source was Mexico, and they would not cross the busy Interstate 10 highway. The lions had migrated into the Eagle Mountains of south Hudspeth County, the Chinati and Sierra Vieja Mountains in southwest Presidio County, and the Davis Mountains in Jeff Davis County. However, lions soon invaded Topper's Sierra Diablo Mountains. They devastated his mule deer population and threatened the desert bighorn sheep that were being reintroduced.

B.A. "Blackie" Wood was crowding eighty years old and had hunted lions all his life. He even caught a few in the 1940s and '50s when there were not many because a concentrated effort was being made to control predators due to the large numbers of sheep and goats in the area which are particularly vulnerable to all predators, especially lions. There was no hope of eradication because they are cunning like the coyote. Most of the ranchers only hoped to control them and keep them moving so that losses would be kept to a minimum in any one area. Blackie and Topper made a great hunting team and caught a large number. But lions were coming in faster than they could catch them, so they began to widen their hunting territory to include the Eagle and Beech Mountains. Topper soon had a good pack of hunting dogs, each with its own name, and he could recite each one's faults and good traits. I asked where the lions were coming from since they wouldn't cross the Interstate highway. He answered that they had learned to live with civilization.

Topper Frank and the Cow on Fire

Topper Frank was manager of the Sierra Diablo Ranch north of

Van Horn. I was pregnancy palpating and chalking. Paul Spitzer, my assistant, was vaccinating for lepto and vibrio.

I don't know why academia has to keep changing the names of diseases, bacteria, anatomy and measurements. They now call vibrio, *Campylobacter fetus*. That's really clever, isn't it? It took me 25 years to educate the ranchers and cowboys to the disease, vibrio. They learned to pronounce it, spell it, and the need to vaccinate for it and then some yeh-hoo has to go and change the name and confuse everybody. It was almost as bad as the change of *cc* to *ml* in liquid measurements. There's no telling how much time I wasted explaining and trying to convince people that they were the same. I don't think some of the Mexican-Americans fully understood. The Mexicans from Mexico didn't seem to have a problem because Mexico was on the metric system.

Scott, Topper's son, was applying the Ivomec Pour-On. This was a systemic insecticide that was absorbed through the skin of the back for the control of parasites.

We had finished about 200 head that were in a large pen directly ahead. They were balled up in a tight group at the far end to which each cow would run as fast as possible to get away from us as soon as she was released. We had finished with a crossbred Brahma cow and released her, but she balked and wouldn't leave the chute. Paul reached out and touched her with a hotshot, an electric prodpole, and she left in a dead run. We watched in amazement as she burst into flames, the solvent in the Ivomec burning. She was headed for the bunch of cows and if she followed the pattern, she would crowd her way into the middle in an effort to get lost from us. We thought she would set the others on fire, resulting in a catastrophe. We stood helpless, fearing the worst. Only Topper had the presence of mind to shout instructions, "Lie down and roll, you dumb cow!" I don't guess she heard, because she didn't even slow down. Fortunately, the solvent was so volatile and flammable that it was consumed before she arrived in the herd, and no others caught fire. Topper later reported the cow only had a little hair singed on her back.

Paul Spitzer would tell other ranch hands about the incident and attempt to demonstrate by pouring some out and applying the hotshot spark. He was never successful. I finally had to put a stop to this, as he was wasting too much high priced Ivomec. Also, I was afraid he might be tempted to try it on a cow and be successful.

A Boy's Pet Turtle

One day I was called to the office of the local physician who was out of his office at the time. The emergency medical team had brought a small boy, perhaps ten or twelve years old, with a turtle hung on his nose. I had a terrible time trying to keep from laughing, and all the others in the room watching were also about to bust a gut.

It is difficult to relate how funny this looked. The boy holding the turtle straight out with both hands to prevent its weight causing more pain. The boy and the turtle looking at each other eyeball to eyeball. The boy squalling like a scalded dog dancing around, first on one foot, then the other with his back and neck ramrod stiff and his eyes big as saucers. The turtle wasn't saying anything or making any move, just holding on, with its neck stretched out farther than I had ever seen. Everyone looked at me and I looked at the boy and turtle. I kinda wished for my dehorning shears to cut the turtle's head off, but that wouldn't have looked good.

I loaded a syringe with Rompun, a tranquilizer drug, that I used on animals but had never tried on a turtle. I was hoping that the old saying about a turtle not turning loose until it thunders wasn't entirely true, because we were in a dry spell. I pulled one of the turtle's hind legs, and with a quick motion I injected the medicine. I don't think the medicine was necessary, as the turtle let go immediately, much too soon for the tranquilizer to have taken effect.

The boy threw the turtle completely across the room and rushed out the door. His mother was close behind. Someone yelled that he forgot his turtle. No answer. We all relaxed and laughed. I picked up the turtle, took it back to the hospital and gave it an injection of Yohimbine which was the Rompun reversing agent, but to no avail. The sleep was permanent.

Aubrey Lange's Helicopter

I was invited to go deer hunting on the Mayer Seven Springs Ranch, previously owned by Willis McCutcheon. Wayne Timmerman, the ranch foreman, Aubrey Lange, a helicopter pilot, and I climbed into a pickup and went off up on top and around to the east side of Carpenter Mountain, which is part of the Barrilla Mountains, to an old homestead.

Wayne suggested that I go up one canyon, Aubrey another, and he would go up a third. We would meet on top of a ridge where the three canyons headed. We met as planned. Neither Wayne nor I had seen a deer, but Aubrey said he had killed a good one down deep in that rough canyon.

We went to it, and it was sure enough a dandy alright. But he was big and a long ways from a road. I suggested we leave him, and Aubrey gave me a look that shot sparks. He didn't think that was a good joke, and I wouldn't have either, if I had been in his place. We halfway carried and dragged the buck up the hillside to a ridge where Aubrey said we could land his helicopter. I was the old man of the group and volunteered to stay and guard while they walked back to the pickup and drove to the ranch for the helicopter. It was a little cold and windy, but it sure beat all the walking they had to do. They finally got back and set downright beside the deer. We tied it to one of the landing skids. I don't know if that is the proper name, but that's what it looked like they should be called.

The 'copter was just a little one he used for rounding up cattle and hunting predators, and I questioned whether it would fly with three men and that big deer, at that high altitude. I volunteered to stay behind and do a little more hunting. Aubrey didn't argue. He seemed kinda relieved, I thought. I prowled around a little, and pretty soon they were back. I climbed in, and we took off. Aubrey circled around, giving me a good joyride, skimming over rimrocks and down canyons. I don't know if he did all those didoes intentionally to give me a thrill or if he was still having trouble with the load.

Big Bend Ranch

John L. Guldemann came to Presidio County working for Ralph Hager who was the foreman for Anderson's Diamond A Cattle Company. The ranch was originally the Fowlkes Ranch. John L. was living at the Cienaga Division with his wife and baby son, Bucko.

He built an excellent set of working pens, especially the crowd chute for the Longhorns. It was made of good, sturdy lumber which was strong but could be sawed easily in case a horn got hung up. The upright posts were staggered so that the horns could slide off as the head was bent from side to side.

Ralph Hager was transferred to the Ladder Ranch in New Mexico which was also owned by Anderson. John L. moved to Saucedo, the headquarters, and assumed the job of foreman of the ranch. He was very capable at this position.

Mr. Anderson had several very interesting experiments at this ranch. One was a Welsh pony herd which was claimed to be the largest in the world, of which I have no doubt. I remember the herd numbering 600 head. Another enterprise was the raising of chukars and pheasants. I don't mean he piddled around with a few like my father did. Mr. Anderson raised great numbers. The plan was to fly in hunters. There was a nice landing strip at the ranch and a nice hunting lodge. The hunters would be stationed in a box with the birds in cages a certain distance away. I don't remember the exact procedure planned, but I think the bird handlers were to be in pits and on command would throw one or more birds in the air. I guess these really would be termed shoots rather than hunts. These never actually took place to my knowledge because of a severe die off of the birds from a combination of Coccidiosis (a protozoan parasitic intestinal infestation) and Salmonellosis (a bacterial infection of the intestines). Each condition is extremely serious, but the combination was devastating.

The Ranch was sold to the State of Texas together with the Longhorn herd which by this time had become certified as Purebred by having a sophisticated test of the genetic material made. The State declared the ranch to be a Natural Area, and plans were made to disperse the herd. A number of animals were sold. John L. personally bought some outstanding individuals when the auction did not sell as well as John L. thought they should. He pastured his cattle on the Ocotillo Ranch which belonged to Jack Brown and his daughter, Becky. Public opinion caused the state park service to change their plans, and the decision was made to keep a remnant of the herd.

The name was changed to Big Bend Ranch State Park with headquarters at Fort Leaton State Park which was included into and under the management of the Ranch. Luis Armendariz of Presidio was the overall superintendent.

I made frequent trips to the ranch while it belonged to

Anderson and later to the State. Most of the calls were to vaccinate the heifer calves for brucellosis and test sale animals for both brucellosis and tuberculosis. The round trip to the Cienaga Division was about 80 or 90 miles and that to Saucedo, the headquarters, was about 180 or 190 miles. Both trips were scenic, and I always enjoyed working with the capable and personable men. I regretted seeing this era pass.

John L. resigned from the Ranch and struck out on his own. He soon leased some country near Mentone in Loving County north of Pecos but the drouth of '94, '95 and '96 caused him to move to Animas, New Mexico. He has gained international recognition in Longhorn circles and in 1998 was president of the National Association of Texas Longhorn Breeders, properly called The Texas Longhorn Registry.

Wind

I never did get used to the strong winds in the spring to the point where it didn't bother me. I did learn to control my outward expressions of emotions somewhat, but in my younger days, I frequently gave voice to my displeasure, especially when dirt and powdered manure filled my eyes, the instrument tray, or an open incision during an operation. The fact is, I would really bellyache from time to time. Often, the older ranchers would chide me, saying that the wind had to blow in the spring for it to rain in the summer. That would shut me up right quick, because rain is our lifeblood. It's everybody's, of course, but in this country, it just seems to make a deeper impression. However, I never did observe the relationship of wind to rain. The winds were bad every spring, but it didn't always rain.

It always seemed to me that the wind was especially strong when it was cold, and the wind chill hurt so bad. On the other hand, it seemed as if it was always deathly still on a hot summer day when a little breeze would be so welcome for our comfort. It is especially needed for windmills to pump water because cattle drink more water in hot weather.

The weathermen are 100% accurate when they predict wind but do a notoriously poor job of predicting rain. They will tell us it is going to rain for several days, and it doesn't. About the time they give up and quit, we start getting a little; then they gain confidence, and as soon as they say it will rain, it stops.

An electric company put windmill-type generators in the Delaware Mountains in north Culberson County just south of the Guadalupes on the Six Bar Ranch. I thought this would be an ideal place, but Mike Capron, the ranch manager, told me it wouldn't work because they cut off automatically when wind speeds reach 45 miles an hour. He said the wind never blows that slowly on that rim.

Before the '70s, small windmill-type electric generators, called wind chargers, were used on some ranches to charge batteries for electric lights. Most used an engine to generate electricity for lights and radio. Television was in its infancy and not available on any ranch I knew of in the fifties. Refrigerators were run by butane at first, and later, by propane.

The Rural Electrification Administration (R.E.A.) began building high lines to provide electricity to the isolated ranches in the 1970s in this area, although in more thickly populated areas it had been going on for several years.

The wind was especially important to operate the windmills which were needed to pump water, as they were the main thing that allowed this area to be utilized for grazing. There was very little permanent surface water, which was limited to water holes, wet weather springs, the intermittent streams, and the man-made water holes we called dirt tanks.

In places where electricity was available, a number of electrical submersible pumps were installed for a more reliable water supply. A few solar cells have been installed for electrical generation that seem to work fairly well for shallow wells.

Ted Harper

During the last few years of the screwworm problem in the late 1950s, most cases in cattle were treated with the product, Smear EQ 335. This contained the chemical insecticide, Lindane, and a pine oil product as a carrying agent. In the early 1990s Ted's ranch dog became infested with ticks, so he dipped his hand in the product and smeared it on his dog. It killed the ticks and almost killed Ted. This insecticide had been banned because it was slow to decompose. The product Ted was using was probably 30 years old or more, and some volatilization of the pine oil had probably occurred which may have resulted in a more concentrated product. Ted said that in the screwworm days, he had often gotten it on his hands without a problem. However, I doubt that he had ever actually dipped his bare hands in it as he had this time. Of course, Ted being older may have had something to do with the toxicity.

Ted had hip replacement surgery when he was crowding 80 years of age. He did very well as he was a thin wiry man, and people with this conformation seem to recover the best. When the doctor released him to go home, Ted asked if it would be all right if he rode his horse. The doctor said it would be, just not to get thrown off. Ted told him that he had never got thrown off a horse on purpose in his life and didn't plan on beginning. Ranch life went along pretty normally for about ten days when his old gentle saddle horse got a hump in his back and threw Ted off. Ted said he landed on his head so it didn't hurt anything, just peeled his head up a little.

Arm Injury

I was testing bulls to go to Florida at the Brite Ranch Double Wells pens. These were new, good, sturdy pipe pens and made so that neither the cowboys nor the cattle could get hurt. Four or five bulls would be loaded out of the crowd pen and into the crowd chute leading to the squeeze. I was reaching between the pipes to draw blood from the tail vein for a brucellosis test, then inject tuberculin for a tuberculosis test in the caudal fold at the base of the tail. I then applied a metal numbered eartag for identification. These were young bulls and had good sharp horns. When the tag was clamped in the ear, they often reacted rather violently by shaking their heads. The horns would go along. It seems as if some of my reflexes kinda slowed down with the years, and maybe that's what happened with this nervous bull because he nailed my forearm to a pipe. The sharp horn penetrated my forearm and went between the two bones. I couldn't move my arm, but the bull quickly moved his head, releasing my arm. I had been working with my sleeves rolled up, so no cloth was poked into the flesh. Apparently he had polished his horns on another bull's side while fighting, so it was a good clean wound except for a little of the usual cow manure dust always present in a pen. I let it bleed good for a little while to clean it out. It did so freely without any special effort on my part. I smeared Furacin dressing on it, then covered it with a gauze pad and wrapped with a Vetrap. I finished the bulls and drove home. It was dark when I got back to town, and the offices of both doctors were closed. I took a couple of antibiotic capsules after growling like a dog and nickering like a horse so I couldn't be accused of practicing medicine on a human.

I processed the blood and did the paperwork before going to bed. I left early the next morning to pregnancy test cows near McCamey. I used my left arm as much as I could, but when it became tired, I would use my right. This would cause it to bleed, and when the blood mixed with the sweat on my arm inside the plastic glove and sleeve, it looked like a lot more blood than it really was. This was a hot day, and, as usual with hot days, sweat accumulated inside plastic gloves in rather copious amounts. Often it had to be drained by raising the arm to let it pour out. A young high school boy was helping who had his sights on becoming a veterinarian. I was told later that watching me that day changed his mind.

The wound healed nicely, leaving very little scar. Jim White III offered to put the ear tags in for me after that. I didn't argue with him. Why, I didn't even fuss at him the time or two he got the tags mixed up.

Chapter 10

Shadows and Hints of Retirement

Heat Exhaustion at Altuda

Late in September in the mid 1980s I was pregnancy testing cows at Altuda for the Paisano Cattle Company. Altuda is usually one of the coldest and windiest set of pens and compares with the pens at the Quebec siding of the Southern Pacific Railroad. We had an early cold spell, and I had drained the water from my tank in the pickup veterinary bed. This was premature, but I was gun-shy for fear of the pipe freezing and breaking. In wintertime I used gallon plastic jugs to carry the water. Depending upon the work, I always carried one gallon and, if circumstances might call for it, I would put in another jug of cold or tap water and two of hot water. This time I had only one gallon. There was no water in the pens, not even a water trough. The cowboys' water was in their pickups that had been left with the trailers at the back side of the pasture where they had started the roundup horseback.

This was a very hot day, especially for late September when I had become accustomed to cooler weather. It was deathly still, not even a slight breeze. John Roberts was in back, in the crowd pen starting cows into the crowd chute. Bubber Mathers and Eric McGuire were scotching the cows with a post behind so they could not back up and punching them forward. Pete Salas was working the tailgate of the squeeze chute and helping punch the cows forward. Ike Roberts was at the front end opening and closing the gate, trapping the head with the neck bar, and working the squeeze part of the Turner squeeze chute. He didn't have time to even light a cigarette. I was pregnancy palpating, working the safety latch on the tailgate, loading syringes, vaccinating for leptospirosis and giving vitamin A injections.

We were working fast and furious. After several minutes of cows trampling on the wooden floor, out came a cottontail rabbit.

Soon, Ike said he could hear a rattlesnake under the chute. He poked under it with a long-handled shovel, and out crawled a red racer snake, which some call a coachwhip.

I had always heard they would kill and eat rattlesnakes often making a noise, supposedly with their mouth, that sounded like one. They were never found together. I assured everyone that the coachwhip had the rabbit charmed and was about to consume it when we started making such a racket and broke the spell.

Ike still insisted he heard a rattlesnake with me insisting it couldn't be. Ike kept poking, and soon a big rattlesnake came out and began crawling back down the chute under the cows' legs, finally emerging at the back end. Ike killed it with the shovel when it coiled in the middle of the little crowd pen, licking its tongue out and rattling furiously. The snake had gone under four or five cows, going between their legs but I guess it was in too big of a hurry to stop, coil and strike a cow because we didn't see any evidence of it. So much for my theory that red racers, rabbits and rattlesnakes don't co-habit a place.

All hands would drink from my water jug except John Roberts and me. I never did catch him at it, but I think even Ike was able to take a swig now and then. John couldn't get to it, and I didn't have time. I never did stop and drink water as often as most men. Also, I was so busy, I didn't think about it and didn't realize I was getting in trouble until I started feeling weak and a little dizzy. By then the water jug was empty. It would have been a major shut down to go for water. We only had thirty or forty cows remaining, so we continued working.

When we finally finished, I lay down under my pickup in the shade while the men sorted the open cows from the pregnant ones and drove them to their respective pastures. When they returned, I had recovered enough to crawl out from under the pickup. We discovered John Roberts was down also, laid out beside the fence. Neither of us had to go to the hospital, but we both had headaches for several days and our thermostats were ruined afterwards. Since then, heat has bothered me, even when I drank water often. It seemed that the direct sunrays in the summer would cause me to wilt.

Blue Norther at the Barlite Ranches

One of my most miserable days, and I have had some bad ones, was at Cell G on the Alta Vista Ranch, part of the Barlite Ranches. A blue norther began blowing a strong northeast wind just as I got there. There was some discussion as to whether we ought to try to pregnancy palpate on such a bad day. However, it is very difficult to change plans at the last minute—extra cowboys had to be hired, horses had to be shod, a cook arranged for and groceries bought. Also, the cows were already in the pen. Charles Guest, the ranch manager, and his cowboys had gathered and penned the 715 head early in the morning. They musta done it mostly by moonlight 'cause it was only just good sunup when I got there. This work had been no small chore because cowboys weren't as plentiful as in earlier days, and most of these were Sul Ross College boys. Sul Ross has an active rodeo club and a well-known range animal science course, both of which attract some good ole country boys.

My schedule was full this late in the fall, everyone trying to get things wrapped up for Thanksgiving and mule deer hunting season. I wouldn't have been able to come back for several days. I had prepared lepto and vibrio vaccines, vitamin A, and Tramisol dewormer injections plus all the syringes and needles that were needed.

I don't remember anyone saying so, but I think all of us were hoping the wind would die down after the first big blow like it does sometimes. This wasn't one of those days. I believe the wind got stronger as the day wore on. I know it got colder.

The squeeze chute was too close to the fence for me to put my pickup for a wind break. The fence was pipe and it didn't slow the wind a bit. To make matters worse, the holding pens and those leading to the chutes were upwind and the cattle milling around kept stirring up dirt, powdered old manure, and hay particles which blew in our faces.

We had no goggles or dust masks. I had tried a few times to use these, but the goggles would get twisted which aggravated me to the point I soon quit trying to use them. I would choke down with the dust masks when exertion caused me to breathe heavily. However, this day I wished that I had them both. I felt I could tolerate them better than the alternative.

I don't know which was the worst, the cold or the wind—but the dust particles were worse than either. It got in my lungs, ears, and nose, but what bothered me the most was the dirt and debris in my eyes. The pain and discomfort of them made the other things insignificant. I kept the vaccine bottles in my pockets to keep them warm, only loading small amounts in the syringes so that the vaccine was not exposed to the cold for prolonged periods. When not actually in a cow, I would hold the needle of the lepto syringe between my thumb and forefinger, because this vaccine and this place is the most vulnerable to freezing.

We stopped at noon to go to lunch. I went by my truck to get a bottle of lidocaine, intending to bathe my eyes with the anesthetic solution. Both bottles had frozen and broken.

The ranch had a nice hunting lodge with kitchen, dining table, chairs, and sofa. The woman cooking had been imported from Alpine and knew the type of meal to feed a bunch of hungry men. She fixed me a cold pack with ice cubes that I kept on my eyes when I wasn't eating. When Charles asked if I was ready to go back to work and I answered that I was, I heard a sigh or two and at least one gasp from the crew.

We finished before sundown and Paul Spitzer, my helper, loaded things in my pickup kinda haphazardly while I tried to start the engine. No luck. The battery was good and strong, but the engine wouldn't kick over. One of the men heard me grinding and brought a can. I popped the hood and he sprayed starting fluid in the carburetor. It worked like a charm and relieved my anxiety. I always carried a can after that, although I hadn't before because the metal vet bed got very hot at times, and I had been concerned it may explode.

Paul told me the next day that he had gone to a beer joint after we got back to town to take on some internal antifreeze. Some of the cowboys who had helped were discussing and complaining what a terrible day it had been to some others. They said that crazy, old veterinarian just kept working. This was in 1989. I was 64, and I guess that did seem old to 21-year-olds. To be frank, I did feel old that night.

The Ribs

The Sierra Diablo Ranch north of Van Horn was fairly typical in that the pens had just about been used up. I had my pickup inside the pen next to the squeeze chute as usual. Suddenly, an ole wild cow was loose in the pen with us. I'm not sure if she busted out or whether a young fellow back there was asleep at the switch. Now, when a boy is not paying attention, he is daydreaming, but when a grown man does so, he is in deep thought.

I was busy fiddling with syringes, needles, and vaccines and filling my soup bucket which was the container for my slickum. There were several cowboys running around hollering and waving their leggins trying to get her to go through a gate. They were at the other end of a rather long pen, and I wasn't paying much attention as this had happened several times before. I should have known better because even a big pen can get awfully crowded with an ole salty cow trying to get in somebody's britches, and this one was a lively rascal.

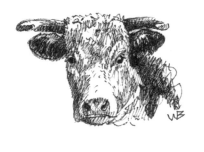

Horned Hereford   Muley (dehorned) Hereford.

They started calling my name, and I looked up just as she hit me in the chest going full speed. She was a muley, no horns, which was lucky for me. I landed up against the chute, doubled up in a knot. Paul Spitzer, my right hand man, came and straightened me out. Topper Frank asked me if I was hurt. As soon as I got my breath and could answer, I told him, no, that if it wasn't for the pain, I probably wouldn't hurt at all. I was able to get to my feet in a few minutes with Paul and Topper tailing me up. I hobbled around a little to shake it off and went back to work. I felt pretty good and thought I had worked the soreness out.

We finished working the cattle after a while. Then Paul and some of the cow hands hooked my portable squeeze chute on my pickup and gathered up all the equipment and supplies while Topper and I discussed worldly affairs. It seems that a difference of opinion developed. This didn't result in an argument, just a heated discussion. Some of the onlookers said we couldn't get up close to each other, because there was a tendency to gesture when making a point. It was speculated that the vocal cords and the hands must be connected because as the voice got louder, the hand and arm movements became more animated. I finally out-shouted Topper and left having won the decision. Paul drove while I navigated. About halfway to Van Horn, I shifted my position and the pain hit. <u>I mean it really hit</u>!! I don't know what happened but I thought perhaps a cracked rib gave way. I had a pretty rough few weeks, hobbling around trying to tell JoAnn I was okay.

Wind at the Arnold Pens

The Arnold pens of the Paisano Cattle Company Ranch are out on a flat with nothing to slow the wind. About 1990 I was there brucellosis and pregnancy testing cows. I had been working all day with a cold north wind blowing dust and powdered manure in my face. This was the only time that I can remember that the debris filling my lungs caused difficulty breathing. This hurt and bothered me worse than it being in my eyes.

It was so bad I didn't have a chance to smoke. I smoked a cig-arette at the noon break, but I don't recall it bothering me at that time. That afternoon I was having so much trouble breathing that I didn't even want a cigarette. This was very unusual because I was a heavy smoker and had smoked since I was 15 years old— about fifty years. I had been a light smoker until I was laid up in the hospital eight months during World War II without much else to do, so I had smoked heavily from idleness.

I may not have realized that I didn't want a cigarette though because the wind was blowing too hard for smoking to be possi-ble. I finally finished the cows. This was one of the few times that I kept looking for the last cow. Ordinarily, I enjoyed this type of practice and the camaraderie that went with it. I think everyone else was anticipating the last cow as much as I was. Although no one was complaining, not even Sally Roberts or Liz Yadon. However, I don't remember ever having heard them complain.

I put my things up, always being careful of the blood samples. I drove out of the pens and down the road a piece and stopped my pickup. I soon calmed down enough to light a cigarette. The first puff shut off my breath, and I snuffed it out. I drove on down the road a little farther and lit another cigarette. It too stopped my breathing, and I discarded it. When I reached the highway, cars were coming from both directions so I took a few deep breaths and tried another cigarette. Same results. There was no coughing, just a complete shutdown of the breathing apparatus. I didn't even want to try to smoke again until the next morning with coffee. I couldn't inhale the smoke. I didn't want another cigarette, but a few days later I tried again and decided I must have developed an allergy to cigarette smoke.

I guess it was true asthma, because I couldn't inhale although I don't remember any residual respiratory problems at that time. I would be alright if I didn't try to smoke. I had tried off and on for several years to quit smoking because of a chronic cough, but I didn't have any luck. I suppose I thought that the satisfaction I got from smoking outweighed the effects. Not a very good excuse for the lack of will power. Actually, I had rationalized for many years that the dust and debris that I breathed in corrals plus the branding smoke and fumes from insecticides were much harder on my lungs than the cigarette smoke. I'm sure that played a substantial part because I worked in dry corrals almost every day from August until December and many other days during the year. Even when it rained, the pens dried out quickly. These were usually long hours of work.

It often bothered me that when I coughed, none of the debris ever came up that I could see. I hoped that it was expelled at times I could not observe it, but a gnawing suspicion existed that perhaps some remained deep in my lungs to produce a chronic irritation.

I knew smoking was injurious, and I seriously doubt that anyone who ever smoked thought otherwise. As kids, we offered another a coffin nail. We surely knew what that meant.

There were times when I considered smoking therapeutic, particularly on long, lonely drives. It helped keep me awake, serving as a stimulant. Other times when I was tense from anxiety, it helped me to relax. I often smoked when I was severely fatigued to give me an opportunity to rest. One of the more important uses was to buy a little time to ponder a case in order to arrive at a diagnosis, contemplate a course of action, or weigh the options of treatments. I thought it looked better to an onlooker than just sitting, doing nothing.

I will have to admit though, that I enjoyed smoking and have few regrets and would probably be smoking yet if my breathing permitted it. However, I would urge anyone to never light a first cigarette and if they did, to stop before the habit became well established.

During the next few years, I gradually had more problems with dust in the pens and especially branding smoke, even though I had quit smoking cigarettes. I began to carry Primatene Mist Inhalers for use when I got into trouble. The problem became so regular that I would take a bronchodilater tablet any time I thought there might be branding or dust.

Heat Exhaustion at Presidio Stockyards

George Jones built a stockyards in 1968 northeast of Presidio. It was past the packing sheds beside the railroad tracks on the north side. I don't know if the pens were built next to the tracks as they curved or if a spur had been built to the yards because many cattle were still being shipped by train.

In 1991 lots of slaughter livestock were being exported to Mexico destined for the slaughter houses in Chihuahua City. These were obvious packers, being fat, barren cows, old crippled ones, bad eyes and spoiled bags. The sheep also were obvious "killers," but I personally could not see why most of the hogs were going because the reason for their being culled was not obvious to me. The slaughter animals required only a minimum health examination of visual inspection for contagious diseases and a government numbered metal eartag for permanent identification.

Soon, better quality cows and bulls began to be presented as slaughter animals. It was plain to see that these were destined for breeding animals and were going to be diverted to ranches. By declaring them slaughter animals, a substantial expense was circumvented. The Mexican government soon realized what was happening so that they began requiring all female and uncastrated males to be given extensive tests and vaccinations.

The bulls 17 months of age or older had to be fertility tested, consisting of not only visual and manual examination of the genitals, but also scrotal circumference and semen evaluation. All cattle had to be tested for tuberculosis, vibriosis and trichomoniasis. Also, they had to be tested for brucellosis, except heifers under 24 months of age, that had been officially calfhood vaccinated for this disease. A problem was encountered in that the vaccination tattoo had to be legible. All had to be vaccinated with an intramuscular injection against leptospirosis and an intranasal vaccination against infectious bovine rhinotracheitis. They had to be examined and treated for external parasites including earticks, then a numbered metal eartag was placed.

The blood for brucellosis testing was required to be sent to the state-federal laboratory in Austin. The vibrio and tricho tubes with the transport media were sent to the Texas Veterinary Medical Diagnostic Laboratory in College Station. The complicated export certificates had to be sent to the federal offices in Austin for approval.

This quickly dried up the exportation, but quite a number of cattle were already in the pipeline. That is, they had been bought and paid for on this side at substantial prices because they were purebred registered, and the demand had inflated the price. When the new regulations went into effect, the purchases stopped and prices fell. The problems of reselling on this side would cause severe losses if they were dumped at an auction, which would have been the logical thing to do if they had been commercial cattle. Many were already in Presidio or on the way.

The stockyards had little maintenance work done on them since they were built and were in poor condition, especially the part where we were working. Perhaps this had been neglected because it was out of the way and out of sight. Boards were broken, with some missing on the fences, and the posts were leaning badly, allowing the crowd chute to spread apart causing the work to be slow and difficult, as some animals would try to turn around. While a few would be successful, others flipped on their backs. The big heavy wooden gates were sagging, making them difficult to open and close.

The squeeze chute was the real challenge. There is no telling how many cattle had been put in it. Very little repair work had been done, and at this point it was irreparable. It was held together with bailing wire, chains and a come-a-long on either side. It was exciting when an animal was in it, as it groaned and moaned, rattled and swayed. I would have to psych myself each time to get enough courage to approach it to process an animal. This necessitated sticking my head, arms and shoulders inside the chute with the animal to perform many of the procedures. It was better than nothing, but only barely. The pens were about six to eight inches deep in powdered manure which reflected the heat of the sun. The only shade was provided by a three-foot tall, dead, cottonwood tree. Not a breath of breeze was stirring. We worked all day finishing around 5:00 PM. Someone said the temperature at the scalehouse was 112° in the shade. I wonder what it was out in the pens. Even the flies had hunted a hole. My pickup was full of them.

I had drunk water fairly often because of some past problems when I did not, but I was barely able to finish. While the men put the cattle back in their respective pens, I crawled under the pickup to lie down since the cab was full of flies and there was no room for me. I may have passed out or just gone to sleep, for the next thing I knew, the men were shaking me and calling my name. I crawled out, feeling a little better.

I was 66 years of age and had experienced heat fatigue or exhaustion a couple of times in recent years. I don't know whether my thermostat was broken or worn out. Either way, I had begun to suffer from extremes of heat or cold. This was a blow to my ego, because I had always prided myself in being able to tolerate both.

The Mexican tradition of an afternoon siesta has been ridiculed, but it is a very logical method of coping with the noonday heat. Therefore, the help readily agreed to my suggestion that we work the next bunch of cattle at night.

A few days later, arrangements were made, and I arrived at 6:00 PM. The thermometer showed 114° in the shade when I arrived and 99° when we finished at 2:30 the next morning. That doesn't seem like much improvement, but actually it was much better because there was no sun blazing down and few flies. Houseflies crawling on your face are aggravating, but the vicious little horn-flies biting hurt. I guess the little night flying gnats and mosquitoes in eyes, nose and ears kept us fighting our heads. I didn't like the mosquitoes buzzing me although most were only window shopping. They didn't bite me very often. I thought I was going to lose my mind in the islands during World War II at first, but I kinda got used to them. They would just drink their fill and move on, not do all that buzzing, or perhaps I became accustomed to it. Now, the American mosquitoes just buzz me a little and rarely bite.

Presidio is always much warmer than Marfa due primarily to the difference in elevation. Marfa is 4848 feet and Presidio is 2594 feet. The bare rocky mountain ranges nearby on either side of Presidio may contribute also.

Ike Roberts

Ike's name was actually Billie, but I never heard him called or referred to as such. He was always Ike. Anyone hearing the name Bill Roberts would have thought they were talking about his cousin in Marfa by that name who was close to the same age.

Ike Roberts took care of the Paisano Cattle Company ranches, both the land and the cattle, for the owners, descendants of Mr. Gage who founded the extensive ranches. One of the descendants was Joan Kelleher, the overall manager, a very capable one, I might add. All members of the family were friendly and congenial, a pleasure to work for and associate with.

Ike was very knowledgeable and industrious. He came from a long line of cowmen. His grandfather had come to the area in the early days. His father, Travis Roberts, was as good as they come and was very interesting to visit with because of his extensive knowledge of the area.

Ike's family consisted of his wife, Sue, a daughter, Sally, two sons, Joe and Tim. Sue was a good cook and fed us well, while Sally, Joe and Tim were good cow hands and hard workers. Ike always had a good crew. The works went well, and I enjoyed them even though some days were pretty long and hard. Sometimes the weather was less than ideal. Ike was one of the many men that I was proud to call a friend.

We were working cattle one day when the wind was blowing. Now, I don't know why I said that because we were at the Altuda pens, and the wind always blows there except one hot September day. The only difference is the direction. A comment was made regarding the wind causing dust pollution which led to a discussion about the Big Bend National Park complaining of pollution from the generating plants, Carbon 1 and Carbon 2, in Mexico at Piedras Negras. The pollution was supposed to be affecting visibility in the Park. I spoke up and said I guess that was right because I could no longer see mountains eighty miles away that I previously could. Ike said, "Doc, you don't suppose 70-year-old eyes have anything to do with it, do you?" I thought of this when I was renewing my driver's license because I was asked if I wanted to be listed as a donor. I thought a little and replied, "Do you suppose someone would want a 72-year-old worn out part?" The lady Department of Public Safety officer looked up at me with a kind of surprised expression on her face. She hesitated a moment, then marked **No** on the application.

Ω

Chapter 11

Reflections

The practice of veterinary medicine was both my vocation and my avocation, as I never lost interest. If anything, I became more interested as I met new challenges and the development of new drugs and techniques.

The emergence or recognition of new diseases or conditions would stimulate me. Also I had to be constantly on the alert for diseases slipping across the border from Mexico where there were few veterinarians, and for many years there were none near the border. I felt that in many ways I was in the vanguard to protect the livestock industry of the United States.

My eventual retirement was caused by COPD, Chronic Obstructive Pulmonary Disease, and heat intolerance, not by emotional or interest burn out.

I was very blessed to practice the profession I loved, live in such beautiful country, work for such wonderful people and make a comfortable living for my family.

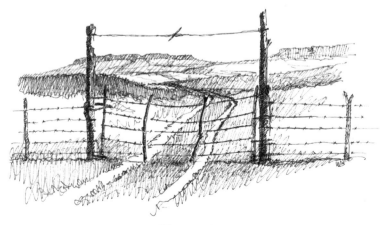

Wire gap gate.